ALSO BY ELIZABETH LEE VLIET, M.D.

Screaming to Be Heard:
Hormone Connections Women Suspect and Doctors Still Ignore

Women, Weight, and Hormones

It's My
Ovaries,
Stupid!

ELIZABETH LEE VLIET, M.D.

SCRIBNER

NEW YORK   LONDON   TORONTO   SYDNEY   SINGAPORE

SCRIBNER
1230 Avenue of the Americas
New York, NY 10020

SCRIBNER and design are trademarks of Macmillan Library Reference USA, Inc.,
used under license by Simon & Schuster, the publisher of this work.

Set in Minion

Manufactured in the United States of America

1 3 5 7 9 10 8 6 4 2

Library of Congress Cataloging-in-Publication Data

Vliet, Elizabeth Lee [dates].
It's my ovaries, stupid!/Elizabeth Lee Vliet.
p. cm.
Includes bibliographical references.
1. Ovaries. 2. Ovaries—Diseases. 3. Ovaries—Cancer. 4. Endocrine gynecology.
I. Title.

RG441. V554 2003
618.1'1—dc21

2003041512

ISBN 0-7432-1056-5

For information regarding special discounts for bulk purchases,
please contact Simon & Schuster Special Sales at 1-800-456-6798 or
business@simonandschuster.com

To my mother, whose suffering planted the seeds of
my inquiry and search for answers

To Gordon, Kathy, and Margaret—my incredible team who
made it possible for me to meet the challenges and deadlines

To those who follow—in hope your health will benefit from our efforts to
sound the alarm and show you the way to change

To God who guided it all

Contents

▬▬▬

SECTION III: Your Ovaries and Your Body

SECTION IV: Getting Well—Your Action Plan

Author's Note:
The Hormone Controversy

Hormones—and their connections in how we think and feel and function—have been my life's work in medicine. The summer of 2002 brought a maelstrom of negative, frightening headlines about "hormones" and "hormone replacement therapy" (HRT). (Recently the term was changed by the FDA to *menopausal hormone therapy*, but we will refer to it by its best-known name.) The headlines screamed that estrogen increased the risk of breast cancer. The National Toxicology Program has added estrogen to the list of human carcinogens. The newsmakers said HRT *causes* heart attacks and strokes, not prevents them. Women are now afraid to consider birth control pills or menopausal hormone therapy. We are made to feel terrified about hormones our bodies make naturally our entire reproductive life. Why suddenly such intense negative focus on estrogen? We don't see such headlines about men's testosterone. What is really going on here?

Negative reports from the Women's Health Initiative (WHI) and Heart and Estrogen/progestin Replacement Study (HERS) hit the media like a nuclear explosion in the summer of 2002. Each of these clinical trials used only one form of estrogen—Premarin—derived from the urine of pregnant horses, and a synthetic progestin—Provera—both hormones not at all identical to anything our bodies ever made naturally, a point rarely mentioned in the coverage. There are many well-studied, alternative bioidentical (or "natural") forms of hormones available, with fewer negative effects. Why does damage found with *one* non-human hormone get applied to all hormone preparations, even though they are chemically as different as night and day? We don't see that happening in any other field of medicine, or with any other class of medications. Why does it happen with women's hormones?

The WHI was presented in the press as a study of "healthy" menopausal women. Healthy? Thirty-five percent of these women were already under treatment for high blood pressure; 35 percent were overweight and another 34 percent were *obese* by the medical definition; 12.5 percent had high enough cholesterol to require medication; 4 percent had diabetes; and 16 percent had a family history of breast cancer. "Typical" American maybe, but not "healthy." Their average age was about sixty-four years, and almost 30 percent were over seventy. This is ten to fifteen years *later* than most menopausal hormone therapies are started. These women, like the older women in the HERS study, already had evidence of heart disease, high cholesterol, and high blood pressure. In the words of Professor A. R. Genazzani, a world-renowned physician-researcher and the president of the

International Society of Gynecological Endocrinology, "We would never choose that kind of combination for our elderly patients with those clinical characteristics." The position paper of the International Menopause Society, published in September 2002, concludes: *"The WHI results, and particularly the data on cardiovascular disease risk, should only be related to the continuous combined treatment of 0.625 mg CEE [conjugated equine estrogens] together with 2.5 mg MPA [medroxy-progesterone acetate], prescribed to elderly, obese women with characteristics similar to those depicted in the WHI study."* In fact, the above comments and WHI findings validate concerns I have raised about Premarin and PremPro in my previous books and medical articles for more than a decade.

Why don't we get a full picture of the studies? Why are the negative results trumpeted and crucial positive findings downplayed or ignored? The press shouted there was a 26 percent increase in risk of breast cancer. What they *didn't* say was that the statistical increase was minute: of ten thousand women taking PremPro, only eight more would develop breast cancer than women not taking PremPro, or only seven more heart attacks. The WHI authors indicated that the average risk in an *individual* woman is 0.1 percent per year for breast cancer or a heart attack. We weren't given that number. The alarmist headlines made it appear that more women died taking hormones. This was not so. Articles neglected to say that the *death rate* from breast cancer or heart disease was *not increased* in the WHI PremPro group.

The focus on fear of breast cancer appears to sell newspapers and magazines. That same fear is also used to sell everything from herbs and soy supplements to new and expensive "designer estrogen" prescription products. Instead of educating women with balanced information, we are bombarded with poorly researched and hastily presented stories with a biased focus on breast cancer to the exclusion of other serious disorders—osteoporosis, diabetes, and cardiovascular disease are prime examples—that kill many times more women every year.

Why is it that *all* you hear about is the *slight* increase in risk of breast cancer that may occur with *some*—not all—types of estrogen-progestin therapy after menopause? There are other links to breast cancer that are far more ominous. For instance, in 1990, researchers in Finland found that women with breast cancer had higher concentrations of pesticide chemical residues *(Lindane)* in their breasts. Women with the highest Lindane residues were *ten times* more likely to have breast cancer than women with lower levels. The blood from all the women with breast cancer was analyzed and had *50 percent more* of this pesticide residue than the blood from women without breast cancer. An analysis of Connecticut women published in 1992 showed similar trends: levels of PCB, DDE, and DDT in the breast tissue of women with breast cancer were 50 to 60 percent higher than in women without cancer. You probably didn't hear much about all this. You need sound facts about other factors in this hormone–breast cancer link before you "throw the baby out with the bath water" on prescription hormones.

As a science-based focus on the international research studies that form the

basis of my clinical work, this book will do much to strip away the myths surrounding hormones and hormone therapy, including such misconceptions as
"Hormones cause cancer," "All estrogens are the same," "All progestins are the
same," and "How you take hormones doesn't matter."

- *Women need straight talk, sound information,* and more of the
  complete story behind the headlines.
- *Environmental endocrine disruptors interfere with function and
  production of human hormones and increase cancer risk.* We need to
  recognize and research, expose and identify these hormone saboteurs
  and toxins that are often ignored.
- *The cookie-cutter approach cannot continue.* One form of estrogen
  derived from pregnant horse's urine has been used in the United States for
  more than fifty years for about 85 percent of all HRT prescriptions—in
  spite of prescription hormones, bioidentical to those made by the ovaries,
  approved in the United States by the FDA since 1976. You wouldn't see 85
  percent of men with heart disease given the same drug at the same dose.
- *Bioidentical human forms of hormone products need to be used* instead
  of horse-derived or synthetic progestins that have very different—and often
  negative—effects in the human body. Examples of current FDA-approved
  products containing bioidentical 17-beta estradiol include Estrace (and
  generic) tablets, Vivelle, Vivelle DOT, Climara, Alora, and Esclim transdermal
  patches; or bioidentical progesterones Crinone and Prometrium.
- *"One-size-fits-all" is not acceptable any longer.* Women are individuals,
  with individual body chemistries. Women vary in response to hormones
  just as they do with all other classes of medicines (and herbs) they use.
  Women desire, and must have, hormone options individually tailored to
  their needs for optimal response.
- *We must measure hormone response with objective tests.* The "gold
  standard" serum (blood) tests for hormone levels are reliable for
  management of infertility in younger women. We must apply these same
  reliable objective tests for management of midlife and menopausal
  hormone issues. Saliva tests and hair analysis simply are not adequate
  for the complexity of women's hormones.

This book answers questions raised by the barrage of alarming stories, sheds
light on the complex puzzle of our female hormones, uncovers new information
about risks to your ovaries, and most important, gives you the tools to effectively
demand optimal care for *your* health and the health of the world you live in.

ELIZABETH LEE VLIET, M.D.
Tucson, Arizona, and Dallas–Fort Worth, Texas
May 2003

Introduction

Have you ever thought to yourself, "What's wrong with me? My body feels like an alien creature. I don't seem to be handling things as well as I used to. I don't feel good. I feel soooo tired. I don't accomplish as much as I once did. I'm not the *me* I once knew. What's going on?"

Something is different. It may have started out with little things: bone-tired fatigue, waking up in the middle of the night, body aches, forgetfulness, going to the bathroom more frequently, more noticeable PMS, headaches coming more often and lasting longer, no interest in sex, feeling blue and anxious for no apparent reason.

You wonder: "Is this all in my head? My doctor hasn't found anything physically wrong with me. He tells me I'm just stressed and need to take an antidepressant and do relaxation exercises. Is this just how it is? I am *too young* to feel this *old!* What is causing this? What can I do?"

Maybe your symptoms are more severe. Maybe you are undergoing medical treatment, seeing various physicians and specialists, taking lots of medication or herbs and teas you can't even pronounce, yet you're still not getting better or finding answers that make sense. You may still be thinking, "My doctor says there's nothing wrong . . . I must be imagining all this after all."

NO. The problem is *not* in your head. These problems can be very real, and are often caused by endocrine changes, changes in the workings of your body's hormones. Menstrual cycle effects on women's physical and emotional health have been described in medical literature since the time of the ancient Greeks. Today, we have extensive science to explain these connections, how they occur, and what to do when problems arise. That's what this book is about—helping young women who are not yet in the classic age range for perimenopause or menopause—understand what ovaries and the hormones they manufacture do to keep you well and healthy.

During more than twenty years of medical practice, I have evaluated countless women of all ages—from nine to ninety—who had been referred to as "crazy" by other physicians. So many women, even though different in age, have described the same physical and emotional experience at similar times of their menstrual cycles that I began to look at these ovarian hormone patterns more closely. I wondered what symptoms were triggered by the changing hormones of the menstrual cycle.

When I started this work in 1983, few physicians took "premenstrual syndrome"—PMS—seriously. My background in internal medicine and my interest in endocrinology, especially the effects of hormones on the brain, gave me a framework in which to think about and track symptoms. Fortunately, I also had formal specialty training in psychiatry at Johns Hopkins, one of the top programs in the country that focuses on the biological underpinnings of behavioral and mood syndromes. With this background, I could begin the detective work to uncover the mood, behavioral, and physical symptoms that appeared at predictable times of the menstrual cycle, then disappeared the rest of the month. If a woman's symptoms were clearly cyclic, at similar times of her menstrual cycle each month, I reasoned that such symptoms were *more likely* to have endocrine, or hormonal, triggers. I was convinced this pattern was *different* from similar problems suffered by women who experienced their mood or physical symptoms most all the time—such problems, occurring on a sustained, day-to-day basis, are more typical of true primary psychiatric syndromes. After having treated thousands of women and checking their cycle-specific ovarian hormone levels, I now see the enormous problem created for women by a health care system that ignores these hormone effects.

Why is it that more American doctors don't check women's ovarian hormones? For one thing, in the United States, gynecologists have been the primary physicians providing health care to women with hormone issues. But most of the emphasis in OB/GYN settings is on the *reproductive* effects of our hormones rather than the effects on other body systems such as the brain. In addition, gynecology is a surgical specialty, so doctors spend most of their residency training learning surgical skills for both delivering babies and for treating structural problems of the female reproductive organs. My friends in gynecology are quick to tell me that their training didn't focus much on the nuances of hormone management, or on how hormones affect the body above the waist!

Internal medicine, on the other hand, is a specialty that teaches doctors to take detailed medical histories of the patterns of symptoms, and then measure various lab tests to determine what is out of balance when the symptoms appear. An example would be diabetes. Internists look at the pattern of symptoms— abnormal weight gain, increased thirst, increased trips to the bathroom to urinate, and increased appetite for sweets, to name a few. Then they measure glucose and insulin levels at set times relative to meals, as well as do several other tests. All of this information is then used to make decisions about medications. Internists are also taught to *recheck* blood tests after starting new medications to monitor a person's response and to determine a proper dose.

So I, too, was accustomed to this approach in evaluating problems described by my patients. Was it diabetes causing the depressed, lethargic mood? Check the blood glucose level and see if it is consistently too high. Was it hypothyroidism causing the depressed mood, slowed thinking, and memory loss? Check the level of thyroid stimulating hormone (TSH) and see if it is out of the optimal target range. These were the kind of objective tests that I used to clarify the medical problems my patients described. But then I began to notice how women's symptoms occurred at the same time in the menstrual cycle, and then they got better. I was struck by this recurring pattern, and began to wonder whether their problems were being caused by the predictable changes in the hormones produced by the ovaries. I researched the medical literature to learn more about hormone effects beyond our reproductive system. I was excited to find a wealth of research about how ovarian hormones affect the brain, altering mood, sleep, and a host of other targets in the body. I began to measure ovarian hormones at different times of the cycle.

That's when the "Aha" lightbulb went on! Women were too often being told by their doctors—most without any formal training in psychiatry—that they were just depressed, anxious, or stressed. I determined that most of these women did not have a psychiatric disorder, nor were they "imagining" their symptoms. With lab tests I could show my patients that their ovarian hormones were in fact significantly out of balance at the time their symptoms were happening. Remember, *psychological* symptoms from effects on brain pathways can be caused by *physical* changes such as low or fluctuating hormones. These endocrine causes of mood and behavioral symptoms are *not* the same as purely psychiatric disorders. Together, my patients and I would then begin the quest to find treatment options for the underlying cause of the problem.

Unfortunately, doctors are not adequately trained in the role of ovarian hormones beyond their obvious reproductive function. The mind/body effects of ovarian hormones are basically ignored until the onset of menopause. It is a staggering fact that systematic measurements of the unique female endocrine system are completely absent in most medical workups and testing procedures for women. Expensive, and often less effective, medications, some with risky side effects, are typically the only approach offered to these women. So vast numbers of women with hormone-related health problems suffer needlessly, in spite of the availability of safe, effective options.

"Gender based medicine" is the current buzzword used in place of "women's health." But even this model, as currently practiced, fails to advocate testing of the very hormones that make us biologically female or male. It obviously isn't truly *gender based* if it ignores assessment of the basic biology of our male and female hormones. In my view, this is our next frontier in medical care for women.

Taking Care of the Ovaries: Whose Job Is It, Really?

Our current specialty-based health care system is incredibly fragmented: Neurologists check your headaches; rheumatologists check your muscle pain; orthopedists check your bones and joints; psychiatrists treat depression and anxiety; and otolaryngologists check your ears and sinuses. Endocrinologists are trained to diagnose and treat "hormonal disorders," particularly diabetes and thyroid disorders. They typically do not view the ovaries as "their area." Instead, they focus on the thyroid, parathyroid, pituitary, adrenal gland, and pancreas (diabetes). Endocrinologists often say that ovarian problems are for gynecologists to treat. But obstetrician-gynecologists deliver babies, address surgical gynecological problems, and provide annual pelvic and Pap exams. It is a surgical, not an endocrine, specialty. At the gynecologist's office, a woman may be told that her nonreproductive symptoms, such as mood swings, insomnia, or low energy, are not "gynecological," and she should see a psychiatrist. But psychiatrists typically don't check hormone levels in their treatment of mood or anxiety symptoms. No one looks at this piece of the picture.

So when it comes to the nonreproductive effects of ovarian hormones . . . *whose job is it?* Thus far this crucial question remains unanswered. There really is no identified specialty that focuses on the ovaries, the hormones they produce, and their multiple connections and effects on the nonreproductive functions of a woman's body and brain. Even many "women's health" specialists don't check ovarian hormone levels!

To illustrate the problem, I recently came across an award-winning endocrine website written by physicians for consumers. The ovaries were not even listed as an endocrine organ! Every other endocrine organ in the body was listed: pituitary, thyroid, adrenals, pancreas . . . but the ovaries were missing. It seems clear enough that if a man lost his testosterone, as abruptly as women lose estradiol with menopause or hysterectomy, he wouldn't feel normal. Yet very few doctors would tell a man that "it's just stress" if he'd lost the function of his testicles due to aging, injury, disease, or surgery. Just as testosterone is the powerful hormone that "sets" a man's biology, the ovarian hormones "set" the patterns of a woman's biology and affect every function in her body and brain.

Ovaries just can't be removed, have wedges cut out, tied off, suppressed, or otherwise impaired with impunity. The hormones they produce are major metabolic regulators that affect every cell and tissue in the body and brain. There are far-reaching consequences throughout the body if a woman's ovaries aren't up to par in their hormone production. These are very real health problems that, left unrecognized and untreated, can have devastating effects. It is time to recognize the hormonal connections critical for a woman's well-being, discuss the causes of premature ovarian decline, and explore the appropriate medical tests and safe, effective treatments. From your teens onward, you need to become informed about your body, about what your ovaries are and what they do besides help you have a baby. You also need to know the early clues that indicate a decline in these important ovarian hormones. You need to understand the symptoms, the serious health problems, and the conditions that affect ovarian hormone production, as well as what treatments are available and the consequences of your decisions. I believe that if you have this knowledge, then you will be able to make appropriate, intelligent choices to feel better and enjoy this time of your life. As one thirty-year-old aspiring actress said recently during her first visit: "I am tired of feeling so bad and so *old*. I am tired of being told by doctors that I am just stressed and need to slow down. I am tired of not having a life! *I want my life back!* That's why I'm here!"

This book will help you take these steps. We will explore what your ovaries and their hormones do throughout your body, what happens when they go awry, and the many ways these hormones can be disrupted, putting women's ovaries on overload and causing them to "shut down" at earlier and earlier ages.

It *Is* Possible—and Desirable—to Test Ovarian Hormones

Ovarian hormone levels are almost never checked unless a woman *demands* it be done. Even then, many doctors refuse and say "it isn't necessary" or "it's too expensive." I disagree with both statements. Doctors also say "there is no way to check your hormones" or "hormone tests aren't reliable." Neither statement is true. In fact, we have a multibillion-dollar infertility industry in this country that is based on measuring ovarian hormone levels. Infertility specialists have been reliably measuring women's ovarian hormones with blood tests since the 1960s. If they did not, they would not succeed in helping infertile women get pregnant. If we can reliably check blood tests for women's hormones when they are trying to get pregnant, why can't physicians use the same tests to help answer *other* health problems? In my view, the health needs of other women are just as important as the needs of those trying to get pregnant.

Why do I find answers to questions while other doctors don't? One major reason is that I feel it is crucial to include a thorough measurement of women's hormone levels in every health evaluation. My patients tell me that other doctors claim that because ovarian hormone levels vary so much with a woman's menstrual cycle, the information isn't useful. But in medicine, where *everything* in our body changes from one moment to the next, it seems illogical to me that you can't use women's hormone levels because they change! No test in medicine is perfect, and every test we use has variability. Glucose, insulin, cholesterol, and all of our other blood chemicals are varying minute to minute every day of our lives. Yet doctors do not treat anyone for diabetes, female or male, without measuring glucose and insulin levels. Doctors don't treat high-cholesterol problems without measuring the complete blood fat (lipid) profile. If doctors deal with this variation in all other tests, they can learn to deal with the variation in women's ovarian hormones, too.

In my office we work with patients to figure out their health problems. We discuss their hormones levels and take into account the fact that all of our medical tests have a built-in day-to-day, hour-to-hour, minute-to-minute variation. Nothing in the body is static. We explore with our patients how their body experiences change as the hormone levels do, and in my view, this concept is central to creating a truly *woman-centered* health care model.

Your Hormone Web: Effects Throughout Your Body

It's difficult to keep the symptom list short when looking at everything that can be affected by changes in ovarian hormones. Estradiol alone is involved in over four hundred functions in a woman's body. That doesn't even take into account the effects of testosterone, progesterone, and DHEA. Is it any wonder, then, that women have a whole panoply of problems when their ovarian hormones go awry? What do I see most commonly in the women coming to us for consults? Here's a typical list.

- *Fatigue, to the point of exhaustion*
- *Weight gain that's out of control*
- *Loss of sex drive*
- *Difficulty getting pregnant*
- *Heart palpitations, racing or pounding heartbeat*
- *Memory problems, difficulty concentrating, feeling scattered*
- *Headaches*
- *Restless, fragmented sleep*
- *Pelvic, vaginal, and/or external genital (vulvar) pain*
- *Painful intercourse, difficulty having an orgasm*
- *Cyclic, severe acne*
- *Mood swings*
- *Increasingly severe PMS*
- *Painful periods, severe cramping with bleeding*
- *Heavy bleeding*
- *Irregular menstrual cycles*
- *"Irritable" bowel or chronic constipation*
- *Sensitivity to strong smells and chemicals*
- *Worsening allergies*
- *Chronic yeast infections*
- *Thinning scalp hair*
- *Excess facial and body hair growth*
- *Dry skin*
- *Dry eyes*
- *Low body temperature*
- *Aching joints*
- *Muscle pain*
- *Marked pain with urination*

These are not "fun time" symptoms, and this is just a partial list. Any of these problems can have many causes; how, then, do we find out a possible *hormonal* cause if we don't have a reliable measure of ovarian hormones?

How Does This Relate to Me? I'm Too Young for Menopause

We have all been taught to think of menopause, or the end of menstruation, as the only time in a woman's life when the ovaries are no longer producing hormones. In our usual life progression, menopause affects women in their late forties and fifties. Doctors generally don't even consider hormone loss as a possibility in women younger than forty. "It can't be hormonal, you're too young" is a phrase you may have heard time and again when seeking medical care for these problems. But these "mysterious" symptoms, often severe, do plague women in their teens, twenties, and thirties. Young women may experience symptoms one would "expect" in older perimenopausal or menopausal women. Doctors—and most women—don't tend to think about the possibility of hormone imbalances in girls *before* puberty. Yet today, this serious problem is happening more and more in younger women for reasons I'll explain later.

What about hormone problems that occur in young women after a serious viral illness, a tubal ligation, or exposure to environmental chemicals? What about the alarming increase in premature puberty in girls as young as six, seven, and eight years old? These young women desperately need good evaluation now to prevent serious health problems later, problems such as infertility, obesity, insulin resistance, and even early onset diabetes.

There are several different, but overlapping, syndromes that affect your ovaries: premature ovarian decline (POD), premature ovarian failure (POF), polycystic ovary syndrome (PCOS), endometriosis, premenstrual syndrome (PMS) and the "new," more severe form now known as premenstrual dysphoric disorder (PMDD), postpartum depression (PPD), and several types of auto-immune, viral, and inflammatory illnesses that affect the ovaries (oophoritis). These different conditions all share a common feature: The ovaries are not producing an *optimal* balance of estradiol and testosterone, even though they may still be producing healthy levels of progesterone. While there are important medical distinctions among these conditions, *all* are overlooked and undertreated. As a result, they cost women—and society—countless billions of dollars in misspent health care costs, substance abuse, lost productivity in the workplace, and premature disability claims. At a more personal level, they cost individual women in staggering and profound ways: lost quality of life from the adverse side effects of medications and frequent doctor's visits to missed time from work, family discord, and the breakdown of personal relationships. Women should have access to a medical system that is sympathetic to the fact that our hormone fluctuations are critically important, not something to be overlooked or trivialized.

Underlying hormone causes of common health problems for women are not taken into account in health care today. Physicians are even *less* aware of the way synthetic chemicals in our environment may be contributing to serious health problems in younger and younger women. Women are facing a *silent* health crisis similar in magnitude to the environmental damage that Rachel Carson first documented in 1962 with her landmark book, *Silent Spring*. Her efforts focused world attention on the damage from DDT. Today, we face even more health threats from newly developed chemicals, permutations of the old DDT. While these new compounds may satisfy legal limits, they are still present in quantities that can seriously damage our bodies. Women's ovaries and thyroid glands are especially vulnerable to these "chemical disruptors," whether we are exposed in our mother's womb, during infancy or childhood, or as adults. This is a ticking time bomb waiting to explode in health problems for today's young women and girls as they grow older. The health of your ovaries is so much more at risk today than ever before in history as a result of environmental "hormone disruptors."

How did I get interested in exploring this chemical connection? As a biology student at The College of William and Mary, I was interested in the developing field of animal behavior and studied what happened to young animals whose mothers were given various drugs and chemicals during pregnancy. My master's thesis explored different aspects of these issues, based on work done in rats, mice, and hamsters. In the 1950s and 1960s, research had shown that chemicals given to a pregnant female could disrupt sexual behavior, fertility, and reproductive tract development in the developing offspring—for example, female offspring displayed male mating behavior or were infertile; male offspring engaged in female sexual behaviors and had abnormally small testicles. I was fascinated by these ominous findings, but little did I know how significant this would become to my later work in women's health. Over the years, as I have worked with patients to creatively connect the dots of their puzzling health changes, I have gone back to this basic science as well as wildlife studies and new research on human health problems, such as endometriosis, PCOS, and women's cancers. The picture that has unfolded is an alarming one, and one we desperately need to understand better and take seriously.

Hormones Alone Are Not the Answer . . .

Is this book just about taking hormones? Do hormones fix everything? Of course not. Hormones are not the only, or necessarily the best, course of treatment for every woman. There are lots of books on other solutions to relieve symptoms. There are very few books, however, that focus primarily on these *hormone* pieces of the puzzle. That is why I have focused on hormones in this book. I will discuss the pros and cons of various hormone-balancing options, talk about ways to help you find the right type of hormones to minimize unwanted side effects, and help you understand the flaws and misinterpretations of the scientific studies that have created an unwarranted fear of hormones, especially estrogens, in the minds of women young and old.

Diet, lifestyle, and the environment can have adverse effects on healthy ovarian function. Some unsuspected culprits are the overuse of soy supplements, too much exercise, chronic dieting, and exposure to environmental chemicals. Television and the Internet bombard us with "cures" that make the quackery of nineteenth-century health hustlers look tame. And some of these "cures" may actually interfere with women's fertility and normal hormone production. I will explain these, and also talk about the "excitotoxins" in foods and beverages that are potent neurological disruptors of the pituitary-ovarian pathways and can lead to hormone imbalance, particularly in women. Diets high in processed foods, which are loaded with these chemical additives, are a major factor in the increase of ovarian hormone problems that are seen in younger and younger women today, as you will see in upcoming chapters.

Who Am I to Write This Book?

It's My Ovaries, Stupid! builds on my twenty-five years of medical experience, including specialty training at Johns Hopkins Hospital, where the Hopkins reputation and specialty clinics attract patients and unusual medical problems from all over the world. This experience provided the extraordinary depth of clinical exposure that laid the foundation for my later work on the neuroendocrine effects on women's total health. You have the benefit of my many years of professional experience with these hormone issues and the benefit of my training as a physician and, before that, as a teacher of chemistry, biology, and psychopharmacology. In addition, because I am still actively seeing patients in my offices in Tucson and the Dallas–Fort Worth area, I have stayed on top of new developments in the field in order to find better ways to help solve my patients' problems. If the old approaches to treatment aren't working, then we must find other, more effective ways to help women feel better. Getting well again is a process, a journey. For some, it is quicker, for others, slower and more arduous, but it is always interesting and challenging. You aren't just reading theory here; you are reading about approaches I have found that *work*.

There is another dimension to my background that is just as important as the "professional" me. As a woman, I have dealt with these same confusing, capricious, and frustrating hormone changes. None of us are immune to these problems. I connect, at a very personal level, with what you are experiencing. I will share some of my own story as we walk this hormonal road together in the pages ahead.

I make certain, in the treatment approaches we use in our offices as well as what I describe in my books, that those I use and recommend are based on the reputable, peer-reviewed, national *and* international medical literature. I do my own literature research and check original articles and sources carefully. *I do not have any financial interest in any of the products I recommend in my books.* I do not recommend something I would not use myself, or would not feel comfortable recommending to a family member if the need arose.

Is this book for you? Take the self-test that follows. Then let's get started on understanding your "marvelous and maddening" hormones, and what they do.

Self-Test: "Is This Me?"

Take this self-test to see what health problems you may be experiencing that may be linked to your ovarian hormones. As you read further, I will provide explanations and helpful options so you can begin to feel better! But first, write down your answers below.

Answer the following questions honestly with a yes or no. Then total the number of yeses and nos and write the totals below.

___I feel tired and barely have energy to get through a normal day.

___I have trouble sleeping through the night and do not feel rested when I wake in the morning.

___I feel more irritable and edgier than is usual for me.

___I have angry outbursts that seem out of proportion to events.

___I feel nervous and tense, especially a week or so before my period.

___I feel depressed, especially a week or so before my period.

___I have crying spells for no apparent reason.

___I have more mood swings than I used to.

___I am gaining weight even though I haven't changed my eating habits.

___I have lost more than ten pounds without trying to diet or change my eating habits.

___I crave sweets/chocolate/carbohydrates more than I used to.

___I crave salty or fatty foods.

___I drink more than one alcoholic beverage a day.

___I find myself craving alcohol and have a hard time resisting it.

___I drink more than one soft drink (colas, etc.) a day.

___I eat processed and prepared foods daily or quite often.

___I have trouble with chronic constipation or diarrhea.

___My muscles and/or joints ache, or are frequently stiff.

___I have more allergies than I used to.

___I am sensitive to perfumes and chemical smells (i.e., get headaches, feel dizzy, can't think clearly, or have other symptoms when around strong smells).

___My menstrual cycles are more irregular.

___My menstrual flow is much lighter/much heavier than is usual for me.

___I have been skipping a lot of menstrual periods lately.

___I have gone more than two months without a period.

___I have tried to get pregnant and haven't been successful.

___I don't have my usual sex drive.

___I have trouble having an orgasm.

___I am losing hair/my hair is getting quite thin and brittle.

___I feel lethargic, sluggish, and slowed down a lot of the time.

___I frequently have problems with my memory and concentration.

___I have trouble making decisions, feel as if my thinking is scattered, or have trouble focusing.

___I have swelling of my hands or feet.

___I have more headaches than I used to.

___I have been having palpitations or racing heartbeat, especially around the time of my menstrual bleeding.

___I have dizzy spells.

___My skin is itchy/dry/feels as if there are ants crawling inside.

___My family/I use pesticides at home, either inside or outside.

___I/We use chemical cleaners for bathrooms, kitchens, carpets, and such.

___My mother took/may have taken DES or other hormones during pregnancy.

Total number   YES____ NO____

If you have answered yes to more than four or five of these questions, you may be experiencing the damaging effects of the endocrine disruptors around you, or you're having premature ovarian decline causing lower than desirable levels of estradiol, testosterone, and other key hormones.

Your Road Map to This Book

I have done my best to write *It's My Ovaries, Stupid!* in simple terms to make the medical explanations and "chemical soup" easier to understand. It may sound complicated at times, but women are smart, savvy, and persistent when it comes to their health. Many women tell me they like to understand the science that explains their experiences. They feel their observations are validated when the science acknowledges what they have been going through. I also find that women who are experiencing puzzling health problems are hungry for as much information as possible, and feel frustrated when books are too sketchy or superficial in their descriptions. I have provided details and background that I think will be useful to empower you in your quest for better health.

I am also writing this book in hopes it will be helpful to those in the community of health professionals who are genuinely interested in improving health care for women, and who want to understand the crucial ways that our ovary hormones affect systems and functions throughout our bodies.

I have arranged the text in a logical progression of information, starting with the basics.

Section I, "Body Basics," describes how the ovaries work, what they do, what their "life cycle" is, how they interact with other hormone systems, and how to recognize symptoms of faltering hormone production. Your ovarian hormones are like a tapestry of pathways interwoven throughout your body, affecting every aspect of your health. You need to have a clear understanding of how they work throughout your life.

Section II, "Ovaries at Risk," contains chapters on the dietary, environmental, and lifestyle "toxins" that put your ovaries at risk, as well as the wide variety of medical conditions, illnesses, and surgeries that can cause hormone imbalances.

Section III, "Your Ovaries and Your Body," shows how the imbalances in ovarian hormones can result in a bewildering array of health problems affecting just about every system in the body—from hair loss, brittle nails, and eye changes to anxiety, insomnia, memory loss, low energy, and loss of sex drive, to name just a few!

Section IV, "Getting Well—Your Action Plan," shows ways for you to improve your health. I have given you a list of tests you may request from your doctors, the hormone levels that should be tested, and when in the menstrual cycle it is most meaningful to have them done. I also explain what the numbers mean, and the differences between "optimal" and "normal" levels and ranges. Then I discuss what hormonal and other medication options you might consider, along with mind-body strategies that will help you regain your energy and zest. I teach you ways to clean up your home and work environment to eliminate toxic chemicals that affect you and your family and describe ways to improve your lifestyle choices so that you don't unwittingly sabotage your fertility or overall health.

Appendix I contains a list of medical abbreviations and definitions of medical terms, and Appendix II provides references mentioned throughout the book, listed by chapter. I have also included a list of resources to give you additional tools to make intelligent decisions about your health and find solutions to the problems you may be experiencing.

One comment about the references: I have included many *older* studies to show just how long many of these connections have been known. Some of these well-done studies go back to the 1970s, and a few even earlier, which is why it is even more incomprehensible to me that thirty or forty years later doctors *still* don't address these issues in women's heath care. Finding these older references took a lot of effort, which many readers will not have time to do. But that's why they are here; don't think that because they are "old" they are no longer valid. These "basics" still hold true today, even if they have been overlooked. I have also included cutting-edge, up-to-the-minute references to illustrate how our knowledge is increasing and the old "myths" are being shattered. A good example of this is the study by O'Meara and colleagues published in May 2001 that showed about a 50 percent *decrease* in risk of recurrence of breast cancer in women who chose to go back on estrogen (or estrogen-progestin) therapy *after* being diagnosed and treated for breast cancer. This is the *opposite* of the current teachings.

I have made frequent use of patient stories, firsthand experiences, and feedback from the women who have visited our offices for comprehensive evaluations. Each one is a real person with real struggles. While I have changed the names to protect their privacy, I have accurately portrayed their symptom descriptions, lab results, and the treatment approaches we used. After reading these stories from patients just like you, I hope you won't feel quite so alone and frightened. Women today are demanding answers and sound approaches to help solve problems. It is my hope that this book will guide you to the help you need to feel your best. Hormones are not to be *feared;* they are Mother Nature's miraculous gift to keep our bodies and minds vibrant and healthy!

SECTION I

Body Basics

1

When Ovaries Go Awry:
Women's Lives, Women's Stories

Introduction

The various permutations of hormone syndromes I listed in the Introduction—from premature ovarian decline (POD) to premenstrual syndrome (PMS) and polycystic ovary syndrome (PCOS)—are hitting younger women for many reasons. Women today are under much more stress than our mothers and grandmothers and lead very complex, demanding lives . . . burning the candle at both ends *and* in the middle. Yes, such stress does affect the ovaries and diminish hormone production. But women today are also immersed in more chemicals than ever before, with insidious consequences for our hormone pathways. At the same time, however, women are living lives that require a higher level of functioning, both physical and mental, than ever before. Disruptive symptoms or health problems that might once have gone unnoticed when women rarely worked outside the home can now seriously get in your way when you are holding down a full-time job in addition to being a wife and/or mother.

POD and menopause have similar symptoms—restless sleep, crawly skin, and hot flashes. But POD isn't *technically* menopause, because younger women still have follicles that can become eggs. Their menstrual periods are still occurring, even if now lighter and more irregular. Women who reach natural menopause have exhausted their lifetime supply of follicles in the ovary, and are therefore unable to produce optimal levels of ovarian hormones. With no follicles, no ovulation, and low hormone levels, the lining of the uterus doesn't build up to be shed as a menstrual period each month. Menstruation ends, which many women don't mind. What they *do* mind are symptoms that affect their quality of life: insomnia, low energy, loss of sex drive, and foggy thinking, among others.

The following stories illustrate an intriguing variety of the effects hormone imbalance and hormone decline can have on a woman's body. Some are devastating; most caused the patient to seek medical help. All are disruptive and unacceptable, particularly when they hit at a young age.

Women's Lives, Women's Stories

The patterns of hormone decline effects are different for each woman, but a common thread runs through each story: confusion, self-doubt, and feelings of being betrayed by one's own body and by the medical system. What's going on? Do these women just need to get a grip, simplify their lives, take a break, relax? Is this mental or physical? Antidepressants are frequently prescribed for these women, but are they the best answer? Are there other, more specific options to treat the underlying cause?

It's Not All in Your Head

The last seven months have been strange for *Rebecca*. Although she's only thirty-one, her body aches as if she's much older. Her joints hurt; she feels stiff and sore. It's hard for her to get out of bed in the morning. She just doesn't have the same level of energy she used to. In the past she could stay up late and really push herself to get all of her work done. Now it takes her a week to recover from even one late night. She had one ectopic pregnancy, plus an early miscarriage, and she has not been able to conceive again. She has totally lost interest in sex and this is affecting her marriage. She's started to get excruciating headaches and is battling a low-grade depression. She's heard about perimenopause but feels she is too young for that. She is able to go through the motions of her life, but feels as if she's missing out on a lot and aging much too quickly. What's going on? Her doctor said she is depressed and recommended an antidepressant, but Rebecca isn't convinced. She thinks there is more to it. What her doctor doesn't know is that Rebecca's mother had been treated with DES, a potent synthetic estrogen that was once used to help prevent miscarriage. DES affects a baby's development in the womb, leading to ovarian hormone problems in adulthood. This plays a role in Rebecca's problems.

For seventeen-year-old *Cathie*, "that time of the month" has always been a nightmare. Since her periods began at age eleven, she has experienced migraines, vomiting, and excruciating cramps every month with the onset of her menstrual bleeding. Various physicians prescribed a range of medications, including Prozac and beta-blockers, but nothing seemed to help. Cathie and her mother figured that since these episodes always came when her periods started, her hormones must trigger the headaches and cramps. They asked the doctors to check her menstrual cycle hormones, but their requests were dismissed. It seemed obvious to them that there was a connection, and they felt "put down" by her doctors' dismissal of their opinions about a hormone link. Now Cathie is getting desperate. She's missing too much school because of the headaches, and she's on so much medication that it is hard to stay alert when she does attend. When I checked her ovarian hormones, I found clues to what set off her menstrual migraines. Her estradiol on the first day of bleeding dropped to an abnormally low 10 pg/ml (see Appendix I for explanation of medical abbreviations). She didn't need so many medications every day; she needed to have a way to keep her estradiol from dropping so sharply and setting off the headaches.

Peggy sought medical help when she realized that at age twenty-eight she had the same symptoms as her eighty-year-old grandmothers! For the last two years she has felt "foggy" and would forget such simple things as her social security number and her best friend's phone number. At first she blamed her failing memory and emotional difficulties on stress and sleep deprivation. But when her hair started falling out, her skin felt crawly, her menstrual periods became irregular, the flow became very light, and her constipation got worse, she realized something else must be happening. Her food allergies were also getting worse, so she gave up foods with wheat, dairy products, sugar, or stimulants, but this didn't seem to help. She decided it was time to see her doctor. He said her symptoms were caused by stress and for her to get more rest and scale back her workload. How could she? She had two young children, a full-time job, and an ailing grandmother to care for. She had handled stress before and didn't have these problems. She was certain something else was going on.

Peggy realized that she never had these problems before her tubal ligation following the birth of her second child. She also noticed that her periods were lighter and her cycles shorter. Though her friends say they feel tired, they seem to be handling their life demands much better than Peggy feels she is. "What's wrong with me?" she wonders. "Is this all in my head? I tried seeing a new doctor, and she didn't find anything physically wrong with me. She tells me I'm just stressed and to do relaxation exercises. But I think there is something else. I think getting my tubes tied must have affected my hormones, but my doctor says that can't happen. . . . I wonder how I find out?" Peggy was correct: Tubal ligations can decrease blood flow to the ovaries, resulting in lower hormone levels. Her blood levels of estradiol and testosterone were extremely low. Her doctors missed it because they didn't check her hormone levels.

Leah, a twenty-six-year-old, was experiencing similar symptoms to the others I described, but hers had a different culprit. For two years Leah had been on a synthetic progestin, Depo-Provera, for contraception. She felt as if her life was "going down the tubes" with loss of energy, depressed mood, loss of sex drive, and irritable, angry feelings much of the time. She said, "I saw the title of your book and it was me! My main concern right now is just feeling better. I had a happy life until all this hit me. This is hard on my marriage. It's hanging on by a thread."

Depo-Provera is a synthetic contraceptive that contains no estrogen. This progestin can cause irritable, depressed, negative moods, typically suppresses the ovarian cycles, and decreases all ovarian hormone levels. But this wasn't quite the situation with Leah. Her estradiol levels were significantly below optimal levels, which is an effect of the Depo-Provera. Her ovaries were still producing a healthy rise in progesterone, typical of that seen with ovulation. The cyclic rise in progesterone from her own ovaries was added to the negative side effects of the Depo-Provera. Her total progesterone/progestin load was much too high relative to her *very low estradiol* for the second half of her ovarian cycle. The E:P ratio was all wrong. The progesterone/progestin dominance was the primary trigger for her severe PMS, headaches, and terrible mood swings. Needless to say, she changed to a different contraceptive!

These stories clearly demonstrate that we cannot just focus on age and then assume someone is too young to have hormone problems. All of these younger women had low hormone levels or abnormal ratios of estradiol and progesterone that caused very disruptive symptoms.

The Hidden Epidemic: What Is Happening to Young Women Today?

Premature ovarian decline (POD) is the early phase of decrease in ovarian hormone production, primarily affecting *estradiol,* our most active form of estrogen. In some women, this early phase also shows a decline in testosterone as well, even though progesterone and follicle stimulating hormone (FSH) may still be quite normal. There isn't a formal "medical" definition of this phase, and there is no well-accepted diagnosis or insurance code for it. Doctors today don't check hormone levels, so they don't recognize it exists. I have checked these levels. POD *does* exist. This is real. You are not imagining these changes.

Over the past twenty years I have systematically checked ovarian hormone levels in thousands of women of all ages, in different phases of the menstrual cycle. I can clearly document that this early phase of ovarian decline exists. Earlier researchers have also described this pattern, but it does not get much attention in today's health care. I have called it *premature ovarian decline* (POD), and I will explain in a moment how it differs from the formally accepted diagnosis of *premature ovarian failure* (POF).

Our "standard" teaching was not based on any systematic tests of ovarian hormone levels correlated with women's symptoms; it was based on the observation that some women developed irregular cycles. The problem is that very few physicians ever looked back to see what came *before* the irregular cycles to trigger the changes. POD, in the women I have tested, is characterized by estradiol levels typically less than half the normal, optimal healthy level for a young woman still in her reproductive years. Progesterone is usually maintained in the healthy ovulatory ranges until much later in the course of ovarian decline. Contrary to what most doctors have been taught, it is *not* progesterone that declines first. There may also be lower than normal testosterone levels, higher levels of markers of bone breakdown, high or low DHEA levels, and the adrenal cortisol levels are *higher* than would be expected. It isn't *adrenal* exhaustion; it's your *ovaries*!

What I did differently that helped me uncover the early stages of this process was explore the detailed health history of women *prior* to their cycles becoming irregular. What had happened in their lives before they developed these menstrual changes and bothersome symptoms? Had they been sick with a virus? Had they been through serious situational stresses? Did they have any other illnesses, surgery, new medications, new supplements, occupational or environmental chemical exposures? Did they start smoking cigarettes or using alcohol, marijuana, or cocaine? Did their mothers take DES or other hormones during pregnancy? Had they been exposed to pesticides? Did they drink excessive amounts of soft drinks? What was their diet like? Most of the women I see are able to identify many pieces of their health puzzle. No one else took them seriously or thought their observations were important. I value my patients' insights, and I use their observations to guide me as I think through their problems and decide what tests we need to reach a diagnosis.

One reason many doctors don't take women's hormone questions more seriously is the popular idea that pregnancy cravings and PMS mood swings are comical. The topics of sitcoms and mainstream jokes, we don't think they are real. For many women, "that time of the month" lasts only for a few days with little significant disruption. For other women, however, symptoms are more severe. We should not tell these women to "just accept it" when there are a number of straightforward approaches to help them feel better. Why shouldn't women's menstrual cycle symptoms be given as much attention as other health issues? Why shouldn't doctors use their medical knowledge to develop individualized treatment options? Health care can no longer afford to ignore women's ovarian hormones and the role they play in the health of our entire body.

In addition to a detailed medical history, I check hormone levels at specific phases of the menstrual cycle and correlate these levels with symptoms, and with what we know to be optimal levels for a fertile cycle. Doctors are taught that estrogen doesn't decline until *after* women lose their ovulatory cycles. With even a cursory review of these test results, this turns out to be incorrect. In all these years of testing, I don't think I have seen anyone with symptoms clearly occurring with the menstrual cycle who had a truly normal, optimal level of estradiol. To me, it is incomprehensible to insist that it isn't necessary to check ovarian hormone levels, especially today when we know how intertwined these hormones are with the function of every other organ system, including the brain. This doesn't mean that all of these women need treatment, but those with symptoms disrupting their quality of life *and* who have abnormally low hormone levels deserve effective help rather than one Band-Aid medicine after another.

For women with POD, I also do detailed thyroid testing, including thyroid antibodies. Although medical wisdom says that menstrual disruption is frequently caused by thyroid problems, I find that the usual thyroid tests often do not detect subtle abnormalities that affect the ovaries. I go a step further and look for evidence of autoimmune thyroid disorders by also checking the thyroid antibodies. Elevated thyroid antibodies can cause enough thyroid gland dysfunction to affect your ovaries, even if the TSH is still normal (see Chapters 9 and 17). Some women have both a thyroid disorder and ovarian decline; some have only one. Many women think they have a thyroid disorder but actually have an *ovarian* problem with significantly diminished estradiol production. The loss of optimal estradiol leads to multiple symptoms and quality-of-life-robbing syndromes. Over time, low estradiol leads to increased risk of serious problems such as infertility, PCOS, fibromyalgia, chronic fatigue, vulvodynia, depression, panic attacks, migraines, loss of sexual function, high cholesterol, high blood pressure, arthritis, diabetes, heart attacks, stroke, and others. It's important to know *which* you have, a thyroid disorder or POD, since health risks and treatments are different for each.

POD is a phase we must learn to recognize and address early to avoid these preventable health problems among young women. I will describe these further in Section II. It is important for you to take charge of this problem now, while you are young enough to prevent permanent damage to your ovaries, your fertility, and your overall health.

Premature ovarian failure (POF), or premature menopause, refers to the actual end of menstrual periods before the age of forty-two. POF is characterized by an FSH greater than 20 mIU/ml and low ovarian hormone levels characteristic of menopause; these just occur at a younger age than is average for natural menopause. POF is a devastating condition that has profound consequences on every dimension of a young woman's life, emotionally and physically. It has many causes, such as early loss of follicles in the ovary, autoimmune illnesses, viruses or chemicals that damage the follicles so they cannot function normally. POF causes infertility, a dramatic increase in bone loss, lower sexual responsiveness, chronic insomnia, headaches, allergies and immune changes, abnormal weight gain, marked fatigue, and, often, depression and memory problems. Later in the process, if not properly diagnosed and treated, it leads to more severe health consequences, including diabetes, early heart attacks, strokes, and early death. POF has many causes, as you will see.

POD and POF are two different conditions, but they are linked by the fact that the ovaries do not produce the proper amounts or balance of estradiol, progesterone, and testosterone needed for the body to function and for you to feel your best, which are typically the levels also needed for fertility. There are subtle differences between these two conditions, but if you are a young woman experiencing the loss of your ovarian hormones, it is ultimately less relevant what name you give it. The symptoms rob you of your quality of life and your ability to function at peak performance.

What are the differences between POD, POF, perimenopause, and menopause? I will explain this in more depth in Chapters 2 and 3, but here are some basic differences. Menopause is a natural progression of the aging process. We are born with all the follicles, or potential eggs, we will ever have. We lose follicles with every menstrual cycle. When we get older, and all the follicles have been used, we no longer make ovarian hormones and menstruation ends. We call this menopause. Perimenopause is the stage prior to the end of menstruation, when we still have some follicles but not enough to keep our cycles regular or to ovulate each month, or enough follicles to make optimal levels of ovarian hormones. POD and POF refer to conditions in which women still have their follicles but the ovaries are not working properly. They don't make optimal levels of the ovarian hormones, even though follicles are still available to do so. Again, it may not be critical what you call it. The fundamental issue is *what* hormones are you making, *how much* are you making, and whether those amounts are what your body needs.

The Hidden Epidemic: What's Different Now?

Precocious puberty. Girls developing breasts at age six or seven. Childhood obesity. Adolescent obesity. Infertility. PMS. PCOS. Postpartum depression. Postpartum psychosis. Diabetes epidemic. Eating disorders. Drug use. Attention deficit disorders. Hyperactivity disorders. Learning disorders. Autism. These topics have been making headlines on TV and magazines for the past few years. Why are they all so common now? What's happening to cause this? Is there something different for women of the twenty-first century than for our grandmothers and great-grandmothers? Yes. There are hidden saboteurs of your health, and I want you to know what they are and how they affect you.

You, and millions of other young women today, are growing up in a sea of chemicals in the foods you eat, the beverages you drink, and the environment you live in, both indoors and out. Your grandmothers and great-grandmothers never faced the threat of these massive numbers of chemicals, most of which were developed during and since the industrial boom after World War II. Your mother may have been exposed to many of them, but because of her age, it is likely that much of her exposure would have occurred *after* puberty, which is a less critical time for these adverse health effects.

Younger women, however, have been exposed to these ubiquitous chemicals as early as the womb. They are called *endocrine disruptors,* and they are hidden dangers to your ovaries, your thyroid, your fertility, and, ultimately, the health of all your body systems affected by these crucial hormones. You have been steeped in these chemicals since conception. And like a teabag that has been steeped too long, these chemicals can leave bitter aftereffects, insidiously affecting many aspects of your health, from your brain to your womb. The long-term potential damage is greater when your brain, ovaries, and other endocrine organs are exposed to these chemicals during critical periods of your development in infancy and childhood. Studies of both animals and humans have shown that the developing young in the uterus are far more vulnerable to chemical endocrine disruptions than are adults.

What exactly are endocrine disruptors? They are chemicals that have the ability to attach to hormone receptors throughout our bodies, and disrupt any one or more of several possible pathways, including: blocking of our own body hormones; producing abnormal responses at our hormone receptors; duplicating or mimicking normal hormone responses; interfering with the normal hormone signaling mechanisms our bodies need in order to work normally; and/or interacting with hormones and/or receptors to produce an exaggerated, or possibly even toxic, hormone effect. Even though these compounds are considered "endocrine disruptors," some effects are positive, such as the reduction of cholesterol caused by various plant-based estrogenic compounds found in many grains and soy. Others, such as pesticides that act at hormone receptors, are seriously toxic to the body and your fertility. Many are known carcinogens and can cause an increased risk of various types of cancers. Still other types of endocrine disruptors, such as genistein, found in soy, have mixed effects: It is beneficial at some concentrations but at other concentrations it has significant adverse effects, such as stimulating growth of breast cancers.

We now know from animal studies that miniscule amounts of hormonelike substances and other chemicals have a profound impact on a developing fetus. For example, studies from around the world show that these chemicals disrupt brain function, cause abnormal sexual and mating behavior, damage the developing structures of the reproductive system, alter function of the immune system and thyroid gland, and damage the ovaries in women and the testicles in men, just to name a few of the disturbing findings.

So how do you get exposed to these chemicals? Endocrine disruptors are found in the foods you eat, the air you breathe, the water you drink, the soft drinks you consume, as well as in the many household products you use in your home. In fact, the chemicals are dispersed throughout your environment. How do they get there? Some endocrine disruptors occur as by-products of industrial manufacturing and the use of fossil fuels like gasoline, jet fuel, and heating oil. They are spewed into the atmosphere and pollute the air. Then they come back to earth in rainwater to foul the water we drink and the soil in which our food is grown. These endocrine disruptors are insidious. You may not even know you have been exposed until you discover that you can't get pregnant, or you have problems with your menstrual cycle, or find yourself feeling so fatigued and sluggish you can't get through the day, or you begin to lose hair, or you develop serious allergies and chemical sensitivities.

At this point you may be thinking, well if these chemicals are in everything as you say, how can I change that? How do I escape the negative effects? What can I, as one individual, do about it? There are many answers to those questions, which will be addressed throughout this book. But the bottom line is yes, you *can* do something about the problem. Yes, you can take positive steps to prevent serious damage to your health. Yes, there are ways to help you feel better. I will discuss all of these approaches in detail in Section IV, "Getting Well." But before you can take these positive steps, you have to know more about how *healthy* ovarian cycles should work, and what happens to your body as you age. You need to know more about where these chemicals are, how they work, and what health problems they may aggravate. You will then see ways to avoid them and reduce their negative impact on your body. I explain these aspects in Section II, "Ovaries at Risk."

In the cases I presented at the beginning of this chapter, all of these women got their lives back on track and are doing well. In most cases, it was a matter of addressing hormonal imbalances, primarily low estradiol levels, and in some cases thyroid imbalances. There are good solutions to all of these problems. It all starts with proper testing, good detective work tracking symptom patterns together with laboratory information, common sense, diligence, persistence, and an innate curiosity to solve the mystery. In Section IV, I will talk more about ways to do this, and show you how to develop your own health action plan. You, and those who love you, deserve it.

So, let's now turn to Chapters 2 and 3 and take a look at how a healthy young woman's body works, what your ovaries and their hormones do for you, and what happens to your hormonal cycles as you age. I'll help you keep your ovaries—and the rest of you—healthy and energetic!

2

Your Ovaries: An Owner's Manual

Introduction

One of the delights of the study of medicine is learning about all the wonderful and miraculous things in our bodies that create us and keep everything going, balancing, responding, and accommodating as we live each day. The process is so perfectly orchestrated and intertwined that one has to marvel at *what* we are as well as *who* we are. We are all so similar, but at the same time, so different, with the most minute subtleties making us distinct from other creatures, and different from each other. As a woman I continue to marvel at the intricacies of our bodies and our rhythms. We are constantly in flux yet in balance, and while our ovaries define us as female from the very beginning, they are so much more than an "egg factory."

Our ovarian hormones play many roles in our overall health and well-being: maintaining bone and muscle strength; keeping our brain sharp; maintaining sleep; overseeing immune function; regulating blood pressure and heart function; and of course, stimulating our sexuality—not only its reproductive function, but our sexual thoughts, feelings, and actions. Our ovaries are inextricably involved with our entire endocrine system, with the hypothalamus, pituitary gland, parathyroid, thyroid, adrenal gland, and pancreas. Each of these glands secretes its unique hormones, which interact with ovarian hormones in many ways, as you will see in upcoming chapters. Our ovaries also have receptors, or docking sites, for chemical messengers that are made in the immune and nervous systems. Ovaries and their hormones are intimately linked to all of our other body systems.

The ovaries are not our most attractive internal organs. They are dullish gray, pitted, lumpy, irregular in shape, and a little larger than an unshelled almond. The ovaries are partially attached to the uterus by arteries, veins, and connective tissue, yet they are also semi-floating in space in the pelvis. Their real connection to the uterus, the fallopian tubes, hover nearby, barely touching the ovaries.

All of this looked so organized in the junior high school health books, yet those drawings did not do justice to the complexity of it all. Some body systems may be more "mechanical" and therefore easier to understand, but I see our ovaries, along with the brain, as more "art" than "science." Everything is delicately balanced, exquisitely sensitive, and closely intertwined. Our ovaries hang in there month after month, year after year, part of a beautifully coordinated hormonal symphony.

Most of us think in terms of eggs when we think of our ovaries, so let's begin there. Our supply of eggs begins forming virtually at conception. By about Week 20, we will have built our maximum number of eggs, approximately 6 to 7 million. During the next fifteen to twenty weeks before birth, we will do away with about 5 million. We don't know what determines which follicles stay and which go; some just quietly burst their membranes, die, and are reabsorbed into the bloodstream. At birth, we have approximately 20 percent of our eggs left, and by puberty we have approximately 20 percent of that last 20 percent, still somewhere between 200,000 and 400,000 follicles. At each ovulation we can lose 20 to 1,000 eggs, usually toward the smaller number. The biblical phrase "many are called, few are chosen" (Matthew 20:16, KJV) applies here. The average woman today who has fewer pregnancies will have approximately 400 to 450 menstrual periods in her lifetime. Earlier generations of women may have had as few as 50 menstrual cycles because they had multiple pregnancies, often beginning in their teens. They also had many years of breast-feedings that suppressed ovulations, and they died at much younger ages, often before they even reached menopause.

We probably learn about our menstrual cycle first from our older girlfriends, then our mothers, and later as we sit through health classes at school. Once we have passed the test for a class, however, we often don't pay much more attention to what's happening with our monthly fluctuations. We become more aware of having periods, and whatever premenstrual problems we might experience, but we usually don't focus on the specifics of which hormone is doing what at any given point.

During early childhood, before age three or four, an area of the brain called the *hypothalamus* occasionally releases small bursts, or pulses, of reproductive hormones to support early female development. Then the hypothalamus seems to take a sabbatical from its female cycle management role until age nine or ten, on average, when it then resumes its command central role. Around this time—age eight to ten—the adrenal gland gears up production of the adrenal androgens. It is the adrenal androgens, not the ovary, that trigger the growth of pubic hair. By age eleven or so, the hypothalamus is fully up and running.

We don't yet know with certainty all the triggers for the onset of puberty and periods. Menses generally begin about midway through the physiological process of puberty, when a girl reaches approximately 100 pounds in body weight and about 25 percent body fat. These "magic numbers" seems to signal the brain that the body has sufficient fat as reserve energy, about 87,000 calories, to support a pregnancy, which requires approximately 80,000 calories. We see further evidence for this "set point" of weight and fat percentage as heavier girls begin menstruating earlier than thin or athletic girls with less body fat. It may be that the brain is responding to the hormone leptin, which comes from the fat stores, or there may be other chemical messengers that govern this process.

At any rate, the hypothalamus begins sending out gonadotrophin releasing hormone (GnRH), and when that level gets high enough, it stimulates the pituitary to release follicle stimulating hormone (FSH) and luteinizing (literally, "yellowing") hormone (LH). These two will continue their work together for the rest of your menstrual life. The long-awaited signal goes out to the ovaries; they rev up and send out the sex hormones that stimulate breast development, put fat on the hips, and widen the pelvic bones. FSH and LH wake up the follicles that are to become eggs (ova). Your early menstrual cycles may be a bit erratic while all the systems are getting organized, but usually, within six to twelve months, the rhythms are humming along in a flow that will carry on for another forty-some years.

The menstrual cycle itself is a dynamic process, part of the complex and carefully timed procedure of fertility. We mark the "beginning" of the cycle with the sloughing of the uterine lining (bleeding) from the previous month's cycle. The brain senses the fall in estradiol and progesterone levels to their low point; it signals the pituitary gland to start the cycle all over. The pituitary first sends out FSH to stimulate new follicles ("egg cells") to grow and start making estrogen, mainly estradiol, again. This primes the follicles to develop for ovulation and stimulates the growth of the lining of the uterus. Progesterone is at a very low level throughout the first half of the cycle, and doesn't start rising significantly until after ovulation. Each month about twenty or so follicles in each ovary start to expand and ripen. On Day 10 or so, one of these is somehow chosen, and it becomes the dominant follicle. Occasionally, more follicles will develop, which can lead to twins, triplets, or other multiples. When the FSH gets to its highest point of the cycle, this rise signals release of the egg, in the process we call ovulation. If multiple eggs are released it appears to be due to a higher FSH level than usual.

The dominant follicle, destined to become the egg, prepares for ovulation by growing a bubblelike sac to protect itself, and forces its way to the surface of the ovary. The other follicles recruited at the beginning of the cycle seem to know which one has been picked, start to shrivel, then die, and are reabsorbed into the bloodstream. The chosen follicle matures and grows, producing significant amounts of estradiol that trigger many changes, including the rapid growth and thickening of the uterine lining (endometrium). The thickening of the endometrium helps prepare the uterus for the arrival of a fertilized egg. When the levels of estradiol reach about six times the usual level, the hypothalamus again nudges the pituitary, and this time it cuts back on the release of FSH, which keeps any more eggs from developing. Meanwhile the fallopian tubes wave their fimbria, delicate hairlike fronds similar to the beautiful soft corals I have seen scuba diving. Anticipating the egg's arrival, the fimbria begin to brush the surface of the ovary looking for the large follicle that delivers the egg. From Day 12–14, the LH signal arrives from the pituitary and tells the egg it's time to pop out. When this happens, many women feel a brief, sharp prick of pain we call mittelschmertz.

The rise in estradiol also changes the cervical fluid, which functions much like seminal fluid does in men. Sperm need a friendly, alkaline, nutrient-rich environment in which to survive during the long journey from the vagina, up through the uterus, and into the fallopian tube. Women only need these estrogen-triggered changes in cervical fluid at ovulation in order to protect sperm from an otherwise acidic vagina. The cervical fluid changes quickly, often within a few hours or so, after the rapid rise in estradiol just prior to release of the egg. To further the preparation for fertilization, the cervix changes its position, hugging the uterus closer, and becomes softer and more open to receive sperm.

Meanwhile, the egg literally bursts from the ovary into the vast openness of the pelvic cavity. The arms of the fallopian tubes are waiting and waving, with their hairlike projections, to quickly move the egg into the funnel of the fallopian tube. Fertilization, if it occurs, normally takes place in the fallopian tube, not in the uterus. The follicle has still more work to do after the egg is released. Just after the egg pops free, the cells lining the cavity in the follicle begin filling with cholesterol, turning all soft and yellow, and become the *corpus luteum* (or "yellow body"). The corpus luteum generates more estradiol and starts pumping out progesterone to stimulate an even lusher thickening of the lining of the uterus. Everything is ready to receive the fertilized egg that should soon be coming down the fallopian tube.

For the first forty-two days or so, the mother's ovarian hormones are essential to the survival of the fetus, until it gets its own hormone support system built, the placenta, which takes over the synthesizing of estrogen and progesterone. Even after the placenta takes over, however, the corpus luteum continues producing progesterone to prevent further development of eggs in the ovary, and continues sending hormones out to the mother's body. If the egg misses contact with a sperm, for whatever reason, within about ten days following ovulation, the corpus luteum gives up, stops all hormone production, begins to shrivel, and dies. Both estradiol and progesterone fall abruptly, but it is the drop in progesterone that triggers shedding of the uterine lining to begin your menstrual bleeding. The whole process begins again, and another cycle is under way.

The box on page 16 provides a shorter, more medical summary with important definitions and terms to keep in mind as you read further.

Some of the midcycle symptoms I often hear described by patients are "twinges" or a dull achiness, which is probably caused by the swelling of the follicles in each ovary in the race to be the chosen one. The brief cramps at midcycle are likely the result of irritation of the abdominal lining caused by leaking blood or follicular fluid from the rupturing egg follicle and/or the contractions of the fallopian tube. In the luteal phase, many of the symptoms you experience are related to metabolic changes triggered by progesterone that prepare the body for pregnancy. I will talk more about those later, but you already know them well, I am sure!

As we get older and our follicles become depleted, egg production stops. We no longer have our ovarian "hormone factory" to produce enough estrogen and

THE MENSTRUAL CYCLE

1. We start with the *menstrual phase* of the cycle. It begins on the first day of menstrual bleeding. Actually, this is the end of the last cycle, but we arbitrarily choose to call it Day 1 since it can be easily marked by the bleeding. Estradiol and progesterone levels are at their lowest point. Optimally, a healthy level of estradiol at this phase is 80–90 pg/ml. Progesterone is typically less than 0.5 ng/ml.

2. The *follicular phase* is next, named for the developing follicles. The lining of the uterus (endometrium) is growing, or proliferating, rapidly now, so we also call this the *proliferative phase.* Estradiol rises to its highest peak of the cycle, then drops again sharply just before ovulation. Follicular phase estradiol levels average about 200 pg/ml; the ovulatory peak is 350–500 pg/ml. Progesterone is still low, usually less than 1.0 ng/ml.

3. The follicular phase is typically when women experience optimal physical and sexual energy, sound sleep, upbeat mood, sharp thinking, mental clarity, sharp concentration and word recall, optimal immune function, to name a few of the common descriptions from my patients.

4. The *luteal phase,* named for the hormone-producing corpus luteum, occurs following ovulation. We also call this the *secretory* phase of the endometrium because the uterine lining thickens to prepare for pregnancy. Progesterone peaks at 10–25 ng/ml on about Day 20, and estradiol hits a second, but lower, peak of 200–300 pg/ml. This is the cycle week in which PMS typically gets worse as progesterone levels increase. I find that women with PMS typically have progesterone levels that rise normally, but their estradiol is usually below about 150 pg/ml.

5. The *premenstrual phase* occurs around Day 26–28 on average in a twenty-eight day cycle. Both estradiol and progesterone levels begin to drop if there is no fertilization, and fall more sharply about Day 26. The drop in progesterone is the trigger for shedding the uterine lining, which we call menstruation.

6. The cycle begins again, and repeats, beginning with #1.

progesterone to support menstruation. The end of menstruation is called *menopause.*

But the menstrual cycle is only part of the job description of the ovaries. As a "female" organ, they have multiple responsibilities. Ovaries are the primary producers of progesterone, testosterone, and our estrogens, especially the primary premenopausal active form, 17-beta estradiol. Very small amounts of

THE MENSTRUAL CYCLE HORMONE RHYTHM

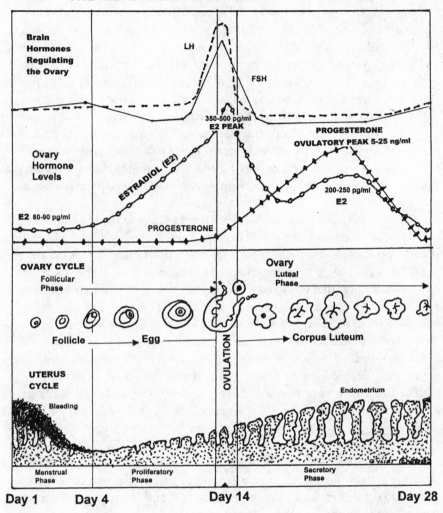

© Elizabeth Lee and Gordon C. Vliet 1995, revised 2003

testosterone, other androgens, and progesterone are also made in the adrenal glands, and our body fat also makes androgens and significant amounts of estrone. Estrone is another estrogen also made by the ovary and is less active than estradiol. It serves as our reservoir, or storage, form of estrogen, and is the only form of estrogen present in measurable amounts after menopause. That's why overweight women are said to have "too much estrogen." They may actually be low in estradiol but have excess estrone, an important distinction that can make a huge difference in your health risks and one we will explore in detail a little later.

Your Ovary as Hormone Factory

Hormones are a major heading included under a bigger umbrella called *steroids*. The basic chemical structure is four rings of carbon atoms. There are literally thousands of varieties of steroids and steroidlike hormones throughout nature, and they all have the cholesterol molecule as their basic building block. Cholesterol serves as a building block for many hormones, including all the estrogens, progesterone, and testosterone, as well as vitamin D. The body can make its own cholesterol from the fat in our diet, provided you eat the right amount of fat. If you eat too little fat, you can't make cholesterol, or your ovarian hormones. If you eat too much fat, this will shift the hormone balance toward more estrone, the remaining form of estrogen after menopause, as well as male hormones that interfere with the normal production of your biologically active premenopausal estrogen, estradiol.

The word *hormone* was coined in 1905 from a Greek word meaning "to excite or to arouse." Certainly the power of hormones in the body was evident long before we understood so many of their specific actions. For instance, the ancients knew that castration removed something of maleness, even if they didn't know exactly what it was that was gone. *Eunuchs* were men castrated to provide guards for harems of kings and sultans in ancient times. Since the eunuchs no longer had their male sexual urges, they were "safe" to guard the women. In seventeenth- and eighteenth-century Italy, castrated men were known as *castrati*. Their high-pitched, feminine voices and ability to hit the high soprano notes were greatly desired in opera houses before women singers were allowed.

The function of a hormone is to circulate in body fluids (primarily in the bloodstream) and arouse or urge targeted body tissues to do, or not do, that which they are supposed to. In short, they are messengers, chemical communicators carrying messages to and from all organs of the body. They serve to connect one organ's function with others. We would die if we did not have this signaling system to keep our organs functioning in a balanced, integrated, and coordinated manner. In a woman, the secretion and interaction of hormones throughout the body is an exceptionally complex process. Because of the intertwining of the glands of the endocrine system, if the ovaries aren't functioning properly *any and all* of the body's systems may show the repercussions of losing these powerful messengers.

The converse is also true: If other endocrine systems are malfunctioning, this causes suppression or failure of the ovary's ability to produce hormones and develop eggs normally. These hormone systems are closely linked. This is another reason the "endocrine disrupting" chemicals I describe in Chapters 4 and 5 are such a threat to our entire hormonal balance and function.

The list on page 19 shows some of the many changes that occur with every menstrual cycle. It is truly incredible to see how many different functions are changed with the ebb and flow of our ovarian hormones every day of our cycle. I hope this list gives you an idea of how profound are the relationships between your changing ovarian hormones each month and every other part of your body.

Body Changes Affected by the Menstrual Cycle

- *Body temperature*
- *Blood glucose regulation*
- *Breast size, texture, skin/nipple color*
- *Energy levels and sleep patterns*
- *Neurotransmitter production*
- *Basal metabolism rate*
- *Estrogen levels in blood and urinary metabolites*
- *Progesterone levels in blood and urinary metabolites*
- *Levels of brain hormones and neurotransmitters*
- *Bile pigments (to digest fat)*
- *Thyroid and adrenal hormone production*
- *Red and white blood-cell counts*
- *Fluid balance*
- *Skin color, texture, permeability*
- *Respiration functions: CO_2, O_2*
- *Blood pH*
- *Memory and concentration*
- *Citric acid (vitamin C) content of mucus*
- *Brain wave (EEG) patterns*
- *Heart rate and rhythm*
- *Balance, fine-motor coordination*
- *ESR ("sed rate") measure of inflammation*
- *Pupil size and reactivity*
- *Platelet counts*
- *Blood levels of adrenaline*
- *Body weight*
- *GSR (galvanic skin resistance)*
- *Pulmonary (lungs) vital capacity*
- *Blood protein levels and amounts*
- *Vaginal mucus characteristics*
- *Vaginal cytology (cell types)*
- *Visual, auditory, olfactory acuity*
- *Serum bicarbonate*
- *Pain threshold*
- *Feeling state and behavior*
- *Concentrations of vitamins A, C, E, and B group*
- *Cervix changes: size, color, position*
- *Urine volume, pH, specific gravity*

How Do Hormones Trigger Actions?

Hormones have "docking sites" we call *receptors* made of proteins and located either on the surface or within the cells themselves, usually in the nucleus. Cells throughout the body are like little manufacturing plants, making the chemicals the body needs to function. Hormones may act like purchasing agents in some instances, or as team facilitators in others. Hormone actions can be faster than the blink of an eye as when acting at receptors located on cell membranes, or they can promote action more slowly as when they act on cell nuclei to direct production of specific enzymes and proteins. Receptors, in untold numbers, are found throughout the body.

Estrogen, for instance, has receptors in the brain, bladder, bones, teeth, muscles, blood vessels, skin, breasts, uterus, eyes, heart, and colon. In any given cell, there may be thousands of receptors, in some many more. Perhaps that is why it doesn't take much to get a major response. It has recently been determined that there are two types of estrogen receptors, *alpha* and *beta*. Some tissues of the body have alpha, some have beta, and some have both.

There can be such a wide variety of symptoms when estradiol levels decline because so many different organs and tissues have these receptors designed to work properly only when activated by estradiol. It has many functions and very complicated interactions with other hormones. Estradiol is a powerful and very active hormone!

Since our scientific understanding of women's hormones and their many receptors has expanded greatly, why is it so difficult for women to get doctors to address the hormone connections they themselves have observed in the patterns of their symptoms? How is it that I "find" these connections when other physicians have not? I think part of the answer lies in one's mind-set. Most physicians still don't think through all the physiological hormone connections linking symptoms that appear to be separate, such as fatigue, headaches, moodiness, and loss of sex drive. The mind-set still seems to be that each symptom has a separate cause and needs a separate evaluation, and a separate medication. Another common mind-set is that such a cluster could "only" be linked with a diagnosis of depression.

My mind-set, however, is that I am looking first for a common denominator in physiological changes that could explain several, if not all, of my patient's symptoms. In other words, I try to find a unifying explanation rather than separate causes and multiple diagnoses. Then I explore treatment options that help alleviate multiple symptoms with the fewest number of medications. The more medications used, the more likely there will be side effects and drug interactions that could complicate the picture.

In addition to the mind-set of the physician, there is also the time it takes for new research to become incorporated into office-based clinical practice. Although hormone receptor research and the hormone effects on every organ system in the body are widely discussed in major medical journals, it is new information that is not often filtering down and finding its way into the practicing physician's office as quickly as we would like to think. A 2001 government survey found that it takes an average of *seventeen years* for new research findings to become commonly accepted in the average doctor's clinical practice.

In addition, research publications often have little information on how to put these new findings into practice, or give few practical guidelines on how these new findings affect women's body systems and produce the clinical problems women describe to their doctors. It takes creative thinking, sometimes "outside the box," to connect the dots between various research findings in a variety of specialty fields with how the body works, patterns of symptoms, lab results, and what to *do* to solve clinical problems. That is what we call the "art" of medicine. It takes time, patience, and a give-and-take relationship with one's patients. Today's insurance-dictated five-minute office visits for most doctors have undermined their ability to engage in creative thinking and the "art" of medicine. Doctors have been forced to focus simply on established protocols and standard approaches. Migraine headaches? Take Imitrex. Insomnia? Take Ambien. Depressed mood? Take Prozac. PMS? Take Zoloft. A hormone connection between all of these? "It's too expensive to check hormone levels." So doctors don't do it. As a result, they miss the fact that underlying all of these seemingly disparate problems could be low estradiol.

I found these connections because I looked for them and checked hormone levels over the years of working with women. Time after time, I found that if I restored the estradiol to more optimal ranges, my patients would come back and tell me that they no longer had trouble sleeping and had stopped the sleeping pills, or that their mood was so much better, they no longer needed the antidepressant.

A typical example of my unifying approach happens when I see a woman who has suffered from migraines. In addition to all the usual history and workup identifying the typical triggers like foods, stress, weather changes, and so on, I ask detailed questions about the relationship of the headaches to her menstrual cycle. If a woman tells me she has a regular migraine every month when her period starts, it makes sense based on the science that shows falling estradiol has effects on serotonin, blood vessels, and pain pathways that can set off the migraine just as bleeding begins. One approach I use for headache sufferers is to teach them to use an estradiol skin patch to avoid the drop in the estradiol level and prevent the headache from beginning. Using estradiol patches this way doesn't stop the menstrual flow, which is triggered by the fall in progesterone. It seems such a logical approach for a migraine that always comes with menses. Of course, if the estradiol patch does not work, I try other approaches. Women frequently tell me that their migraine headaches are relieved, or are less frequent and or less severe, when we find a way to keep the estradiol steady. I consider this a crucial first step with menstrual migraines. I can always go to the standard medications later, if needed.

There are other ways our new understanding of hormone receptor action and specificity determines medical approaches for individual women. Science has shown that the docking of a hormone at its receptor is greatly affected by having just the right molecule size and shape. In my writings and talks, I use the analogy of hormones being "keys" that fit into their special receptor like a "lock," switching that receptor "on" or "off." In reality, it is much more complicated, but this visual image is still helpful in understanding why the right molecular key is important. Differently shaped molecules may actually block or interfere with proper hormone action. If the molecular "key" is not exactly right, it may fit in the lock but not turn, so it can't "open" the action of that cell or pathway.

For example, when we replace estrogen for a young woman who has had her ovaries removed, it becomes important what type of molecular makeup the substitute estrogen has. Do you want an exact duplicate molecule of what your body used to make, or would you settle for a mixture that gives you many more, and many different molecules . . . some of which your body has never made and doesn't quite know how to use? This second option has been offered to most women in this country for the last fifty years, even though it may not now be the best choice for optimal energy and well-being. This is the major reason so many women feel that a hysterectomy left them miserable. It usually isn't the surgery that's the problem, it is the lack of the exact molecular replacement of the hormones your body used to make, and matching the amounts to your individual needs. One size *does not* fit all.

Let me explain a little more: 17-beta estradiol is the naturally occurring, human, primary estrogen made by the ovary before menopause. If a young woman has her ovaries removed before menopause, she would likely want to replace what was lost and just use 17-beta estradiol. Make sense? The primary prescription product used in this country, however, is derived from pregnant mares' urine (Premarin) and contains mostly horse estrogens (*equine estrogens*). Equine estrogens, or equilins, are actually many compounds that are foreign to our bodies and have various chemical additions that make them different from our own 17-beta estradiol. Consequently, the equine estrogens don't fit the body's receptor sites in exactly the same way, which means their effects can be very different. This is one reason why women taking Premarin often say their memory isn't as good, or they don't sleep as well, or they gain weight, or they don't have their usual energy. Small changes in the molecule can make a big difference in the way a particular estrogen works in your body and, especially, your brain. This same concept will be important as we look at ways the molecules of endocrine-disrupting environmental chemicals can mimic, block, or intensify hormone actions in your body.

There are other important differences between the equine estrogens and our own natural 17-beta estradiol. Equine estrogens attach very strongly to estrogen receptors and can block or interfere with the attachment and action of our own estradiol. It also takes much longer for the body to metabolize the equine estrogens because our body doesn't have the enzymes necessary to break them down.

This means they last a lot longer in the body than our estradiol does. For example, if you take Premarin and then stop, it may take two to three months for all the horse estrogens to be cleared from your body. This is especially true in the breast, where the equine estrogens are very strongly attached to the receptors and build up over time the longer you take Premarin. If you use 17-beta estradiol and stop, your body's metabolism clears it away in only a day or so.

There's another reason that women taking Premarin say they feel different, and not "back to my normal self." The mixture of equine estrogens in Premarin provides a high level of total estrogens but does not provide enough of the human 17-beta estradiol that most women need to feel their best. Typically, with a standard dose of Premarin, even though the overall horse estrogen levels are high, the critical 17-beta estradiol levels may only get to the 30–50 pg/ml range. This is a long ways away from the 100–200 pg/ml range typically circulating over a healthy menstrual cycle. Estradiol patches or pills easily provide levels of 100–200 pg/ml to restore what has been lost.

Hormone Power: Incredible Potency from Your Ovaries

Estrogen

You may get a better grasp on the subtleties of estrogen effects if you consider how powerful these hormones are. Many hormones are measured in as little as a billionth of a gram, called a *nanogram* (ng). Estradiol, for example, is measured in picograms (pg), or one *trillionth* of a gram. In her beautifully written book *Woman: An Intimate Geography*, Natalie Angier paints this amazing visual image: To get *one teaspoonful of estradiol* you would need to drain *all* the blood from the bodies of 250,000 premenopausal women. Each of those bodies also contains approximately a teaspoonful of sugar and two tablespoons of salt. To get a teaspoonful of estrogen you'd have to deal with a hill of sugar and a mountain of salt. And they try to tell us testosterone is the "power" hormone!

We think of estrogen as the quintessential female hormone, but "it" is really fifty or more different compounds, some more potent than others. Our three primary human estrogens are *estrone* (E1) and *estradiol* (E2), both made by the ovary and body fat, and *estriol* (E3) manufactured by the placenta during pregnancy. Many of the other estrogenic compounds in that fifty-plus group come from the metabolism of our three major estrogens as they are broken down into a variety of compounds. Some are inactive; others are still hormonally very active.

It can get quite involved, so I decided it would be much more practical to focus on E1, E2, and E3. They differ in their chemical makeup, when they play a role in a woman's life, the primary site where they are synthesized, and what they do in our bodies.

Estrone (E1). Estrone was the first human estrogen identified—in 1929—when scientists were doing a random search of pregnant women's urine looking for the hormones of pregnancy. It is made in the ovary, body fat, and liver; it is called E1 because it has only one oxygen-hydrogen group attached (estradiol has two, estriol has three). Estrone is important to us as a reservoir source of estrogen. It is known as the postmenopausal estrogen because it can be made from androgens and stored in body fat with the help of an enzyme called *aromatase*. Aromatase converts androgens like testosterone and androstenedione to estrone, and then to estradiol. Estrone plays a role, along with androgens, in the change in our body shape from pear to apple, as shown in the diagram, page 53. It is the only remaining source of estrogen after menopause if women are not taking estrogen replacement therapy. While it provides at least some estrogen effect, it doesn't have exactly the same actions and benefits we see before menopause with estradiol, which is the major reason why women's bodies look so different, and have different health risks, after menopause.

Estradiol (E2). The primary and most active estrogen from puberty to menopause, estradiol affects over four hundred functions in our body, and receptors are located in virtually every organ. Estradiol is made primarily in the ovary, via the aromatase pathway, so when we run out of our follicles or our ovaries are removed, we no longer have a way to make adequate amounts of estradiol. Earlier, I described the levels of estradiol that correspond with feeling your best. In pregnancy, both progesterone and estradiol levels rise rapidly in the first trimester. Then progesterone decreases sharply at the sixth to eighth week, while estradiol continues to rise and remain high throughout pregnancy. Progesterone does not rise again until about the thirty-fourth week of gestation, just in time to prepare the body for delivery. Estradiol is rising from early pregnancy until the very end, peaking at around 20,000 pg/ml for the last few weeks before delivery. If you have been pregnant, think about how you felt the last six weeks compared to the beginning and middle months. When did you feel your best? That will give you a clue as to which hormone affects you with the most positive feelings, physically and emotionally. If you pay attention to the changes in how you feel at different points in your cycle, you can again see some of the physical and psychological differences between estrogen and progesterone.

Estriol (E3). This is a much weaker form of estrogen, and it is made by the placenta during pregnancy. Estriol receptors are primarily concentrated in the vagina, hair follicles, and skin, and may help to account for the skin and hair "glow" that women often notice during pregnancy. Hundreds of studies over the last fifty years have found that estriol has very little estrogenic action at bone, brain, heart, and other critical sites where estradiol plays crucial roles and has multiple actions. Estriol does not appear to play a significant role at times other than pregnancy.

The body makes smaller amounts of estradiol in other areas of the body via the same aromatase pathway I described above, and it uses estradiol nearly everywhere. For example, research has shown that our bones make small amounts of estradiol critical for a healthy, strong skeleton. Our blood vessels make and use estradiol, the brain makes and uses estradiol, and even muscle tissue makes both estrone and estradiol by the aromatase pathway. Women who are physically active and have more muscle mass often have better estradiol levels than less active women with less muscle mass. Clearly, we are only beginning to understand all the ways the body makes and uses estradiol to keep all our systems humming along efficiently.

Women with endometriosis have always been thought to make too much "estrogen," but the very latest research findings show that the excess estrogen isn't actually being made throughout the body. It is occurring *in the endometriosis implants* themselves. These little areas of uterine lining tissue scattered like buckshot throughout the pelvis actually become their own miniature estrogen-producing factories. They contain the enzyme aromatase, which enables the implants to use androgens from our adrenal glands (androstenedione, and smaller amounts of testosterone) to make estrone and estradiol. The two estrogens produced inside these endometrial implants in the pelvis "feed" the implants to grow more. Rather than having an estrogen-dominant condition throughout the whole body, as is most commonly described, endometriosis patients we have evaluated actually have much *lower* than normal serum estradiol levels and have the myriad symptoms from low estradiol.

Another interesting aspect of the aromatase pathway is that, as we get older, it becomes more efficient in making estrone from conversion of androstenedione in fat tissue. The more body fat women have, the more aromatase, and the more estrone is made. This is partly why the balance of estrogen shifts from about 1:1 estradiol to estrone before menopause to far more estrone present after menopause, the ovaries no longer make estradiol but our body fat is still making more estrone. After menopause, women have a greater than 1:1 estrone to estradiol ratio unless they are taking HRT. The more overweight a woman is, the higher this ratio of estrone becomes. This is important because higher estrone levels are a risk factor for high blood pressure, diabetes, and endometrial and breast cancers in women. In case you wondered whether men make estrone in their fat tissue, they do; it is by the same aromatase pathway as in women. This may help explain why, as they get older, men have less of the active testosterone: They have higher estrone as they gain body fat.

We know that estradiol levels decline in the years leading up to and after menopause. As this happens, our estrogen balance shifts to about 2:1 estrone dominance. Women with PCOS or Syndrome X, due to excess body fat, will have an even greater estrone dominance *before* menopause. Why is this important? Because even being 20 percent overweight as you age causes about a 40 percent higher level than in thinner women. As I commented earlier, higher estrone levels, along with fat around your middle, increases your risk of diabetes, early heart attacks or strokes, and your chance of developing breast or uterine cancers.

Progesterone

Another major ovarian hormone is progesterone. The name means "pregnancy-promoting," or "pro-gestation," hormone. It was first identified in the

1920s in the yellow-bodied corpus luteum of the ovary by researchers seeking to identify the hormones made by the ovary. Progesterone is made primarily after ovulation by the corpus luteum, from the "building block" molecule cholesterol. Until ovulation, progesterone blood levels are typically less than 1 ng/ml; after ovulation, levels rise to 8–25 ng/ml by the peak, about Day 20 of your cycle. If there is no ovulation, there is no corpus luteum to make progesterone, so there is no rise in progesterone. This is why you may not have many typical PMS symptoms if you don't ovulate.

The rise in progesterone in the second half of your cycle prepares for metabolic changes the body will need to make to support a pregnancy: increased appetite, increased thirst, breast engorgement and more rapid proliferation of the breast cells, and suppression of the immune system, among others. Progesterone also triggers insulin to shift toward more fat storage for the fuel needs of a growing baby. The progesterone effects on the insulin-glucose pathways trigger more "blood sugar swings" and reactive hypoglycemia in the luteal phase. This is why you have more sweet cravings during your premenstrual week. Researchers at Tufts University found a 12 percent increase in appetite and metabolic rate in the high-progesterone phase of the cycle. So you are not imagining it: You really are hungrier. Mother Nature wants you to eat more if you are going to be pregnant.

Progesterone also relaxes the smooth muscles of the intestinal tract, so that the waves of contractions (peristalsis) are decreased. This slows the movement of food through the GI tract. The metabolic effect is that the digestive system has more time to work on breaking down foods and is able to absorb maximum nutrient value for mother and baby. The low fiber content of the typical American diet, on average about 10 grams of fiber daily, rather than the 30 grams we need, makes the progesterone effects of premenstrual bloating and constipation even worse. We feel sluggish and fat. Other common complaints when progesterone is high are feeling headachy, lethargic, depressed, irritable . . . and having no sex drive! These same feelings can occur in your own cycle, or when you take high amounts of progestins in birth control pills or HRT.

Progesterone and its metabolites have a tranquilizing effect on the brain, much like our current antianxiety medications. For some women, progesterone feels like a sedative, and they don't like the groggy feeling. For other women, the "slowing down" effect of progesterone feels "wonderful" and "soothing." They feel "relaxed" or "more centered." Still others experience full-blown "depression," severe fatigue, or lethargy. These women say, "I don't have any get-up-and-go"; "I withdraw"; "I can't get out of bed"; "I don't have any energy." You can see how a hormone that calms and tranquilizes might be an evolutionary advantage in the early stages of pregnancy. Being calmer at the time the egg is implanted helps to keep it from being jostled out of the uterus. This facilitates early development of the embryo. At other times, however, many women don't like feeling sedated and slowed down.

PROGESTOGEN, PROGESTERONE, OR PROGESTIN?

Definitions to Guide You

Progestogen is a general term that describes any chemical substance that has the metabolic effects in the body to sustain a pregnancy and activate the progesterone receptor. There are a number of types that fall into this category:

- *Progesterone* is a biologically natural pregnancy-sustaining hormone (progestogen), produced by many species. In women, progesterone is made by the corpus luteum after ovulation, although a very small amount is also produced by the adrenal gland and by the ovary. Its primary role is to stimulate the metabolic, functional, and structural changes needed for a woman's body to adapt to, and sustain, a pregnancy as well as undergo delivery.

- *Progestins* are man-made chemicals that are more potent than progesterone because of a different chemical structure that gives them some actions similar to progesterone as well as some different actions. Progestins may be derived from progesterone, called *progestational progestins,* such as Provera; or they may be derived from testosterone, called *androgenic progestins,* such as norethindrone (common brands are Aygestin, Nor-QD, or Micronor). Progestins in the Provera group are more likely than testosterone-based progestins to cause depression, weight gain, headaches, and low libido. Progestins have many important medical uses, such as contraception or suppression of endometriosis and fibroids, that the lower potency of progesterone cannot do as reliably.

- *Progesterone USP* is a chemical molecule made in the laboratory to be *identical* in all respects to the natural hormone made by the ovary. It begins as building blocks found in soybeans and wild yams; it is then purified and processed through a series of chemical changes that require enzymes we don't have in our bodies. It has been available in injectable form since the 1940s and is now available as a tablet (Prometrium) or vaginal gel (Crinone). Progesterone USP is also used by compounding pharmacists to make individualized prescriptions in many forms, including tablets, suppositories, and creams. Because it is identical to the natural molecule, many women find that it has fewer unpleasant side effects than progestins such as Provera. Some women, however, feel terrible on natural progesterone and prefer the synthetic progestins.

Since women respond differently to these various types of progestogens, it is best for you and your physician to decide which is best for you based on your medical needs and your response to the various different options available. There is no one "right" answer for every woman.

There is much misleading information claiming progesterone is the "mother" hormone because it comes at the beginning of a chemical pathway, and is the one from which all the other hormones, including testosterone and estradiol, are made by the body. This point is then used as a sales pitch urging you to buy progesterone creams to treat PMS and other problems. Many women's health books do not accurately portray what is going on in your body, or where and when these reactions take place.

First of all, most of the conversion of progesterone to the end products of testosterone and estradiol require the presence of enzymes in *fully functioning* ovaries. If you had a hysterectomy with the ovaries removed, it is obvious you no longer have these ovarian-"converting" enzymes. If you still have ovaries, they may not produce optimal levels of your key hormones, especially after severe viral illness, hypothyroidism, a tubal ligation, prolonged stress that disrupted your cycle, or any one of many other possible causes of ovarian decline. If your ovaries aren't functioning normally, or if you have reached menopause, then you are not able to convert a load of progesterone into estradiol and testosterone. So you end up getting much more progesterone than you need, and not enough of the others, leading to all kinds of adverse effects on metabolism, brain, and immune function, to name a few.

I think the important point here is that Mother Nature gave us a series of steps for the body to go through to get to the end result. You can't assume that loading up on one building block at the beginning of the process means you will be making all the same molecules the body makes when your ovaries are working optimally. Another metaphor may help to explain what I mean. Think about the many stages of growth and development that have to occur for a baby to become a child, then an adolescent, and then an adult. Think of progesterone as the "baby" in our hormone development process. It can't carry out all the functions of the "adult" hormones, estradiol and testosterone, until it has been shaped and altered by the changes of this *entire series* of chemical reactions. Progesterone can't be made into testosterone or estradiol directly; it *has* to undergo intermediate changes to become the molecules that are the direct building blocks for testosterone and then estradiol. This is just like our life process: We can't fully function as an adult until we have gone through the life stages (infancy, childhood, adolescence) that shape and equip us to be an adult.

Without our ovaries to facilitate this "development" of the "baby" progesterone into "adult" testosterone and estradiol, we are stuck with a molecule that doesn't have the specific shape to activate the receptors for normal function. Remember what I described in earlier chapters: Each of these molecules acts like a different "key" in various receptor "locks" throughout the body, so the proper shape to the molecule key is crucial to create the desired effects in various parts and organs of our body.

The bottom line here is that progesterone will not replace the symptoms and problems accompanying declining estradiol or testosterone levels. Period.

Scientists have discovered ways to make various estrogens and testosterone, as well as the synthetic progestins, in the laboratory, from plant compounds. Today, all of the pharmaceutical-grade estradiol, testosterone, and progesterone come from precursor molecules in wild yams and soy that are then chemically converted in the laboratory to make bioidentical hormones. Our bodies, however, do not have the enzymes needed to change the plant building blocks into the same molecules our bodies make, so eating lots of soy or yams simply will not supply your body with the identical molecules of hormones you need.

One of the major problems in finding a way to prescribe "natural" progesterone is that when taken orally, it is quickly deactivated by stomach acid. In the 1960s, a process called *micronization* was developed by which large hormone molecules could be made tiny enough to be absorbed before being broken down by stomach acid. Unfortunately, by the time the technology had solved the problem, physicians had become accustomed to using Provera, which was cheaper and also reliable. Micronized progesterone was widely used in Europe, but not much in this country, except by compounding pharmacies for PMS and other special needs. It was not until Prometrium and Crinone were approved by the FDA in 1998 that there was wider acceptance of the micronized progesterone over the synthetic progestins like Provera.

Testosterone

The third primary hormone of the ovaries is what is popularly referred to as the *male* hormone, testosterone. This hormone is part of a larger group of hormones called *androgens* that bind at androgen receptors throughout the brain and body. All androgens are made from cholesterol by the female ovary, the male testes, and some by the adrenal gland. They are also made in limited quantity by body-fat tissue, muscle, the liver, skin, and brain, using precursor molecules made in the ovaries and adrenals.

Just as men require some estradiol in their system to function, women require testosterone. Men's optimal testosterone levels are 600–1,000 ng/dl, or even more, while an optimal testosterone range for women is 40–60 ng/dl (the units we usually use). For an interesting and surprising comparison, however, 40–60 ng/dl would actually be *400–600 pg/ml* if we use the same units we use for estradiol. Perhaps you never realized that during the years from puberty to menopause women have higher testosterone than estradiol! For the rest of the book, I will stick with the conventional units ng/dl used in the United States.

Testosterone has many benefits. It helps you keep and build your muscle mass, which burns more calories than fat tissue, and it helps you build bone and prevent osteoporosis. Women lose approximately 50 percent of their testosterone production by the time their ovaries decline at menopause, and the adrenal glands also begin to reduce their testosterone and DHEA output. I don't know of many men who would like a 50 percent reduction of their testosterone. But remember that, as a woman, you need to have the right balance of estradiol *with* your testosterone to see all the positives and not so many negatives.

Testosterone activates the brain's sexual circuits in both men and women. Your sexuality is an important dimension of your life, and many of my patients ask, "How do I get my libido back?" Just as it is hard to light a campfire using wet matches, it is hard to arouse the sexual circuits in the brain without the metabolic fuel they need in testosterone. So, if your doctor suggests seeing a sex therapist, have your hormone levels tested first! You need your basic body chemistry functioning properly before psychological and relationship therapies can be effective.

A hysterectomy and removal of the ovaries before natural menopause causes a rapid drop in testosterone that is a big shock to the body. Other causes of ovarian damage I describe throughout this book can also lead to loss of testosterone, although not as abruptly as the loss that occurs when the ovaries are surgically removed. Without optimal testosterone, you have loss of sex drive and other negative effects. Your energy level drops, you lose muscle mass and bone density, you may feel depressed, have achy joints, or have an overall loss of your sense of well-being.

If you had a hysterectomy but your ovaries were not removed, you'll still have a decrease in your hormone levels within just a few years after the surgery, as your ovarian functions falter. This decline doesn't "wait" until you reach that magic age of natural menopause, as doctors have mistakenly thought. I explain how this occurs in Chapter 8. If you take only estrogen after a hysterectomy, the amount of free active testosterone falls even further because of the increase in sex hormone binding globulin (SHBG). Many women lose interest in sex at this point and have lower energy levels. It is not due to depression or the effects of the surgery. It is the loss of your key hormones.

You may not need an antidepressant, as doctors commonly recommend, and in fact these medicines are likely to reduce your sex drive even further. You first need a serum blood test to determine your testosterone and estradiol levels. Most physicians don't realize that a decline in estrogen production also means a decrease in testosterone production, partly because the precursors are no longer being made by the ovary. Taking DHEA supplements won't help increase your testosterone, since it is in the ovary where most of the enzymes and pathways exist to convert it to testosterone or estradiol.

When the ratio of estradiol to testosterone falls during perimenopause, the usual androgen effects are unmasked: facial hair, thinning scalp hair, deepening voice, the male pattern of middle-body fat distribution. There are even more adverse body changes, including an increase in blood pressure and total cholesterol, a decrease in HDL ("good") cholesterol, and an increase in LDL ("bad") cholesterol. Up go your risks of heart disease, hypertension, and diabetes. The right balance of estradiol and testosterone is key to feeling your best.

The Hormone Cycle of Your Breasts

One of the often overlooked aspects of the menstrual cycle is the way hormonal fluctuations cause changes in the breast. Some are visible and you feel them, others are microscopic, so you are not aware of them. There are estrogen receptors in the tissue of the breast that respond to rising hormone levels to stimulate both growth of the ducts and the breast connective tissue. Most women notice that their breasts change each month during their cycle. The significant difference comes in the luteal phase, when your breasts feel larger and full or swollen. The rise in progesterone at this time of the cycle causes increased fluid retention, as well as more growth, or proliferation, of the breast lobular tissue, in preparation for a possible pregnancy. These changes cause the breasts to increase in volume and become sensitive or, at times, even painful. These same changes also occur in the early stages of pregnancy, when the progesterone levels also rise rapidly.

Estradiol in the first half of the menstrual cycle causes the growth of breast cells, but the rise in progesterone in the second half of the menstrual cycle *triggers even more rapid and greater proliferation* of the breast than estradiol does. This is one reason that you now hear more concern about possible increased risk of breast cancer when *combination* hormones are given. Doctors and health writers seem to only focus on "estrogen," overlooking the basic physiology of progesterone and its potentially negative effects on the breasts, as well as other body systems.

A significant number of women, as high as 70 percent in some studies, complain of breast tenderness and/or breast sensitivity the week before menses. There are also a number of women who experience more intense breast pain, called *mastalgia,* which can vary from uncomfortable to debilitating. The best research to date points to an imbalance in the ratio of progesterone to estradiol and/or an excess of prolactin, a pituitary hormone that stimulates lactation. Studies also show that breast pain changes in a pattern that follows hormonal changes in your life, by age, by stress level, and, for some women, by diet. We know that much of this goes away with menopause, when hormone levels fall significantly. I often explain to women on hormone replacement therapy (HRT) that they can tell when their estrogen or progesterone levels are too high, because their breasts will become too tender as a result of excess amounts of *either* hormone. HRT can actually help relieve the discomfort of mastalgia by normalizing the hormone ratios. If breast pain or discomfort is hormonal, it will most likely occur with your cycle and in both breasts. If you have any concerns about breast pain and a possible relationship to other problems, you should consult your physician. If the pain is in one breast only, or noncyclical, I also recommend you have this checked.

In menopause, the loss of estradiol results in a decrease in breast tissue, and an increase in the fat cells. The breasts become less dense because of the increase in fat, and they are softer and flatter. For women on HRT, a more premenopausal breast density and fullness are typical.

Hormone Cycles and Your Body

There are many ways that the hormonal changes of your menstrual cycle may contribute to symptoms and changes in your health. This book will go into more detail about these hormone effects on your brain and body, but here are a few brief illustrations of how profound these connections can be. For example, falling estradiol can trigger migraine headaches, regardless of your age. Falling estradiol at your period's start can cause a spasm of the arteries that serve the heart, called *coronary vasospasm*. Many physicians, and even many women, are uninformed about these hormonal connections, and Georgia's experience shows how devastating this can be.

Georgia, a thirty-eight-year-old mother of two young children, had just had her *third* heart attack. Both her first and second attacks, the first at age thirty-six, had occurred right with the onset of her menstrual period. She was in a coma in the ICU, and her relatives had been notified that there was little hope she would survive. She had no evidence of cardiovascular disease or arteriosclerosis plaque blocking her arteries. For some time, her physicians had dismissed her chest pains and palpitations, always appearing at the onset of menses, as being "psychological," caused by the life stress of being the mother of young children. Like many women, she was referred for a psychiatric evaluation and treated with antidepressants, antianxiety medications, and a placating attitude. Sadly, when women's symptoms seem unusual, busy doctors often find it easier to "refer out" rather than take the time to go into more depth or do more tests. This is especially true in offices where managed care plans force doctors to see between fifty and sixty patients a day just to stay open.

Ironically, it was not an invasive cardiovascular treatment or powerful medication that saved her life. Rather, it was a family friend who recommended to the woman's husband that he read my book describing the dilating effects of estradiol on blood vessels, thereby improving blood flow by relaxing the smooth muscle tissue of the blood vessels, enhancing the delivery of oxygen to the heart muscle. He did, and the doctor agreed to give the estradiol patch a try. This noninvasive, natural hormonal therapy saved her life. Today, a year later, Georgia is back home, able to be a normal mom to her children, and getting her health back.

I used the protocol I developed during my years of practice to measure hormone levels at specific times during Georgia's cycle. The tests confirmed what she had suspected all along: Her heart problems were not caused by anxiety and stress but by important hormone shifts and imbalances related to her menstrual cycle. During her menses, falling estrogen levels caused constriction of the arteries supplying the heart muscle, and the decreased oxygen triggered her heart attacks. In addition, her estradiol levels were abnormally low and became dangerously low at certain times in her cycle. Adding the estradiol patch raised her level, caused the blood vessels to dilate, and increased the life-saving blood flow and oxygen supply to her heart muscle. None of her doctors had considered that low estradiol could cause her heart problems. She was so young and still had regular periods. To Georgia and to me, the fact that her heart attacks only occurred with her menses, coupled with lab tests that showed lower than normal estradiol and excess testosterone, identified the problem: a severe ovarian hormone imbalance. She now pays meticulous attention to her hormone therapy, which has saved her life.

Another patient, *Linda,* age twenty-three, had a history of three serious, and nearly fatal, suicide attempts, each time at the onset of her menstrual period. Although various physicians and psychiatrists had evaluated her, no one had ever asked where she was in her cycle when these self-destructive feelings hit her. No one had thought to do simple blood tests at the key times of her menstrual cycle to see if her hormone levels dropped precipitously when she had these difficulties. During her last hospitalization, physicians told Linda's parents that she had permanent brain and liver damage from the drug overdoses and the loss of oxygen during the coma that followed. Her parents were devastated.

Finally, a *nonmedical* therapist recognized the menstrual cycle connection, and recommended a consultation with me to see if this young woman's hormones were a factor. The biggest clue for the therapist and Linda was the connection between the suicide attempts and the onset of her menstrual bleeding. She did not have such suicidal thoughts at any other time of her cycle. When I evaluated her, I carefully went over her history of both the mood and physical symptoms. I checked her hormone levels, and found that she had a form of exercise-induced premature ovarian failure, a result of her strenuous training as a dancer and her constant dieting. Several years later, she is alive and healthy on a steady hormone regimen to restore her ovarian hormones and provide stability from the terrible mood swings and suicidal "crashes" each month. She is no longer on antidepressants. She has returned to the dancing she loves, and has achieved a healthy balance in her training schedule. She now understands what her rigorous training and inadequate nutrition did to her ovaries and is beginning to rebuild the bone she lost earlier. Brain and liver damage? Based on current test results, these problems have been resolved. She says, "My mind feels sharp and clear again. I have my energy back." She went on to graduate school and is now working full-time.

A Guide to Your Other Hormones

The brain and body are interconnected by an incredible array of chemical and electrical circuits, each one interacting with and affecting others. The brain has a multitude of ways to direct the orchestra of the body. In women's bodies, the entire process is even more complex, with the menstrual cycle changes causing brain-body systems to continuously adapt to the internal and external environments. While men have a fairly steady production (*tonic* pattern) of testosterone all month, women's brain and body are designed to work with a *cyclic* pattern of ovarian hormone rise and fall.

Since we will be talking throughout this book about other hormone systems and their interactions with the ovaries, I have given you this diagram and table of our other major hormones. There will be more on the role of the ovarian hormones and the thyroid, adrenal, brain, and pancreas hormones in upcoming chapters.

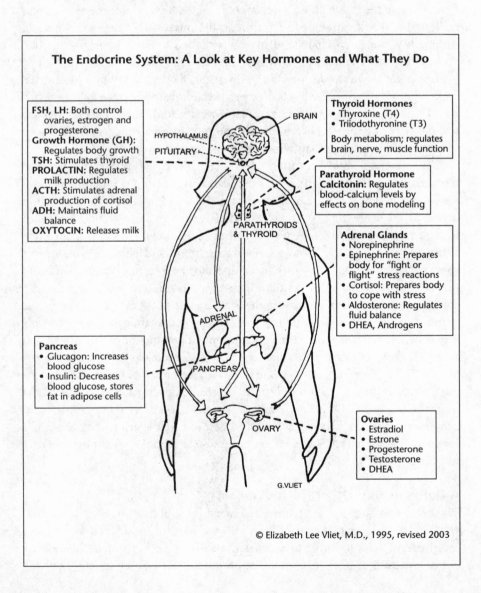

The Endocrine System: A Look at Key Hormones and What They Do

FSH, LH: Both control ovaries, estrogen and progesterone
Growth Hormone (GH): Regulates body growth
TSH: Stimulates thyroid
PROLACTIN: Regulates milk production
ACTH: Stimulates adrenal production of cortisol
ADH: Maintains fluid balance
OXYTOCIN: Releases milk

Thyroid Hormones
• Thyroxine (T4)
• Triiodothyronine (T3)
Body metabolism; regulates brain, nerve, muscle function

Parathyroid Hormone
Calcitonin: Regulates blood-calcium levels by effects on bone modeling

Adrenal Glands
• Norepinephrine
• Epinephrine: Prepares body for "fight or flight" stress reactions
• Cortisol: Prepares body to cope with stress
• Aldosterone: Regulates fluid balance
• DHEA, Androgens

Pancreas
• Glucagon: Increases blood glucose
• Insulin: Decreases blood glucose, stores fat in adipose cells

Ovaries
• Estradiol
• Estrone
• Progesterone
• Testosterone
• DHEA

BRAIN
HYPOTHALAMUS
PITUITARY
PARATHYROIDS & THYROID
ADRENAL
PANCREAS
OVARY
G.VLIET

© Elizabeth Lee Vliet, M.D., 1995, revised 2003

Our Hormones and Their Actions

I. STEROIDS	PRIMARY ACTIONS
Cortisol	Many metabolic actions, especially to store more body fat; produced in higher amounts under stress and suppresses normal immune function due to anti-inflammatory actions
Aldosterone	Regulates fluid balance by stimulating kidneys to retain sodium and water and excrete potassium; contributes to excess water weight gain when progesterone levels are high in second half of menstrual cycle and stimulate more aldosterone secretion
Androgens (DHEA, others)	Enhances sex drive, produces male features in women (e.g., facial hair, male body shape), stimulates appetite, contributes to middle body and waistline fat gain when levels too high
Estrogens (three)— Estrone (E1) Estradiol (E2) Estriol (E3)	Female secondary sex characteristics; key role in menstruation, pregnancy, and over four hundred other crucial functions throughout the body and brain, including increased metabolic rate, improved insulin sensitivity and carbohydrate tolerance; plays a role in body temperature regulation
Progesterone	Helps maintain pregnancy, many metabolic effects including increased appetite, increased fat storage, and reduced sensitivity to insulin; high levels give sedative, analgesic effects at brain; may produce depressed mood, decreased libido
Testosterone	Produces male secondary sex patterns; triggers sex drive and arousal in both males and females; many metabolic effects (bone and muscle growth, increased metabolic rate, etc.); also enhances mood and energy level

Our Hormones and Their Actions (cont.)

II. AMINES	PRIMARY ACTIONS
Thyroid hormones—thyroxine (T4) and triiodothyronine (T3)	Stimulates body metabolism by increasing cell energy release; increases heart rate, heat production, and brain activity; helps maintain normal regulation of metabolic pathways, normal growth, and function of nervous and musculoskeletal systems
"Adrenaline" hormones—norepinephrine (NE) and epinephrine	Fight-or-flight (stress) hormone; prepares body for emergencies by increasing heart rate; acts on brain to lift mood (or in excess, to cause anxiety) and increase alertness; dilates arteries to key organs to provide more oxygen, glucose, and nutrients

III. PEPTIDES AND PROTEINS	PRIMARY ACTIONS
Insulin	Lowers blood sugar (moves glucose into cells to be used for fuel in muscle or stored in fat cells); stimulates fat storage and protein synthesis
Glucagon	Raises blood glucose (glycogen breakdown and glucose release from liver, gluconeogenesis)
Somatostatin	Mild effect to raise blood glucose
Parathyroid (PTH)	Major role in increasing blood calcium levels, stimulating bone breakdown; calcium release
Calcitonin	Involved in regulating blood calcium levels by inhibiting bone breakdown; calcium release
Thymosin (thymus gland)	Major role in development of immune system
Adrenocorticotropin hormone (ACTH)	Stimulates part of the adrenal gland to make cortisol
FSH	Stimulates ovaries; activates and promotes follicle growth to produce estrogen
LH	Triggers ovulation, formation of the corpus luteum, secretion of progesterone and estrogen

III. PEPTIDES AND PROTEINS (cont.)	PRIMARY ACTIONS
Growth hormone (GH)	Oversees entire process of normal body growth; stimulates formation of more muscle and less body fat; declines during menopause with loss of estradiol; improves with estrogen therapy
TSH	Stimulates the thyroid gland to release T3 and T4; will be *high* in *hypo*thyroid conditions and *low* in *hyper*thyroid conditions
Prolactin	Stimulates breast enlargement during pregnancy and regulates milk production after delivery; increases appetite and body fat to support nursing; often elevated in PCOS
Antidiuretic hormone (ADH)	Prevents dehydration by stimulating kidneys to increase resorption and retain water
Oxytocin	Stimulates uterine contractions during labor, helps trigger milk release after delivery
Melatonin (pineal gland)	Regulates sleep cycles, body rhythms; promotes fat storage by increasing appetite, especially for carbohydrate foods (for example, to prepare for winter hibernation); plays a role in winter depression (SADS) syndromes that are characterized by low energy, weight gain, daytime sleepiness, depressed mood

© Elizabeth Lee Vliet, M.D., 2003

In Summary

Our wondrous, at times infuriating, hormonal ebb and flow occurs every month and has widespread effects on brain-body processes and on our psyche. Every cell participates in the flow of our menstrual rhythm. Cyclic changes occur in almost all body functions as the levels of female hormones rise and fall. Science is discovering at an amazing rate how these hormonal shifts interact with the endocrine, immune, metabolic, cardiovascular, respiratory, musculoskeletal, reproductive, urinary, and nervous systems. When you understand the specific effects and roles of each of the primary female hormones, you see how beautifully orchestrated the female endocrine system is for bringing new life into being. From an evolutionary standpoint these hormonal actions make sense for the tasks they govern in our body and for sustaining our survival as a species.

All of these physiological changes then affect how we respond to the external world and the impact of external stresses on our brain-body pathways. We are not at the mercy of our hormones. If we understand what is happening, we can learn to "go with the flow," so to speak, in positive ways, rather than make things worse with uninformed or misinformed lifestyle choices. I want us to better understand women's physiological changes and not confuse the *physiological* with the psychological. We desperately need more gender-specific research so that we can effectively manage our complicated lives in a body that is much more complex than a man's.

Our hormonal cycles are not limits for what we can do with our lives. What limits us is that most doctors don't fully use the available medical research on hormonal cycles to address our unique health needs. It is often easier to prescribe an antidepressant than to measure and interpret women's hormone levels, and then design an individualized treatment approach. And drug companies spend billions of dollars on ads convincing doctors and consumers that we need a different pill for every symptom. My goal is to give you the information you need to overcome such obstacles and get the health care you need, tailored to your body and your unique hormone balance.

3

Your Ovaries and Their Life Cycle

Introduction

Our ovaries travel a remarkable journey from gestation to the waning days of our lives, with a number of important stages during their life cycle. I want you to have a guide to these phases, because it is crucial to understanding why there are so many ways to disrupt optimal hormone production. The dietary excitotoxins and chemical endocrine disruptors (see Chapters 4 and 5) can act at any of these stages to damage our ovaries and our overall health. Illness, lifestyle habits, and surgical interventions can also have a critical impact. Knowing what is happening at each stage will help you to understand how the disruptors affect you, and what you can do to help avoid problems.

Before Puberty

You are born with all the eggs/follicles you will ever make. By puberty you will probably have 300,000 or so left to start your periods. Today, more women are delaying children until their thirties and forties, and having fewer children. By forty, the average woman has only 5,000 to 10,000 follicles remaining. A number of follicles are "recruited" each cycle, of which one or two are used. The others are lost, leading to a decrease in follicles with every menstrual cycle. Many factors, such as illness, environment, and stress also contribute to the loss of follicles. So if you are not trying to get pregnant, what is the problem?

Follicles and maturing eggs produce estradiol, the most active form of estrogen. As you lose follicles, estradiol levels decline erratically, causing disruptions and problems throughout your body. Declining estradiol brings on many of the classical symptoms of menopause. Usually, menopause is only associated with older women, but these symptoms can occur in younger women if follicles are damaged or prematurely lose the ability to produce adequate amounts of estradiol. Younger women experiencing these problems are often undiagnosed. The good news is that there are simple blood hormone tests to measure and diagnose premature hormone decline.

As you read the life cycle of the ovary, think about your body now and the changes you have experienced. These are your clues for checking hormone levels.

Puberty: The Awakening of Our Ovaries

American girls generally enter puberty between ages nine and fourteen. If puberty occurs earlier than this, it is called *premature* (or *precocious*) *puberty*.

The first stage of puberty—called *thelarche*—is signaled by the beginning of breast development. This stage is followed by *adrenarche*, so called because it is triggered by the release of adrenal androgens, with the appearance of pubic hair, axillary hair, oily skin, and acne. *Menarche* is the beginning of menstrual periods. The first menses usually occur when the breasts are more defined, typically around the age eleven and a half to thirteen. The average time span from the first stage of puberty to the first menses runs about four years.

From 1850 to 1950, the average age of menarche decreased approximately 3 months every decade as a result of better nutrition. The average age of 12.8 years held fairly steady until the 1990s, when we began seeing girls develop breasts and menstruating at much younger ages. Menstrual onset also varies by race, diet, weight, percentage of body fat, light exposure, and the presence of certain diseases. Recent research suggests it may be more the ratio of body fat to weight, rather than just weight. African-American and Hispanic girls tend to start menstruating earlier than Caucasians. Thin girls tend to get their periods later than heavier girls. Girls with diabetes tend to have a delayed menarche. Blind girls, who do not have significant light stimulation of brain centers, tend to have an earlier menarche than girls with normal vision. There is also a genetic clock that sets in motion a chain of events.

Puberty is triggered by a series of hormone reactions. It starts with the hypothalamus increasing secretions that cause the pituitary gland to release increased amounts of gonadotrophins into the bloodstream. Gonadotrophins are hormones that stimulate activity in the gonads (ovaries in females, testes in males). This causes the ovaries to produce elevated levels of estradiol, which leads to visible signs of maturing, such as developing breasts, pubic hair, underarm hair, and often a change in the timbre of the voice. These secondary sex characteristics are typically followed by a growth spurt. Such changes usually occur two years earlier in girls than boys and are why girls at this age are often taller. Internal changes are also occurring due to the influence of pubescent hormones. The walls of the vagina become thicker, and the uterus becomes larger and more muscular. The pH of the vagina also changes from alkaline to acidic due to the increase in vaginal and cervical secretions.

Early in puberty, menstrual flow is usually very light, and comes with little warning. Periods may be irregular at first but usually become regular within the first two years. The ability to conceive and bear children (fertility) occurs when ovulation begins. It is difficult for many adolescent girls to know when they are fertile since both ovulation and the menstrual cycle can be erratic. This is one reason (among many) for accidental pregnancies, so it is important to always use some form of contraception if you are sexually active. You can even get pregnant, although it is less likely, if you have sexual intercourse on the bleeding days of your cycle or have missed periods due to stress, illness, poor eating habits, or intensive athletic training.

Most of the physical changes occur during the early years of puberty, but behavioral changes and social expectations dramatically change throughout adolescence. Prior to puberty, the body's growth focuses on becoming taller and stronger. With puberty, the hormone changes in women and men prepare the body to reproduce. These physical changes are a portion of the complex process of growing up. Adolescence is a time for psychological and psychosocial growth, when social adjustment and maturation are added to our physical changes. These emotional and social transitions are less defined and less orderly than the physical ones. This unpredictability leads to the "turbulent teens." Thankfully, we eventually transition into mature young adults.

Your menstrual cycle is a normal process of being a woman, and there is no reason to curtail your normal activities during your period. But it is helpful to pay attention to your monthly cycles and patterns of physical and emotional changes such as headaches, bloating, tiredness, changes in mood, body aches, food cravings, acne or minor breakouts, cramps, tender breasts, constipation, cold sores, and even nosebleeds. Paying attention to your body signals and understanding your unique responses during your cycle will help you recognize changes triggered by hormone shifts. Keeping a menstrual response calendar can be helpful in understanding your patterns, which in turn will help you head off more severe symptoms. It is important to have regular exams after periods have begun. A pediatrician or primary care physician will probably do these during the adolescent years. If you become sexually active, it is especially important to have a pelvic exam and begin annual Pap tests. This may be the time to establish care with a gynecologist. Take your menstrual tracking records, or a calendar if you have one, to your doctor. This is an important component of your medical record, and your doctor should appreciate this information.

I have described the more "typical" onset and stages of puberty. But what about girls who enter puberty far ahead of the average age? What happens then? Why be concerned about early puberty?

Premature Puberty—Health Risks When Puberty Comes Too Soon

Look around at malls and schools and in your community. More girls today are entering puberty at younger ages. Girls only five, six, and seven are developing breasts. It's as if we have a whole generation of girls who are hormonally accelerated. During the 1800s, girls on average began to menstruate at about age seventeen. By the mid-1990s, however, about one in five Caucasian girls *by age eight* were showing breast buds and pubic hair, the beginning signs of puberty; *50 percent* of African-American girls now reach puberty *by age eight;* another 15 to 20 percent of African-American girls have hit puberty by *age seven.* This is a staggering change. In the few studies that have been done to date, Hispanic girls show patterns of early puberty closer to those of African-American girls. There are many serious reasons why this is happening. What future health problems lie ahead for girls who enter puberty so young?

Physical. There are a number of emerging health risks in girls with early puberty: increased risks of PCOS, adolescent and adult obesity, diabetes, endometrial and breast cancers (from longer exposure to estrogenic chemicals that are ubiquitous in our environment, as well as our own body estrogens). Premature puberty also increases the likelihood of becoming sexually active at younger ages, with increased risk of sexually transmitted diseases (STDs) and unplanned pregnancy. We see an ominous trend with girls ten to twelve becoming pregnant and even younger girls with sexually transmitted diseases (STDs).

Researchers worldwide are looking at these important issues. Dr. Dimartino-Nardi at Montefiore Medical Center in New York evaluated African-American and Caribbean-Hispanic girls with premature increases in adrenal androgens, and found that both ethnic groups were obese, had high insulin levels with insulin resistance, elevated androgens, and subtle decreases in their "good" cholesterol (HDL). Many of these girls also had a strong family history of Type II diabetes mellitus. Dr. Dimartino-Nardi found that girls with premature adrenarche who remain obese are at risk of developing polycystic ovary syndrome (PCOS) as they go through puberty. The girls with elevated androgens and insulin resistance *before puberty* continue to have obesity, insulin resistance, and high androgens after puberty. They develop classic symptoms of PCOS related to the high androgens and insulin: irregular menses, excess facial and body hair, and severe acne. This sets up a lifetime of health problems.

Premature adrenarche and early puberty can be a risk factor for continued obesity for certain girls, and an early stage in the progression to the adult metabolic disorder we call Syndrome X. We must get better at early identification of girls at risk for these conditions so we can develop interventions to prevent later health complications.

A recent study found that levels of growth hormone binding protein (GHBP) are significantly higher in girls with premature puberty and middle-body fat. This leads to less *free*, active growth hormone (GH) available to stimulate the building of bone and muscle. Less muscle mass creates a vicious cycle of more body fat, followed by more insulin resistance, that in turn helps store more body fat, and then even less free growth hormone to build bone and muscle. This is a crucial factor in overweight children getting even fatter.

Early puberty and a high percent of body fat work together to increase a girl's risk of later developing breast cancer through exposure to estrogens, particularly estrone, at an earlier, critical window of time in development. Early puberty and being fat is even more of a concern when you add the increase in breast cancer risk as a result of environmental exposure to the many hormonelike chemicals (see Chapter 5). London researcher Dr. B. A. Stoll and colleagues wrote in 1994,

Earlier onset of menarche and tallness in adult women are mainly confirmed as risk markers for breast cancer. Recent . . . studies have reported abdominal-type obesity and higher circulating levels of insulin, testosterone, and insulin-like growth factor 1, to be further risk markers for breast cancer. There is evidence that abdominal-type obesity is recognizable in girls even before puberty, and disparate studies have shown it to be correlated with earlier onset of menarche, insulin resistance leading to hyperinsulinemia, and an abnormal sex steroid profile.

Other studies over the years have shown that the longer the breast is exposed to abnormal hormone ratios, especially if there are higher than normal levels of insulin, the higher the risk of breast cancer. If earlier onset of puberty in some girls produces these same changes, then we are simply being prudent to be concerned about a later breast cancer risk.

Psychological. Girls (and boys) between ages six and ten enter the psychological stage we call *latency.* This is a stage when both sexes retreat into their own world, avoiding the other sex almost like the plague. You know this age: Girls hate those "creepy" boys and boys think all girls have "cooties." This is a critical developmental stage for both sexes. Girls especially need these years to develop confidence and a strong sense of self, separate from a role defined by boys or men. They need this phase of their lives to develop close friendships with other girls, to develop social skills and a sense of mastery in school and activities—especially sports—that help them successfully navigate the turbulent years of puberty.

If the physical changes of puberty come too early, it gives girls confusing signals—their body is attracting boys like flies to honey, but their psyche is still in latency, not wanting anything to do with boys. Their body looks like that of a young *woman,* but their mind is still that of a *child.* Our society already pressures children to grow up too fast. When the body is filling out and accelerating into puberty before the psychological "work" of latency has been completed, it can wreak havoc with later psychological, social, and academic adjustment.

If girls don't have enough time in the latency years to develop an adequate sense of self before they are pulled into relationships with boys, they have difficulty defining their sense of independent identity. They become further defined by how they *look* rather than by who they *are.* It becomes more and more difficult to develop positive self-esteem. Many social pressures already make it difficult for today's kids to feel good about themselves, so the psychological consequences of early puberty compound an already serious problem. These are issues we all need to address, since they contribute to the medical consequences of early puberty.

Sociological-cultural. There are other ominous pitfalls for girls whose sexual development comes too early: These girls are teased by boys their own age but get increased sexual overtures from older boys. Girls who sexually develop too early experience more sexual harassment, increased risk of date rape, and an earlier vulnerability to accidental pregnancy. Girls who look seventeen but are really twelve are under much more pressure from older boys to engage in risky behaviors like smoking cigarettes or pot, drinking alcohol, and experimenting with street drugs. Younger girl teens are even more susceptible to all this because of the taunts from boys their own age. The dangers of these cultural pressures are quite real and require supportive solutions that go beyond the medical health issues I listed previously.

Theories on the Causes of Premature Puberty

What is happening to cause this widespread problem of premature puberty? It is no longer only a rare case seen in specialty centers for pediatric endocrine problems. Doctors across the country see this in their offices daily. Is it a uniquely American phenomenon, or is it happening in other countries for the same reasons it is happening here? Let's look at some of the culprits.

Environmental chemicals. The problem is not limited to the United States. Studies done in numerous countries have found that children's normal progression of sexual and reproductive development is being affected by exposure to the hormone-disrupting chemicals that permeate our food chain and water supplies worldwide. These hormone-mimicking compounds, or *persistent organic pollutants* (POPs), are *everywhere.* Many of these compounds also pass through the placental barrier and expose the developing baby in the mother's womb. They are concentrated in our body fat and breast milk because of their high fat content, and are then passed to infants during nursing. This is a primary reason that various studies have shown a correlation between breast-feeding infants and an early onset of puberty. Most scientists think the benefits of breast milk for the baby outweigh the risk of exposure to these environmental chemicals, but no one can say with certainty because these issues are just beginning to be studied more aggressively.

These chemicals—DDE, PCBs, bisphenol-A, and a host of others—have profound effects on the brain centers that regulate everything from sexual development to metabolism and body weight. They have known adverse effects on the development of puberty in animals. Ominous findings are being seen in humans as well, confirmed by studies now being published worldwide. The number of these endocrine disruptors is increasing rapidly, and they are not limited to pesticides. Several different compounds used in the food industry, in plasticizers, and in dental restorations are also estrogenic. The few studies that have investigated their effects on humans all indicate that there are significant concerns for our health, including major disturbances in sexual development and brain function (see the complete references listed in Appendix II).

We are still learning sad lessons from the 1968 accidental poisoning of two thousand people in Japan. Rice oil was contaminated with PCBs leading to a condition called *Yusho disease.* A similar PCB poisoning in Taiwan was called *Yu Cheng disease.* Both of these conditions had many damaging effects on skin and eyes, but researchers also found symptoms of endocrine disruption: altered menstrual cycles and abnormal immune function. In a May 2001 summary of the consequences of these poisonings, Dr. Aoki said, "The most tragic aspect of

Yusho and Yu-Cheng diseases was the exposure of children to PCBs. In the case of Yu-Cheng, children exposed to PCBs in utero and (in breast milk) were reported to have poor cognitive development. Intellectual impairment was also observed in children born to women who had eaten fish contaminated with PCBs in the United States."

Several important observations relevant to the mechanisms of Yusho have been made from animal studies. For example, some PCBs cause the thymus gland to shrivel and also adversely affect androgen metabolism. Animal studies show exposure to PCBs during fetal development causes profound disruptions in thyroid hormones along with other changes, including abnormalities in brain development, that appear to lead to the higher incidence of learning and attention disorders in the children.

There is strong scientific evidence that these same chemicals are altering critical metabolic pathways that can clearly add to the existing problem of childhood obesity (see Chapter 5). Any chemical exposure that damages the thyroid and its hormone functions during development in the womb or during breastfeeding will have a profound impact on children's ability to maintain normal body weight as they grow. Dietary excess with the junk food so prevalent in our culture is a huge factor in the epidemic of obesity among children. But I don't think *all* the blame rests there.

We can no longer afford such simplistic explanations for obesity in children by saying they are fat because they eat too much and don't exercise enough. That is only the tip of the iceberg. The enormous part still lies below the surface of our awareness: the profound degree of chemical pollutants in everyday life that disrupt critical thyroid and sex hormone pathways and functions in our body. We may not yet have the final "proof," but as you can see, the evidence is staggering. We can no longer afford to ignore the warnings that we see in animal populations all over the world. We are sitting on a time bomb that is beginning to explode on this current generation of children. Like the canary in the mine, the animal population is giving us warnings that we would do well to heed before we sacrifice an entire generation of children. I recommend that you read "Children's environmental health risks: a state-of-the-art conference" (see review in March–April 2001, *Archives of Environmental Health*).

Dietary excess. We live in the age of "super-sizing," not only food and beverage portions but our bodies, too. We live in a culture of *excess everything:* excess calories, excess fat, excess sugars and simple carbs that promote more fat, and excess "couch potato" time in front of TVs and computers. How does this contribute to the earlier onset of puberty? As I described earlier, we have known for a long time that reaching a certain amount of body fat for girls plays an important role in signaling the brain to begin menstrual cycles. Overweight girls tend to begin to menstruate at younger ages, while girls who are very thin or anorexic have later onset of menstrual periods, many times as late as seventeen or eighteen years of age.

- Researchers from the University of Liege in Belgium found a higher incidence of early onset (precocious) puberty in children who had immigrated to Belgium from developing countries where they had been exposed to organochlorine pesticides. These children had higher blood levels of p,p'-DDE (a breakdown product of the organochlorine pesticide DDT) than did a similar group of native-born girls growing up in Belgium where use of these pesticides had been banned years ago. The researchers concluded that precocious puberty could be triggered by early childhood exposure to these endocrine-disrupting pesticides. They recommended further studies to understand the impact of these environmental contaminants on children.

- A study that appeared in the April 2000 issue of *Journal of Pediatrics* summarized the levels of PCBs and DDE in 594 pregnant women and their effects on development of the children born to these women. Female children exposed to PCBs hit puberty earlier than their unexposed peers and, by age fourteen, tended to weigh on average 5.4 kg (11.8 pounds) more than girls who had not been exposed. For a fourteen-year-old girl, almost 12 pounds of extra weight can be quite a lot—certainly from a psychological standpoint, as well as a medical risk. Boys exposed to the highest levels of DDE (a potent estrogenic breakdown product of DDT), were on average 6.9 kg (15.2 pounds) heavier than their unexposed peers but did not show signs of earlier puberty. With our epidemic of childhood obesity, an additional factor that *increases* body weight in children should be taken seriously.

- In 1973, more than four thousand individuals in Michigan were exposed to high levels of the endocrine disruptors called *polybrominated biphenyls* (PBBs) due to accidental contamination of the Michigan food chain. Emory University researchers from the Rollins School of Public Health studied the effects of PBB exposure on age of menses onset in the female children born to mothers who had been exposed. They found that breast-fed girls exposed to these high levels of PBB (greater than or equal to 7 parts per billion) in utero, had onset of menses approximately one full year earlier than girls who were not breast-fed. Girls who were bottle-fed were, on average, 12.7 years old at onset of menses, right at the national average. This suggests that there was more delivery of PBBs in breast milk (high in fat) than what occurred from just passing across the placenta. PBB exposure during gestation and breast-feeding was associated with an earlier pubic hair stage in breast-fed girls, but the researchers did not find a significant change in the time of onset for breast development. They concluded that onset of puberty could be affected by PBBs both before birth and during breast-feeding, but a greater adverse impact occurs when chemical contaminants in breast milk are added to a baby's exposure in the womb.

- Another study further illustrates the connection between breast-feeding and chemical exposure. Dr. Schantz and colleagues from the Institute for Environmental Studies at the University of Illinois measured blood levels of organohalogens (PCBs, PBBs, DDT, DDE, etc.) in a group of Michigan women and children. Of the possible sources they checked, breast-feeding was the greatest source of exposure for children. For adults, the length of time they had lived on a silo farm and how much PCB-contaminated Great Lakes fish they had consumed were the most significant factors in determining the concentration of these chemicals in body fat and breast milk. DDT was present in 93 percent of the mothers and 66 percent of the children, with DDE accounting for 89 percent of the total DDT in serum. PCBs were detected in 86 percent of the mothers, with a high mean serum concentration of 9.6 ng/ml; approximately 42 percent of the children had serum PCB levels at a mean of 6.8 ng/ml. PBBs were detected in 25 percent of the mothers, but not in the children.

- A 1986 study by Drs. Rogan and Gladen of PCBs and DDE in the breast milk of over eight hundred women in North Carolina found higher levels of the chemicals in their first lactation; the levels of contaminants decline as more time was spent breast-feeding and with the number of children nursed. These striking declines indicate the child's exposure because the chemicals are carried out of the mother's tissues into the breast milk as it is formed. A firstborn child who is breast-fed will have a higher exposure to these chemicals than will the next babies. Almost all samples of breast milk showed detectable levels of both chemicals. DDE was measured at higher levels for older women, black women, cigarette smokers, and women who consumed sport fish during pregnancy. Higher levels of PCBs were found in older women, women who regularly drink alcohol, and women having their first pregnancy. This study is especially significant because there were such detailed measurements of chemical levels in umbilical cord blood, placenta, maternal blood and breast milk, as well as because such a large number of women and children were studied over a long period of time.
- Earlier studies of chemical residues in body fat of infants and young children in Germany found that the concentration of organohalogens in children with high breast milk intake was significantly higher than in those with low intake of breast milk.
- We haven't made much progress in the last decades: In Spain, along the Mediterranean coast, extensive farming areas using large amounts of pesticides lie alongside residential areas. Samples of fat from children living around these farm areas contained a total of fourteen pesticides, including Lindane, HCH, heptachlor, aldrin, Dieldrin, endrin, Endosulfan, o,p'-DDE, and o,p'-DDD, among others. All of these substances mimic and/or interfere with the action of our body's estrogens. Drs. Olea and Olea-Serrano said, "After more than four decades of pesticide use, little is known about their adverse effects on health. There is a need to address the potential risks associated with the current contamination of water, soils, and foods in many agricultural areas."

Sociological pressures. Sexualized messages and images besiege girls and boys at younger and younger ages. Such immersion in provocative, often erotic, images may also contribute to changes in brain chemistry that trigger the onset of puberty signals in the pituitary. If you think this is a strange idea, just remember that seeing someone eat a chocolate chip cookie can make you salivate, or watching a horror movie makes your heart race—so for all of us, seeing things around us will trigger physiological changes in the brain and body. We also know that women who live together—in families, in college dorms, in residential high schools—will typically begin to menstruate together. This phenomenon has been described for centuries, as in *The Red Tent* by Anita Diamant (St. Martin's Press, 1997), a story of Jacob's wives and their experiences in the menstrual tent in biblical times. This menstrual synchrony seems to occur from a variety of olfactory and environmental cues that stimulate the brain-ovarian pathways to entrain, or synchronize, menstrual cycles. It may not be so far-fetched to think that constant exposure to visual sexual images may also contribute to brain changes that accelerate sexual development.

The Ovary Life Cycle Continues: Our Fertile Years

Your menstrual cycle tends to regulate itself by late teens or early twenties and you can generally count on it to be a regular length throughout your twenties and into your early thirties. By twenty-five, we have usually reached the peak of our fertility and the peak function of our circulatory, respiratory, and digestive systems to meet the demands of pregnancy with the least stress on our body. Hormone production is more predictable, helping keep the cycles regular. Estradiol levels are high in the first half of the cycle, fall around ovulation, and then rise slightly in the second half of the cycle when progesterone production dominates. Testosterone levels remain fairly constant throughout the cycle.

Our late teens and twenties are a time when one third of sexually active individuals will contract a sexually transmitted disease (STD), so protection such as condoms is important. I recommend that you establish care with a gynecologist when you become sexually active, whenever that age, and have annual Pap smears as well as testing for STDs.

By your mid-thirties, you may begin experiencing a small change in your menstrual flow. By your late thirties or early forties, your flow may become noticeably lighter and last for fewer days. Your cycle length may become either longer or shorter. This is a time when women notice more pronounced premenstrual mood, energy, and appetite changes that we know as premenstrual syndrome (PMS), or as more severe cases, called *premenstrual dysphoric disorder* (PMDD). At this stage, women may often experience the wide variety of effects of estradiol decline: worsening migraines, fibromyalgia, bladder problems, vulvodynia, loss of lean tissue, increasing fat stores, and other annoying symptoms that worsen with our pre- and perimenopausal years.

Estradiol is the first ovarian hormone to decline. It is a misconception that this is a time of progesterone decline and estrogen dominance. Women in this first phase of ovarian decline typically still have normal ovulatory progesterone levels even though estradiol is typically lower than it should be. This imbalance in the estrogen/progesterone ratio may cause PMS symptoms to occur for the first time, or increase the severity of existing PMS. Current studies in reproductive medicine worldwide discount theories that a decline in progesterone precipitates PMS.

The Waning of Our Ovaries: New Insights on Stages of Ovarian Decline

The decline in hormone production that takes us from full reproductive capability to menopause is typically called the *climacteric,* with recognized subsets of premenopause and perimenopause. This decline in estradiol and progesterone commonly begins between the ages of thirty-five and forty, as the number and/or quality of remaining follicles decrease. It begins much earlier in some women.

The standard medical teaching is that premenopause begins with anovulatory menstrual cycles (cycles that do not produce an egg) and the loss of progesterone rather than estrogen. This standard "wisdom" is primarily based on *observations* of women's menstrual patterns, however, rather than on actual systematic hormone levels being done to show objectively what is happening at each phase of the process. It is difficult to "observe" if there is no egg being produced each month, so this is why most doctors don't have a good understanding of what is actually happening to your hormone production. We need more reliable objective measures. I have been tracking and checking cycle-specific hormone levels for many years, in thousands of women, and then correlating them with symptoms. The objective data shows how incorrect our standard teaching can be.

In the women I have tested, I find significant decline in ovarian estradiol levels that *preceded* the onset of anovulatory cycles and loss of progesterone. *It is my contention that an unrecognized estradiol decline is the first step in our bodies' move toward menopause.* I have discussed my observations with many reproductive endocrinologists trying to help infertile women become pregnant. They do regular checks of ovarian hormone levels to achieve pregnancy, and see the same patterns of estradiol decline I find in my patients. Infertility specialists do not address the types of problems I see in my practice as effects of waning ovarian hormones, because their focus, appropriately so, is on helping women get pregnant. But many women who struggle with infertility also experience some of the problems I see in my patients as a result of lower estradiol and testosterone: increasing PMS, headaches, muscle-joint pain, fatigue, weight gain, insulin resistance, bone loss, immune problems, low sex drive, bladder and vaginal problems, and a host of others.

In the box on pages 56–57, I divided our current standard definition of "premenopause" into Stage 1 and Stage 2 of ovarian decline that come before perimenopause. I propose that we "reclassify" these stages, based on patterns that emerge from systematic hormone testing, correlated with women's symptoms:

Stage 1: Declining Estradiol

This occurs when your estradiol level begins to decrease but you still have normal menstrual cycles. In what we call the "normal" or usual time frame, this stage would generally begin in our late thirties or early forties. In this phase, progesterone is generally within normal ovulatory ranges, but estradiol has declined below optimal levels, which makes PMS symptoms worse. One of the first symptoms of lower estradiol is multiple awakening during the night, with difficulty getting back to sleep. Our dreaming phase (REM sleep) is altered, and you may notice that you don't dream as much as you used to. Because sleep is now more restless, you wake up feeling tired.

Other early signs may include fuzzy thinking, memory loss, mood swings, fatigue, muscle and joint pain, headaches, increasing allergies, more sensitivity to strong smells, vulvar pain, and loss of sex drive, among others. Women are usually able to recognize these as hormonally related changes because of the cyclic pattern in which they come and go. Often doctors say, "You're 'too young' to have hormone problems," or "You're still menstruating, so your hormones are fine." This stage I call premature ovarian decline (POD) (see Chapter 1 for more detailed information), and here is where I find so many women are underdiagnosed, undertreated, and left seeking answers in alternative medicine because their symptoms are not recognized by most doctors.

One of the reasons for this lack of recognition at this early stage is that doctors are taught that women who are still menstruating must have "normal" hormone levels. But my detective work to find out why my younger patients have these menopauselike symptoms shows that bleeding patterns are not an accurate marker of hormone levels. Any of you who struggle with infertility know: You can have regular periods yet still not get pregnant. You have to *measure* the ovarian hormones at specific times of the menstrual cycle to see if there are healthy amounts of all the crucial hormones, and in the optimal balance.

Most of my supposedly "premenopausal" patients are still having regular periods, and yet their estradiol levels are far lower than what we now know from menopause research is needed to preserve bone and maintain healthy brain function. The best analogy is that we measure glucose levels to diagnose and monitor diabetes. Women with menstrually related symptoms deserve the same attention to detail we give other health problems.

Stage 2: Beginning of Anovulatory Cycles

This is the beginning of classically defined premenopause. In our "normal" model, this phase would generally begin in our mid-forties, but like all the other phases can occur much earlier. There will be cycles when ovulation does not occur because follicles don't develop properly and estradiol is not produced normally in the first half of the cycle. This then means progesterone doesn't rise as expected in the second half of the cycle. PMS doesn't usually occur if there is no ovulation or rise in progesterone. Levels of FSH and LH are typically still low and haven't risen to the menopausal range. Fewer ovulatory cycles result in estradiol levels continuing to decline, and this is the time you may experience hot flashes and night sweats, especially with the drop in estradiol when your period starts. Your periods typically become irregular, or may skip.

Often common symptoms, from mild to more severe, include insomnia, further memory loss, inability to concentrate or focus, feeling depressed or anxious for no clear reason, and worsening pain syndromes. In this phase of life, you could find yourself with urinary leakage or feelings of urgently having to go to the bathroom, vaginal dryness, painful sex, and feeling that your get-up-and-go got up and went. Part of this energy decline may be due to declining testosterone levels as well as the loss of estradiol. Lower levels of both hormones can rob you of your sexual drive and interest and also make it much harder to have an orgasm because clitoral nerve endings are less sensitive as we lose estradiol and testosterone.

Perimenopause

This stage is classically defined by rising FSH and LH levels as the brain struggles to increase the falling estradiol levels. The amount of estrone, produced primarily by body fat tissue, is rising relative to the decreasing estradiol. Since it doesn't act quite the same way as estradiol does, estrone doesn't keep your body functioning at your previous level. This is why you may notice more "brain fog" and mood changes, as well as more fat around your waist.

You will still have periods, but they now become more erratic and most cycles will likely be anovulatory. You may skip periods now as well. Bleeding is typically lighter and shorter in duration, but it can also become heavier and longer in duration some months. The color of your flow changes, too; it is more likely to be brown rather than a healthy bright red. You may also notice worsening menstrual cramps. Fibroids and ovarian cysts tend to occur more frequently. As a result, hysterectomy is recommended for many women, although there are a number of nonsurgical options to help control or prevent many of these problems (see Chapter 16).

Simply said, at this phase of your ovary life cycle, your periods will most likely be erratic, with changing bleeding patterns. If menses come more often than every three weeks, or if you have heavy bleeding, you should talk with your gynecologist to discuss options. A word of caution: With cycle irregularity and erratic ovulation at this phase of life, you could find yourself with an unexpected pregnancy. If this is not desired, then you still need to use contraception until you are clearly menopausal, with an FSH greater than 20 mIU/ml.

Menopausal Stage

This final stage may seem out of place as part of our "reproductive" cycle, since we are no longer able to get pregnant, but it is the stage that brings our ovary life cycle to completion. The average age in the United States for natural menopause is between forty-eight and fifty-two, but this is just an average. Ten to thirteen percent of women experience true menopause between ages forty and forty-seven. Another estimated 1 percent, or several million women, will undergo complete menopause, or premature ovarian failure, before age forty. Premature ovarian *decline* is a gray area between the two, in terms of FSH and hormone levels. When menopause comes so early, it can be quite a shock. It is a physical shock to your body to lose these important metabolically active ovarian hormones at too young an age, not just an emotional blow of feeling old before your time and feeling the loss of your fertility. Early onset of menopause has many causes, which we'll discuss later. Certainly our genetic makeup is one factor: Studies of women around the world have shown that heredity is a major determinant of when we will reach menopause. It helps to find out when your mother and grandmothers reached natural menopause (unless a hysterectomy created an artificial menopause) to give you an idea of what you might expect.

We no longer menstruate because our follicle supply has been depleted, and we can't make the hormones that trigger our menstrual cycles. The brain senses the decrease in estradiol and sends out more FSH and LH to stimulate the ovaries to produce more hormones. FSH and LH levels rise above 20 mIU/ml, which is our official definition of the menopausal level. But the rise in stimulating hormones FSH and LH is useless because there are no follicles to produce estradiol and progesterone. The low levels of ovarian hormones are now present in steady, noncycling patterns.

With menopause, we lose almost *all* of our 17-beta estradiol production, with levels typically below 30–40 pg/ml. That's a lot lower than the average 100–500 pg/ml of a menstrual cycle, so it isn't surprising that you feel so many body and brain changes! Progesterone levels remain low because there is no ovulation, no corpus luteum, and progesterone is no longer needed to sustain a pregnancy. Women also lose approximately half of their testosterone production. The ovary still produces testosterone and other androgens, though at lower levels, but it is no longer producing adequate estradiol to balance these male hormones. The uneven balance of estradiol and testosterone causes some of the unwanted changes in skin, facial hair, and distribution of body fat. The female "pear" shape (gynecoid) fat pattern around the hips and buttocks suddenly begins moving up toward the middle of the body to become the "apple" shape (male or android pattern), as shown in the diagram on page 53.

In official "medicalese," menopause is defined as *one year from the last menstrual period.* It may seem odd that we wait so long to apply the label. The problem is that our periods get more irregular at the end, so we never know which period is the last one for quite a number of months. We can then look back and

WOMEN'S MIDLIFE BODY SHAPE CHANGES

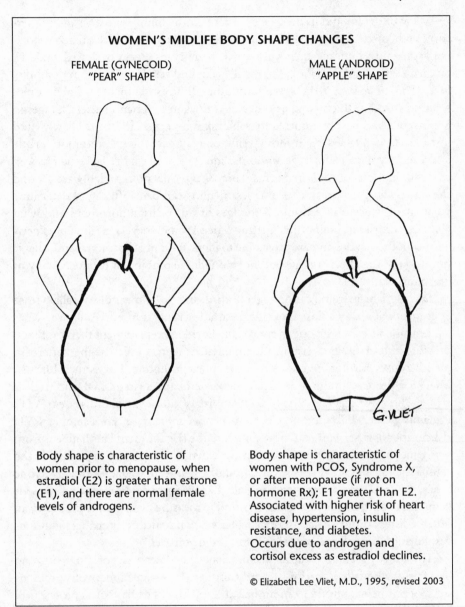

FEMALE (GYNECOID)
"PEAR" SHAPE

MALE (ANDROID)
"APPLE" SHAPE

G.VLIET

Body shape is characteristic of women prior to menopause, when estradiol (E2) is greater than estrone (E1), and there are normal female levels of androgens.

Body shape is characteristic of women with PCOS, Syndrome X, or after menopause (if *not* on hormone Rx); E1 greater than E2. Associated with higher risk of heart disease, hypertension, insulin resistance, and diabetes.
Occurs due to androgen and cortisol excess as estradiol declines.

© Elizabeth Lee Vliet, M.D., 1995, revised 2003

realize "that was it." In earlier years, we also did not have reliable blood tests to accurately measure FSH and estradiol to determine clearly that a woman had reached the endocrinological stage of menopause. One caveat for younger women who are athletes: Intensive training may cause you to stop having periods, but you are not classically considered to be "menopausal" because you still have ovarian follicles. Once you decrease the intensity of your workouts, periods are likely to return.

Many of the symptoms described earlier become more noticeable and bothersome with lower menopausal hormone levels. Women often notice a marked worsening of brain symptoms such as insomnia, memory loss, foggy or slowed thinking, and pain symptoms. Hot flashes may still occur and get worse with lower estradiol levels. For some women, however, hot flashes diminish as the estradiol becomes steady, instead of fluctuating as much as it does in perimenopause. Changes in appearance also become more noticeable: skin becomes drier and "crawly," and loses its elasticity, leading to more wrinkles. Hair gets thinner and more brittle and you may start losing large amounts. You may notice more facial hair as well as loss of hair on your legs and arms. There is typically more weight gain around the waist, and your breasts become less firm. It can be confusing to determine what changes occur as a result of the loss of our ovarian hormones and what changes occur as a result of just getting older. Women have a lifetime of experience with their cycles and are often able to identify what is hormonal and what is not, though the effects of age and hormone loss combine to produce many of our body changes.

Risk of diabetes, colon cancer, osteoporosis, and Alzheimer's disease all increase after menopause as you lose the critical estradiol. Breast cancer risk also increases after menopause even if you never take any hormone replacement therapy. Blood pressure and cholesterol rise in menopausal women, similar to the pattern in men because testosterone effects become more pronounced as estradiol is lost. There is a decrease in the good "HDL" cholesterol and a rise in LDL and triglycerides. These changes combine to increase risk of cardiovascular disease (CVD). Previous gender *differences* now become gender *similarities*. For example, CVD risk for menopausal women is now similar to the risk for men. This happens from being menopausal, regardless of your age when it occurs, and regardless of the cause. The rate of CVD increases as estradiol levels decline relative to testosterone levels, as we see in younger women with PCOS. Since cardiovascular disease is the number one killer of women, it is critical to measure ovarian hormone levels in order to assess your risk of CVD, particularly if you notice body changes that suggest hormone imbalance, regardless of how old you are.

The entire process of ovarian decline may take fifteen years or more, or it can be a fairly rapid fall, occurring at nearly any age. This transition involves dimensions of our being: physical, emotional, and spiritual. The biological process will happen sooner or later to all women who live long enough. Psychological and spiritual changes are more variable, and include learning to see our later years as fulfilling and meaningful, taking stock of our lives and what we want to accomplish in the years ahead, changing priorities for how we spend our time, and exploring our spiritual beliefs. While there may be a sense of loss over no longer being able to bear children, there is also the opportunity for the years after menopause to have a sense of freedom that is equally gratifying.

Some women experience no major physical symptoms at all; they stop menstruating and that's that. Others have a few irksome symptoms but aren't significantly bothered by these changes. Still other women have a very difficult time in the years leading up to menopause with symptoms and health risks that profoundly disrupt quality of life and ability to function well each day. This latter group often describes serious declines in energy level, mental sharpness, sex drive, quality of sleep, and overall well-being. Many will develop chronic debilitating diseases, such as diabetes or osteoporosis, that further sabotage quality of life.

It is important to keep in mind that symptoms of hormonal decline can occur at any age. When I describe the ovaries' "normal" aging process, I am only giving you age ranges for a relative idea of when these changes can occur. Your ovaries are as individual as you are and may not follow the time line as outlined. To put it another way, each woman's body marches to its own drummer. Each woman has slightly different experiences along the way, just as it was with puberty and pregnancy. The stage of life when you notice changes and symptoms, as well as the symptoms themselves, is not necessarily going to be the same as your friends. You may be perimenopausal in your early thirties or you could even be endocrinologically menopausal in your twenties. I have many patients in both categories. Whatever *age* these changes occur, the stages and body markers, or symptoms, are similar, and we may use some of the same treatments. The key is to recognize what is going on at any age, understand why it is happening, and have the knowledge to make informed health decisions that meet your needs.

In my practice, we primarily see women who feel terrible and want ways to regain their energy and vitality. As one woman said so succinctly: "I don't like this foggy-brained feeling, I want my brain back!" It isn't a matter of "medicalizing" menopause when we replace what is lost to restore hormone balance. I help women achieve *their* goals and desires based on our collaborative efforts to assess what causes such disruption in their quality of life. I work to find ways for them to have a smoother transition, avoid the pitfalls and uncomfortable symptoms that can become even more pronounced if untreated or mistreated. Since women are now living thirty to forty years after menopause, our ultimate goal is to find healthy, safe, effective ways to maintain vitality and zest for those years ahead.

The Sixties and Beyond: Postmenopausal Stage

We have seen an impressive increase in the average life span for both men and women in the last century. Thanks to medical technology, new medications, a more plentiful and varied food supply, and better knowledge of disease prevention and lifestyle risk reduction, we are living longer than ever before. While most of us view this as a good thing, it also presents a whole new set of challenges. It is only in the last two or three generations that large numbers of people have lived long enough for us to see some of the brain-body effects of declining ovarian hormones in women and declining testicular hormones in men. Women today may live thirty to forty years beyond menopause.

Worldwide studies have shown that taking estradiol after menopause decreases

DR. VLIET'S MODEL: STAGES OF OVARIAN DECLINE

Stage 1: Declining Estradiol, Normal Cycles
- FSH and LH are within normal ranges
- Estradiol (E2) level is beginning to decrease
- Testosterone may be starting to decrease
- Progesterone is within normal range but may be out of balance with your estradiol, making PMS worse
- Menstrual cycles are still regular and most are ovulatory
- Beginning of restless sleep, fuzzy thinking, memory loss, mood swings, fatigue, muscle/joint pain, headaches, allergies, and other symptoms of low E2

Stage 2: Beginning of Anovulatory Cycles
- FSH and LH are within normal ranges, still less than 10 mIU/ml
- Estradiol level continues to decline; hot flashes typically begin at times of the cycle when estradiol is falling (menses, ovulation)
- Testosterone is typically decreasing
- Fewer ovulatory cycles mean progesterone (P) does not rise during second half of cycle; PMS doesn't typically occur if there is no ovulation and no rise in progesterone
- Menses becomes irregular
- Insomnia, memory loss, depression, and pain syndromes get worse; low libido, leaking urine, vaginal dryness, and loss of energy are common

Stage 3: Perimenopause
- FSH and LH are beginning to rise, typically in the 10–20 mIU/ml range
- Estradiol much lower now over the entire menstrual cycle
- Loss of ovulatory cycles, progesterone decreases further
- Testosterone continues to decline, affecting libido, mood, energy level, and muscle and bone mass
- Periods become much more erratic, cycles are skipped, there may be more bleeding problems due to the changing balance of estradiol and progesterone
- Hot flashes, restless sleep, and fuzzy thinking become more pronounced and regular; other symptoms develop or become magnified

Stage 4: Menopause
- FSH and LH have risen to levels above 20 mIU/ml (the level that defines menopause)
- Menses no longer occur
- Estradiol level is decreased to levels typically below 30–40 pg/ml
- Progesterone levels remain low since no further ovulation occurs
- Testosterone levels decline further, often less than 20 ng/dl
- Brain symptoms (insomnia, hot flashes, memory loss, pain, etc.)

increase as estradiol declines. Other changes occur with loss of estradiol, such as bone loss, elevated blood pressure, decrease in HDL cholesterol, waistline weight gain, hair loss, dry skin, dry eyes, crawly skin, incontinence, difficulty reaching orgasm, loss of sexual interest, and many others

© Elizabeth Lee Vliet, M.D., 2003

the risk of Alzheimer's, osteoporosis, heart attacks, stroke, incontinence, and colon cancer by 40 to 60 percent (see Section IV for more detail on these benefits). You don't need to fear your years after menopause if you integrate healthy lifestyle changes with information from the rapidly advancing science about how our bodies change, and incorporate commonsense treatments outlined later. There are many ways to improve your health and vitality, reduce disease risks, and enjoy a better quality of life for all the years you live.

Premature Ovarian Decline

Now that we have talked about hormones and body changes in a "normal" progression through the life cycle, let's explore premature ovarian *decline* (POD). This is a stage of life when you are transitioning from optimal fertile hormone levels to less optimal levels. It is not the same as true premature ovarian *failure* (POF) because you still have follicles and menstrual periods. POD simply means that your ovaries are not producing ovarian hormones at levels sufficient to maintain "optimal" metabolic function throughout the body, even though your FSH still remains in the premenopausal range. This decline is taking place before you would expect it. You are too young for this, so no one is really looking for it and it is blamed on something else. That "something" is usually labeled psychological, or just "stress," and young women are told to take an antidepressant. For women experiencing premature ovarian decline, a significant portion of the first half of adult life is spent searching for answers. The consequences throughout your body can be dramatic, as you will see in later chapters.

Medical studies show that women who go through premature menopause have a shorter life span. Perhaps because the body has less time with the full benefits of estradiol, including its immune system effects; or it may be that these women have earlier onset of the diseases and conditions such as osteoporosis, diabetes, cardiovascular disease, Alzheimer's disease, and colon cancer as a result of the absence of the critical 17-beta estradiol. To some extent, these same risks can be increased in women who experience the early decline in estradiol as well, although definitive studies are lacking.

There are many clues to declining estradiol; some of the common ones I see in patients can be found in the box on page 58.

CLUES TO DECLINING ESTRADIOL

- Worsening PMS
- Restless sleep, difficulty sleeping especially prior to menses, multiple awakenings during the night
- Loss of energy, feeling too tired to get through the day
- Premenstrual migraines, more frequent migraines
- Increase in tension headaches
- Aching joints
- Muscle soreness, stiffness, fibromyalgia pain syndrome
- Memory and concentration problems that are worse before menses
- Mood swings, episodic tearfulness for no reason, irritability, angry outbursts, and spells of feeling depressed, especially premenstrually
- Worsening allergies, sensitivities to chemicals, perfumes
- Palpitations, especially those that get worse a few days prior to menses and during bleeding days when estradiol is low or falling
- Anxiety attacks, worse around menses
- "Spiking" blood pressure, higher blood pressure than normal
- More irritable bowel problems prior to menses and during menses
- Dry eyes occur early; later, as women lose their estradiol, risk of macular degeneration, cataracts, and glaucoma increases
- Hair gets thinner, more scalp hair loss
- Nails are dry and brittle
- Facial hair increases
- Skin becomes dry, crawly, and looser; less elastic due to decline in collagen; wrinkles start to appear
- Vaginal dryness, pain with sex
- Loss of sex drive, difficulty having orgasm
- Bladder changes: more infections, pain on urination, more frequent urination, urinary leakage
- Posture becomes more slumped as bone is lost from spine
- "Spare" tire around middle—abdominal fat gain
- Food cravings
- Difficulty losing weight, even with diet and exercise

It is obvious from this list that estradiol affects many body functions. In women with POD, loss of estradiol can sometimes be sudden, but more often it is a subtle, gradual change occurring over several years. The change in hormone production may be so gradual that it is virtually unrecognized as you go along, day by day. Your mind and body make adjustments, similar to the way the body adjusts to a gradual loss of hemoglobin in an early anemia, but gradually, you begin to notice you just don't feel like your usual self. Eventually, the decline in estradiol changes the balance of estradiol in *ratio* to testosterone, DHEA, and progesterone to lead to a wide variety of physical and psychological experiences. Some of these may occur for the first time, or take a turn for the worse as the hormone balance changes.

There are many known causes and contributors to early ovarian decline, and even more that we don't fully understand yet. Some of these we can control, some we can't. Good lifestyle habits will certainly help slow and ease the aging process. But when it comes to our ovaries, this is not always enough, and women may need hormonal support. The box on page 60 lists many of the potential causes of POD. Note how varied they are. In later chapters, I will explore these in more depth.

In Summary

Your hormones can be both marvelous *and* maddening—marvelous when they allow us to create new life and function at our best, maddening when they are out of balance or declining. But ovarian hormones are more than just for creating new life; our female hormones are at the core of our being, fundamental to every part and function of our body, mind, and spirit. The patterns of physiological changes that occur each month and throughout the ovaries' life cycle give us observable phenomena that help us to then "connect the dots" and see the hormonal triggers related to physical and mood symptoms. We need to look for these patterns, track them, and then find ways to communicate our observations to physicians.

Although the life cycle of ovaries refers to overall stages of our lives rather than the monthly menstrual cycle we discussed in Chapter 2, one affects the other. As our ovaries age and we approach menopause, or undergo surgery, or experience other problems, our menstrual cycles change, too. The normal ebb and flow of our body changes. Is everything *supposed* to be downhill from now on? Is this just a part of life we must accept? I don't think so. As one woman so eloquently put it: "It was about fourteen years ago that I had my hysterectomy for severe PMS, and they also found endometriosis. I was better after the surgery and managed for a few years, but for the last several, I started having really horrible menopausal symptoms even though I was taking estrogen daily. After reading your books, I finally insisted on getting my hormone levels checked and they found my estrogen was too low . . . but they added testosterone! It is so frustrating. . . . I have learned a lot from all my reading because I had to in order to help myself! But doctors don't seem to want to listen to what I know, even when it is my own body. Every time I try to do something I am up against obstacles, but I keep fighting because I know it isn't right and I stand up for what I need."

I know it is difficult to convince doctors of something they can't see— hormone problems are not visible, like a broken leg. And when you don't feel well over a long period of time and have sought help from multiple doctors only to be told there is nothing wrong, it can leave you doubting yourself physically as well as psychologically. You feel battered, frustrated, and alone. You suspect it is

OVERLOOKED CAUSES OF PREMATURE OVARIAN DECLINE

- Chronic dieting, eating disorders (anorexia, bulimia) that suppress hypothalamus regulation of ovarian function
- Compulsive exercise for weight loss, or the intensive training schedules of competitive athletes that interferes with ovulation and release of follicle and thereby estrogen production
- Cigarette smoking, which damages ovarian follicles
- Tubal ligation, which interrupts normal ovarian blood flow
- Hysterectomy without removal of the ovaries, which interrupts ovarian blood flow
- Thyroid disorders, which interfere both with brain regulation of ovaries and ovarian hormone production and function
- Polycystic ovary syndrome, which leads to excessive production of testosterone and insulin that prevents normal ovulation with normal production of estradiol and progesterone
- Viral oophoritis, which is a viral infiltration that may damage the ovary just as happens with the thyroid and pancreas glands
- Postpartum phase, in which high prolactin levels during nursing suppresses the normal menstrual cycle hormone production and ovulation; with older age at pregnancy, ovaries may not come back into full normal cycles after nursing ends
- Cessation of birth control pills after long-term use, especially high-progestin pills
- Toxic exposures: examples of this in my practice include black widow spider bites, Lyme disease, pesticides
- Hypothalamic dysfunction or suppression due to excessive exercise, chronic dieting, high intake of soy, high intake of excitatory amino acids (such as glutamate, MSG, aspartate, Nutrasweet)

Other Potential Risk Factors for POD
- Mother had early onset of menopause
- Body weight—thinner women have earlier onset
- Vegetarian diet resulting in lower consumption of protein and fat and a generally higher intake of soy products; lower body weight and fat composition
- Malnutrition
- Living at high altitudes
- Never having been pregnant (more pregnancies leads to later menopause)

MECHANISMS OF PREMATURE OVARIAN DECLINE/FAILURE

Loss of Primordial Follicles During Fetal Development
- Genetic abnormalities
- Damage in utero from maternal smoking, alcohol, pesticide, and other chemical exposure

Premature Death of Follicles in Childhood and Young Adult Years
- Chemical exposure: xenobiotics (pesticides, etc.)
- Smoking
- Alcohol
- Marijuana, cocaine, ecstasy use
- Chemotherapy
- Autoimmune disorder—viral, bacterial (mumps ovaritis, herpes ovaritis, chlamydia, Lyme, post–flu vaccine, etc.)
- Radiation exposure
- High altitude

Inhibition/Disruption of Hypothalamic-Pituitary-Ovarian Pathways
- Excitotoxins affecting brain centers
- Smoking
- Alcohol, marijuana and other street drugs
- Certain medications—antidepressants, antipsychotics, and anticonvulsants
- Malnutrition, anorexia, bulimia
- Body weight abnormalities—underweight, obesity
- Stress
- Thyroid disorders, especially autoimmune ones
- High altitude

© Elizabeth Lee Vliet, M.D., 2003

your hormones, yet no one takes you seriously. Many of my patients tell me it is often hard to get their physicians to listen to their observations and pay attention to these hormone-related issues. Many of my patients have done so much research to educate themselves, they often know more about these issues than many doctors!

There are ways to help you get what you need when dealing with health care professionals. If your doctor isn't listening, find one who will. I encourage you to be assertive about getting checked for these potential hormone connections. I urge you to get answers that make sense. There are too many health consequences if you don't. While there are no easy solutions for changing the health care system to be more responsive to women's observations and insights, I do have some suggestions you may consider.

Many women depend on their gynecologist for primary care as well as annual pelvic exams. But you may find, as have many of my patients, that family medicine or internal medicine physicians are more open to the idea of checking hormone levels than are many gynecologists. I think this is related to the fact that medical specialists are more accustomed to using laboratory tests both to evaluate health problems and to monitor response to medications. You may also find that internists and family physicians are likely to be responsive to your written summary of the patterns you notice in relation to your menstrual cycle. It facilitates communication with your physicians if you bring any journals you have kept to track your symptoms as you go through your menstrual cycle.

Don't focus on just treating or "getting through" symptoms. That's a lot like just putting a Band-Aid on an abscess instead of treating the cause of the infection. Look for the underlying causes and make decisions based on what you need for overall vitality and health for many years to come.

It is *your* body, *your* health, and *your* life.

SECTION II

Ovaries at Risk

4

Ovaries at Risk: Surprising Toxins in Your Diet

Introduction

Why is it we see so many more women today suffering from serious health problems, including infertility, arising from premature ovarian decline? Are we overlooking a crucial connection that lurks "innocently" in the foods we are eating and the soft drinks we are collectively consuming, literally by the gallon, every day? I think the answer is *yes*. As you read the stories of the women I have seen for consults, you will see that many have one thing in common: Their ovaries have been damaged by subtle, insidious dietary and environmental "hormone disruptors" that have affected their ability to make the ovarian hormones they need to effectively "run" the cellular engines that make up every organ in their bodies (see Chapter 5 for more on environmental disruptors). Some of these hormone disruptors are common everyday elements in our lives—such as soft drinks and flavor enhancers like MSG. We would never dream that they could wreak such havoc with our ovaries and our hormones.

Soft drinks? "Impossible," you say. *MSG* in all those foods? "Not in a million years."

This chapter may shock you. You may not think it is real. But I am describing *worldwide* research showing adverse effects on men and women and animals and fish and birds and insects and reptiles . . . from all over the planet. Dietary toxins are *very serious* problems and can affect many aspects of your health, from future cancer risk to your fertility now. This is your call to action.

So let's first explore some surprising "ovary damagers" that lie in some unsuspected foods and beverages you probably eat or drink every day.

The Soft-Drink/Fast-Food Menace: Excitotoxins and Hormone Health

How can soft drinks and foods affect our ovaries? The answer may be more astounding, more macabre, and more insidious than the twists of a horror movie. Truth is sometimes stranger than fiction. Let's look at what truth we know about certain types of food additives and sweeteners that fall into a group of chemicals called *excitotoxins.*

Excitotoxins, or neurotoxicants, are chemicals that cause damage or death to nerve cells. Basically, these chemicals stimulate such intense and rapid firing of the nerve endings that the cells run out of their chemical messengers, and then die a few hours later. The nerve cells in the hypothalamus, our master hormone regulator, are some of the neurons in our body most sensitive to this excitatory damage and death. While we are still quietly developing in our mother's womb, the brain cells in the hypothalamus can be damaged by these excitotoxins, but the impact doesn't show up until many years later, when our menstrual cycles begin. While children, we typically consume large amounts of these excitotoxins in soft drinks and other processed foods. The damage to the hypothalamus accumulates each day and each year, and we don't realize what is happening. Again, the most marked consequences of this damage show up later in our reproductive years, when "hormone problems" can begin in earnest.

What Are Excitotoxins and Where Are They Found?

Some of the excitotoxins are natural compounds that occur in plants and animals as amino acids: *glutamate, aspartate,* and *cysteine,* which are the building blocks of proteins. Some excitotoxins are man-made chemicals and are even more potent. One example is MSG, the well-known chemical culprit that causes "Chinese-restaurant headache" syndrome. MSG, or monosodium glutamate, is a flavor-enhancer first synthesized in the 1920s. It is widely used in making all kinds of processed foods to improve taste and make us want to eat more, and more! MSG is made by adding sodium to the amino acid glutamate, and it is the glutamate part of the molecule that does the excitatory damage to nerve cells. MSG-induced damage to the brain has been studied and written about for at least forty years, but the food manufacturing industry has effectively managed to keep this research from broader public awareness.

George R. Schwartz, M.D., described this critical problem in his excellent book *In Bad Taste: The MSG Syndrome* (Santa Fe, N. Mex.: Health Press, 1999). In spite of continuing research showing more damage than first thought, concerns about the overuse of glutamate have not been heeded. Problems have only intensified with the addition of even more MSG-related compounds to an ever-increasing array of foods and beverages. MSG makes foods taste better by causing a chemical reaction in our mouth to keep us coming back for "just one more." We eat more and buy more . . . a manufacturer's dream. No wonder it is added to all kinds of foods. Manufacturers are not likely to stop using these additives anytime soon—the prepared foods market is too lucrative. *In Bad Taste* focuses on the role of MSG in learning and behavioral disorders in children, as well as in degenerative neurological syndromes that occur later in life, but it didn't address the damage to women's hormonal systems that leads to the health problems I describe.

I am taking the already extensive research to a new level in drawing my conclusion: Long-standing consumption of MSG and other excitotoxins can adversely affect women's health and reproductive system via their effects on our brain. Manufacturers won't tell you this, and most doctors don't know it. It is up to you to eliminate these damaging additives from your diet as much as possible.

MSG is only one of the excitotoxin chemicals added to foods. Another man-made example is HVP, or hydrolyzed vegetable protein (sometimes shown on food labels simply as vegetable protein or plant protein). HVP is derived from plants that aren't fit to eat but are high in the excitatory amino acids such as glutamate or aspartate. The plants are processed with acid and caustic soda, dried, and made into a concentrated powder that contains a potent mix of the same *three* known excitotoxins—glutamate, aspartate, and cystoic acid. In spite of the known adverse brain effects of these excitotoxins, HVP is found in much of the food you eat; it is almost hard to find something that *doesn't* have it! It is in protein drinks (an obvious place), but also finds its way into cereals, frozen dinners, diet meals (without it, these meals would taste like cardboard), sauce mixes, soups, salad dressings, diet drink powders you mix with milk or water, to name a few. Again, the research is compelling, but the food industry has fought to keep this hidden from you, the general public. Furthermore, the FDA has failed to warn us of the dangers of these hidden additives in our foods.

Even babies have not been spared getting dosed with MSG. Manufacturers add flavor enhancers to intensify the flavor of baby foods and stimulate babies to eat more. MSG consumption in infancy and childhood makes kids eat more and also alters brain pathways. And then we wonder why we have a nation of obese people and an epidemic of childhood obesity! It wasn't until 1970 that adding MSG to baby foods was finally stopped as an outgrowth of brain research conducted by Dr. John W. Olney. Dr. Olney showed that the amount of MSG in even one jar of baby food was enough to cause permanent damage from cell death in crucial areas of the retina and brain during development. Damage to the ultra-sensitive hypothalamus was especially severe. His studies showed that high-dose exposure to MSG in mice caused the pituitary glands and ovaries or testicles to *shrink* (hypoplasia). That's not exactly what you need! High-dose MSG also caused a major loss of the pituitary secretion of luteinizing hormone (LH) and growth hormone (GH). But even more alarming, *low doses* that were well *below* toxic levels, caused abnormally *high* LH and loss of the normal bursts of GH secretion. As a result, "MSG babies" were short in stature, obese, and had difficulty reproducing as adults. Reduced GH explained the short stature and obesity. Abnormal levels of LH explained the infertility. These same body changes are seen in girls with PCOS, a serious neuroendocrine disorder in young women that often causes infertility (see Chapter 13).

The reproductive disruptions and infertility found in all the animal studies are strikingly parallel to what I see in patients. The combined evidence suggests that excitatory amino acids cause damage to the hypothalamus so that the hypothalamus-pituitary-ovarian pathways can't work properly. This in turn contributes to the many endocrine abnormalities seen in PCOS and other reproductive disorders as women reach puberty. I am convinced that excitotoxins hitting the brain in the womb, in infancy, and in childhood play an insidious role in the increasing problems with ovarian dysfunction, including PCOS and other "hormone havoc" syndromes I see in women.

In a troubling finding, scientists discovered that a human infant's brain is *far more sensitive to damage* from excitotoxins than the brains in *all* other species studied. Unlike animals, human brains have additional development during infancy and childhood, not just while in the mother's womb. The data became so overwhelming about this hidden health hazard to infants that researchers raised the alarm to Congress, which banned MSG additives in baby foods. This was too late for the generation of children born in the forties, fifties, and sixties (actually, many of the baby boomers, including me) who ate baby food laced with large amounts of this additive. I am certain that this is another factor for the high incidence of reproductive disorders and subtle forms of "learning disorders" in adults now between the ages of thirty and sixty. These are the *same* kinds of learning and abnormal hormone effects seen in all the animal species studied.

It is more frightening to realize excitotoxins are still added to baby foods today, in spite of the ban. Banned MSG has morphed into other chemicals that consumers don't recognize, such as caseinate, beef or chicken broth, and "natural flavorings"—all of which may be made from sources high in these excitatory amino acids. Scientists think that the rise in learning disorders, impulse control disorders, behavioral problems, and premature puberty is triggered, in part, by these additional excitatory amino acid additives.

Why are diet soft drinks a particular problem? Because they contain MSG or aspartate, which is found in the Nutrasweet used to sweeten them. And *liquid* forms of excitotoxins are much more toxic to the brain than dry, because they are absorbed faster and produce higher blood levels than when ingested in solid foods. Since their damage primarily hits the hypothalamus and "learning and memory" centers, the effects aren't seen until you are much older, so you don't realize they are a problem. When you look at how many soft drinks an average American drinks every week, you can see there is a serious potential for causing hormonal chaos.

Not only infants and children are severely affected by excitotoxins; adults, too, are hit with their damaging effects. Current studies link the rising rate of degenerative diseases in older people after a lifetime of consuming excitotoxins in food and soft drinks. These diseases—among them Parkinson's, ALS (amyotrophic lateral sclerosis, or Lou Gehrig's disease), Alzheimer's, MS, and other, less common debilitating nervous system disorders—may have additional primary causes, but the evidence is strong that excitotoxins increase brain damage and younger onset of symptoms. These links are described in detail in an excellent book by neurosurgeon Russell L. Blaylock, M.D., called *Excitotoxins: The Taste That Kills* (Santa Fe, N. Mex.: Health Press, 1994).

Common neurological disorders—migraine headaches, some forms of daily "tension" headaches, strokes, and seizures (particularly the more subtle types, such as complex partial, absence-type, and petit mal)—are now linked to these same excitotoxins. I am suspicious that there is also a link between high intake of dietary excitatory amino acids and damage to the pituitary-ovarian hormone production in young women who develop the mysterious chronic fatigue syndrome (CFS) and diffuse muscle pain syndromes. We lack research to confirm this. We do know, however, that dietary excitatory amino acids cause subtle nerve cell damage in hormone-governing centers. Does this then lead to premature decline in your ovarian hormones? Draw your own conclusions as you read on.

Brain Basics: Your Body's Chief Executive Officer and Chief Operating Officer

Our hormones affect our brain directly, and our brain regulates hormone production by endocrine glands throughout the body. Our brain is far too complex for me to find a perfect metaphor for its function. But think of a CEO and COO of a multitrillion-dollar, multinational company. Your CEO brain has to oversee incredibly complex actions, interactions, ramifications, repercussions, and constantly changing information bombarding it from thousands of sources constantly 24 hours a day, 365 days a year. It has to organize, analyze, direct, execute, evaluate, delegate, and coordinate . . . all day long and all night long. Our hormones work as chemical communicators that facilitate the connections among all the body's parts, and help all of these brain functions run smoothly.

EXCITOTOXINS: WHERE THEY ARE FOUND

Man-made: Hydrolyzed vegetable protein powder
Found in nature as amino acids: glutamate, aspartate, cysteine

Name	Where Found
Monosodium Glutamate MSG	Many types of prepared foods
Hydrolyzed vegetable protein: (contains 3 excitotoxins: glutamate, aspartate, and cystoic acid)	Many prepared foods, diet products, frozen dinners
Aspartate (Nutrasweet)	Everything from foods to soft drinks
Glutamate	See above
Cysteine (cystoic acid)	See above

© Elizabeth Lee Vliet, M.D., 2003

MAJOR BRAIN AREAS AND WHAT THEY DO

The *cerebral cortex* is our master "thinker" and overseer for integrating information between the body and the outside world; it is made up of the brain's frontal, temporal, parietal, and occipital lobes.

The *limbic system* is deep in the brain in what we call the *subcortical area*. It is made up of several structures that regulate many functions known as the human "drives" (appetite, thirst, sex, aggression, sleep-wake cycles). The limbic system is crucial to our discussion in this chapter because it encompasses our body's master hormone regulators, the hypothalamus and pituitary, that oversee endocrine regulation, memory processing, mood and emotion, alertness, focus, and movement coordination and helps integrate sensory information, including pain. Pain-carrying signals from the body relating to *chronic* pain come through the limbic center, while *acute* pain pathways bypass the limbic system and go directly to the higher brain centers. This is one reason that chronic pain shatters the stability of our mood and sleep-governing centers, and causes insomnia and depression along with the pain. People suffering acute pain usually do not experience depression or severe sleep disturbances.

The *cerebellum* lies below the cortex and to the back of our head. Its major role is to coordinate movement (with the cortex), balance, and fine-motor control. For example, imbalance seen with alcohol intoxication and the abnormal movements seen in Parkinson's disease result from damage to these movement-control pathways.

The *brainstem (midbrain, pons, medulla)*: These structures regulate our "survival functions," such as respiration, heart rate, and blood pressure in response to all the information they receive from multiple connections in the brain and spinal cord.

The *spinal cord* is a thick band of nerve fibers that connects to the brain at the base of the skull and travels the length of our spine to the low back. It carries all the nerve tracts and the constant flow of chemical messengers from the body to the brain and from the brain back to the body so that our brain and body functions can be properly coordinated.

The Brain's Communicators

Nerve cells have to "talk" to each other for our brain and body to work as a coordinated whole. They connect to each other by branches we call *axons* and *dendrites*. In order for actual messages to be passed from one nerve to another, chemical messengers called *neurotransmitters* travel back and forth across gaps (*synapses*) between the nerve endings. Hormones also act as messengers, helping nerve cells carry their messages. Our hormones also "talk" to nerve cells and to neurotransmitters like serotonin by way of special "docking sites" that we call *receptors,* specific for each type of molecule. Neurotransmitters and our hormones also have docking sites on the cells of the immune system, as well as our endocrine glands, the intestinal tract, and other organs all over the body.

There are many chemical messengers in the body, but I want to focus on those most critical to the interactions between our hormones and the brain: serotonin (5-HT), norepinephrine (NE), dopamine (DA), acetylcholine (ACh), gamma-aminobutyric acid (GABA), glutamate, N-acetylaspartate (NAA). These neurotransmitters scurry throughout our brain and body, day in and day out, relaying and modulating information between cells in different parts of the body. They link our emotional and physical health. These same chemical messengers and pathways are ones that can be seriously disrupted by excitotoxins.

We make these information-carrying molecules from building blocks called *amino acids* found in the food we eat. We need various vitamins and minerals as catalysts and cofactors for the synthesizing enzymes to make the neurotransmitters. If you don't eat a healthy, balanced diet, your body can't make neurotransmitters *or* hormones, or make them work properly. When you drink a lot of soft drinks, the excitotoxins cause even more damage by interfering with your ability to absorb vitamins and minerals.

Your brain's chemical messengers have incredibly diverse roles and functions. Serotonin, for example, turns out to be involved in many behavioral dimensions of our lives, including aspects we previously thought were caused by "psychological conflicts." Pain, sleep, anxiety, and appetite are all regulated by serotonin. We need the right balance: insomnia, anxiety, and overeating can each occur when serotonin is either too low *or* too high. Serotonin imbalances may also cause other behavioral problems, from compulsive shoplifting and gambling to compulsive sexual behaviors, compulsive hand washing, and hair-pulling (trichotillomania).

The *balance* of brain chemical messengers also helps regulate mood: Mania can result from excessive levels of norepinephrine and dopamine. Depression can occur when serotonin, dopamine, and/or norepinephrine are either produced in inadequate amounts or the receptor sites are not functioning properly. The balance of ovarian, thyroid, and adrenal hormones influences the balance of these neurotransmitters, and is one way that low estradiol or low/high thyroid activity can cause a depressed mood. Depression of this type is a biological disorder occurring as a direct result of marked changes in these chemical messengers and an alteration in the receptor numbers and sensitivity. It is *not* a "character" problem or lack of willpower.

Attention deficit disorders are also affected by the balance between serotonin and norepinephrine, as well as by the decline in estradiol and testosterone as women grow older. Abnormalities in dopamine production and function are thought to be the primary disturbances causing schizophrenia and Parkinson's disease. Loss of acetylcholine, accentuated by loss of estradiol, is a primary deficiency leading to Alzheimer's dementia. Irritable bowel syndrome and fibromyalgia are two of many so-called vague medical problems aggravated, if not caused by, serotonin and norepinephrine imbalances set up by the loss of estradiol. So you see, these tiny molecules have powerful effects!

Glutamate is another widespread chemical messenger in the brain, along with its acidic amino acid relatives such as N-acetylaspartate (NAA). Glutamate is an *excitatory* neurotransmitter that is used by about 40 percent of the brain's nerve junctions. Remember, excitatory amino acids stimulate nerve cells to fire. *Inhibitory* amino acids, like GABA, described below, slow down nerve cell activity. An analogy is that excitatory amino acids act in ways like the stimulant cocaine, and inhibitory amino acids act somewhat like the relaxant Valium.

Glutamate plays a key role in learning and memory formation, among other functions. "Learning" results in an immediate release of glutamate, followed later by another release of glutamate during memory processing. We seem to require this increase in glutamate outside the nerve cells in order to properly consolidate, or "store," long-term memory. When glutamate is released from its nerve cells, it is then taken up by special cells called *astrocytes* and converted to *glutamine*, which is then returned to the neurons that require it for their function. Glutamine is then used again to make more glutamate.

The *balance* of glutamate delivered to nerve cells appears to be critical in how well they can function. If too much glutamate is delivered at one time, short-term memory can be disrupted. This is why the concentrated glutamate, and glutamic acid-herbal mixtures, sold in health food stores as memory "boosters" can actually damage memory pathways: They deliver a large dose all at once, which disrupts the normal functioning of the memory pathways and chemical messengers. I strongly recommend that you avoid such supplements, especially since glutamate and aspartate already have such a widespread presence in foods and beverages today. L-aspartic acid, another amino acid in this group, can also block glutamate uptake into nerve cells and interfere with memory processing. Other substances can also damage memory processing if they interfere with either the production of glutamate or with the action of glutamate receptors. Glycine is another amino acid that affects both the normal action and toxicity of glutamate and aspartate. Depending on the amount of glycine in the diet or in supplements, it can add to glutamate damage.

Memory loss can occur when the extra glutamate causes overexcitation, or activation, of nerve cells. There is also evidence that continued overexcitation of glutamate-regulated channels in the brain is one cause of nerve damage and cell death in a number of neurodegenerative disorders such as ALS, Parkinson's, Alzheimer's, and subtle types of seizure disorders, among others. There are many different types of glutamate receptors in the brain, so this is why many different diseases can result from exposure to this one compound.

Whenever there is brain injury such as a concussion, high levels of glutamate are released from nerve cells in the area of injury. Concussions, or blows to the head that do not cause a skull fracture, can cause significant short-term memory loss because brain damage from the blow leads to high levels of glutamate released in the hippocampus, our primary memory center. Strokes, seizures, and high blood pressure also cause extremely high levels of glutamate release in areas of injury as well as a breakdown in the protective blood-brain barrier. People who have had brain injuries should be even more careful to avoid excitatory amino acids in foods and beverages because these chemicals cause even more brain damage.

N-acetylaspartate (NAA) is the second most abundant amino acid in our brain, found mostly in the nerve cells. NAA itself hasn't been found to have specific neurotransmitter effects, but it is important to our discussion of excitotoxins because of what it does and because of how it can be affected by the amount of aspartate, glutamate, and cysteine in our diets. As with glutamate and glycine, the NAA balance available to nerve cells seems to be critical. Low levels of NAA have been found in the brains of people with such severe degenerative neurological disorders as Alzheimer's and Huntington's disease. Excessively high levels of NAA, on the other hand, actually disrupt the formation of myelin, a protective fatty sheath around nerves that helps conduct nerve impulses. Multiple sclerosis is a disease in which myelin is lost and leads to progressive loss of nerve function. I am not aware of any research investigating levels of NAA in MS patients, but clearly this is a critical issue to explore.

As you can see, these deceptively simple molecules have a profound impact on many aspects of our health. Chemicals in our environment and in our diet can disrupt any of these hormones and chemical messengers and cause depression, anxiety, insomnia, and other brain symptoms. In spite of what current advertisements want you (and your doctor) to believe, depression is not *just* a "serotonin deficiency." Nor is it always "psychiatric" in the usual sense. Many causes are "medical": physical-endocrine-metabolic changes that affect the physical function of brain pathways overseeing our moods. Some of these diverse, common causes are listed in the box on page 74.

How Do Excitotoxins Affect the Pituitary and Ovaries?

Now that you know some of the hormones by name and key function, and have had an overview of brain areas and their key functions, let's look at just how excitotoxins wreak so much havoc.

Sensitive Sites, Hardest Hit

The hypothalamus, as mentioned earlier, is the master controller for our hormone systems, body temperature, appetite regulation, body weight, sleep cycles, and a host of other critical functions. It is a brain area extremely sensitive to excitatory amino acid damage. The hypothalamus is so vulnerable because, even in adults, it lacks the protective blood-brain barrier found in the rest of the brain. High levels of offending chemicals in the bloodstream can bathe the hypothala-

THE MANY TRIGGERS OF
MOOD AND ANXIETY PROBLEMS

- Hormonal changes: loss or decline of estradiol and testosterone, imbalance of estradiol and progesterone (especially excess progesterone relative to low estradiol), excess DHEA, thyroid too low or too high, excess or deficiency of cortisol, excess insulin causing low blood glucose, to name some major ones.
- Nutritional factors: deficiencies of key vitamins and minerals; excess or deficiency of amino acids; imbalance of protein, carbohydrate, and fat; dehydration.
- Metabolic imbalances: abnormal glucose regulation, such as rapid rises or falls in blood glucose, or levels that are too low or too high; sodium-potassium imbalances; calcium or magnesium imbalance; and iron deficiency.
- Infectious organisms: viruses and bacteria that damage the brain directly or have indirect effects via damage to the thyroid and ovary hormones that in turn affect our moods.
- Environmental exposures: food additives, pesticides, xenobiotics, heavy metals, molds, and other chemicals. Many of these can disrupt formation or action of neurotransmitters and hormones (for more details, see Chapter 5).

© Elizabeth Lee Vliet, M.D., 2003

mus directly. This is one reason that Dr. Olney and other brain researchers have been so concerned about the increasing use of MSG, HVP, cysteine, and aspartate as food additives.

Another study, this one by Dr. Ralph Dawson, showed that even low doses of MSG produced profound alterations in sex hormone release via the hypothalamus and resulted in marked abnormalities in the onset of female puberty. Mice (remember, they are *less* sensitive than humans) given low doses of MSG had decreased estrogen binding at the hypothalamic receptors, abnormal patterns of LH and LHRH release, delayed vaginal opening, and disturbances in sexual behavior. Even *subtoxic* doses of MSG can cause severe abnormal changes to the hypothalamus and thereby disrupt our entire endocrine "control center." Put another way, it would be like having a computer virus take over your computer's operating system and change all the settings.

I wonder if these food additives might be yet another reason I see some young women who need much higher than usual blood levels of estradiol to maintain their sense of normal mood, sleep, and memory. It may be that a lifetime of soft drinks and "flavor enhanced" foods act in the brain to change the way the estrogen receptors respond, much like a computer virus disrupts computer functions. More estradiol is then needed to counteract the effects of these excitatory amino acids that have disrupted hypothalamus pathways.

With what I know now, I shudder to think about all the MSG I added to foods when I was a teenager, and all the hundreds of "diet" soft drinks I consumed in high school, college, and medical school. I quit drinking them in 1983, and doubt that I've had more than a half dozen in the last twenty years. But the damage was probably already done. I had no way of knowing then, but I suspect this was a factor in some of the ovarian hormone imbalances and weight gain I have had since my mid-twenties. It was in college and the ten years afterward that I really guzzled those diet sodas. That was about the time I really started having menstrual irregularities and weight gain similar to that seen with PCOS. I hate to admit this, but I also smoked cigarettes in college and for a couple of years afterward. Boy, was that dumb. I finally got smart and quit before I was twenty-five. But cigarettes had these same flavor-enhancer chemicals added, unbeknownst to us consumers, and the toxicity of cigarette smoke caused an even greater neurotoxic effect with the excitatory amino acids (EAAs) in foods and soft drinks (see Chapter 6). So I was getting an overload of these chemicals that damage the hypothalamus, and I didn't realize it.

Unfortunately, the damage is not limited to the hypothalamus. Large doses of glutamate, still below the toxic doses, given to animals caused *reduced* production of thyroid hormones and *increased* production of cortisol—two other hormone imbalances that lead to weight gain and also interfere with the normal function of ovaries. Since MSG causes both the *"miswiring"* of nerve pathways and the *"misfiring"* of nerve signals during brain development, it can affect all the endocrine glands the brain oversees. This explains why thyroid and adrenal gland hormones, as well as the ovaries, are altered. When you consider everything the hypothalamus governs, it isn't surprising that we see such diverse damage throughout the body.

Dose Effects: Animals and Humans, Infants and Adults

Remember the point I made earlier: Human infant brains are many times more sensitive to damage by excitotoxins like MSG and aspartate than the brains of all animals studied. This really shouldn't surprise us, since the human brain is one of the most complex and highly organized in all the animal kingdom. Dr. Olney's studies showed that human children get a twenty-fold increase of glutamate in blood levels while the same dose causes only a fourfold increase in mice. That's a huge difference. This fact is overlooked by people who dismiss the toxicity concerns of MSG and aspartate based on the studies in mice.

Keep in mind, too, that the human brain continues to develop throughout childhood, not just while in the womb. The foods we eat and the chemicals we are exposed to during infancy and childhood have additional potential for harm. Walk around a mall today and you see children of all ages with super-jumbo-size soft drinks in their hands. Dr. Olney found that human children often get MSG doses in the range of 100–150 mg per kilogram of body weight just by eating manufactured foods containing these flavor enhancers and hydrolyzed vegetable protein, and his work was done forty years ago when 12-ounce cans of soft drinks were all we had. Today's prevalent 32- and 64-ounce super-jumbo drinks were nonexistent then. And remember, getting EAAs in liquid form from soft drinks is far more damaging than from solid foods because they are more readily absorbed into the bloodstream and reach higher blood levels. Parents have no clue what subtle brain damage is occurring.

Timing of exposure is critical. Mother Nature has carefully choreographed the complex process of egg and sperm uniting and then dividing and dividing to ultimately become an embryo, then a recognizable human infant in the womb. Each day of gestation is important, with certain developmental events unfolding in sequence. Disrupt one step and another cannot occur properly. This is why excitatory amino acids and environmental endocrine disruptors are so incredibly damaging to the brain—they interrupt this normal developmental sequence. That's also why the endocrine disruptors you will read about in the next chapter are often called *gender benders*. Tiny amounts of these chemicals are so powerful they can completely derail the process of gender development, preventing the full complement of male or female characteristics from being displayed at puberty, adolescence, and adulthood.

I mentioned earlier that we are all genetically programmed to be female, and have a female cyclic brain pattern of response—unless the embryo gets the proper signal at the proper time to trigger the testes to start pumping out testosterone. Don't you know men will love finding out they *really* started out as female! If the embryo gets the signal activating a gene on the Y chromosome at just the right time, then testicular testosterone begins to be produced and changes the basic primordial female brain pattern into a male one. The brain pattern is programmed to steady testosterone levels (*tonic* pattern) throughout life rather than the cyclic pattern of sex hormones women have. Fetal tissue that would have become ovaries, uterus, and vagina develops as penis, testicles, and prostate. A similar process occurs in all mammals.

When does this momentous event occur? This critical day—the day a female brain and body is permanently transformed into a male—is Day 56 of gestation in humans. If *anything* interferes with the activation of this Y chromosome on this particular day, it can alter this exquisitely timed sequence of hormone messages and permanently skew the male pattern of brain, body, and hormone development. If environmental or dietary chemicals interfere with Mother Nature's plan on Day 56 in human gestation, a genetic male embryo can be left in a bizarre limbo state—genetically male but with his male body and hormone patterns not operating normally for the rest of his life.

This is one explanation for the rising incidence reported in the last two decades of stunted penises, undescended testicles, and lower sperm counts in male children, findings reported from around the world. Countries still using pesticides banned in the United States (but still exported by the U.S. companies that manufacture them) have the highest incidence of these male abnormalities. Studies on women lag behind. There are similar disruptive effects in female embryos and developing babies, but these are harder to quantify because the changes are more subtle, such as endometriosis and "unexplained" infertility. Women's internal reproductive organs are more difficult to directly observe and quantify, unlike in males where the penis and testicles are visible.

What's the message? Be careful what you eat or drink (or smoke or inhale or spray into and around your body) during these critical early days of pregnancy— you may unwittingly set off a cascade of unwanted consequences.

Other Diet Risks for Your Ovaries: Excess Fats and Sugars

Sometimes we really don't want to know everything we are eating. We enjoy a particular food, we want it, we buy it, it tastes good, and we play ostrich to what might really be there and what it "may" do to us later. But if you consider the role diet plays in disrupting optimal ovarian function, it's time to take your head out of the sand. Excess body fat (as in obesity) as well as too little body fat (as in anorexia) can both cause irregular menstrual cycles, abnormal ovulation, infertility, and a variety of other hormone problems. We have an epidemic of obesity in children today, not to mention the staggering rise in obesity-induced diabetes in elementary school–age children.

Girls are particularly hard hit: Childhood obesity leads to premature puberty, increased risk of PCOS and endometriosis, increased risk of infertility, a later risk of diabetes, and a higher risk of developing breast cancer, even before menopause.

Excess Fats and Your Ovaries: What's the Connection?

Most women don't realize that the average American diet is about 45 percent fat, a culprit in many health problems that affect your ovaries and your overall health. The persistent organic pollutants (POPs) accumulate in fat tissues because they don't dissolve well in water (see Chapter 5). This means the fat of animals and fish, the fats your food is fried in, and even your own body fat become the depository for all these POPs that subtly, but persistently, permeate your body systems and damage important hormone pathways. The more fat in your diet, the higher your exposure to these endocrine disruptors. The fatter you get from the fat in your diet, the more your body becomes a storehouse for these toxic chemicals.

Most women have heard ad nauseam about saturated fats that increase the risk of heart disease. Long before that happens, however, you may inadvertently sabotage your fertility or make endometriosis or PCOS worse by eating a lot of fats. High saturated fat causes increased body fat that increases your load of estrone, which helps the growth of both endometriosis and fibroids. The more you eat, the more likely you are to develop an early onset of insulin resistance, and then diabetes. As you get older, the more saturated fats you have eaten over your lifetime, the greater your risk of heart and blood vessel disease, and the greater your risk of developing breast, colon, and/or uterine cancer. If you want to be around to "worry" about menopause, pay better attention to what you are eating now in your younger years.

What are some of the fat shockers lurking in those tasty foods we enjoy? Getting this list together even makes me feel guilty for enjoying some of them! Most of us don't think about the damage we can do in just a few minutes of indulgence.

STICKER SHOCK: A HIGH COST TO YOUR HORMONE HEALTH

Consider these equivalencies:

- *One* regular soft drink (12 ounces) = 10 teaspoons of sugar (40 grams!), 140 calories

    And most of you probably drink more than one a day! Remember, you're getting empty calories; there's no nutritional value, plus all those excitatory amino acids and artificial chemicals for taste enhancers that can affect the pituitary. Soft drinks also give you high levels of sodium and phosphates that leach calcium from your body, adding to low bone density in young women.

- One bag of potato chips (15 ounces) = 1 cup of oil (150 grams of fat!), 1,400 calories

    This is more than your whole day's allowance of fat, not to mention almost your entire day's calories, all easily consumed by "couch potatoes" in about fifteen minutes! Since the calories are coming from carbs and fat, with practically no fiber, they add up fast and you don't even feel all that full, so you don't realize how much you've eaten in calories or fat. They are also loaded with flavor enhancers, those excitatory amino acids I described earlier.

- One movie-theater popcorn with "butter" (medium, not jumbo) = 8 potatoes, 910 calories, 75 grams of fat

    Popcorn at the movies is an insidious "fat saboteur" because the fat grams are so high, and also because it is usually made with the unhealthy saturated or trans fats. Add to that all the flavor-enhancing chemicals. And it may shock you to know that the carbs in this popcorn are equal to *eight* whole potatoes! You would not be likely to eat that many potatoes at one time! With all these calories, and the average rate of burning about 100 calories per mile of walking, you'd have to park about nine miles away from the theater to walk off all those extra calories you ate! If you like popcorn, try taking a smaller bag of the no-fat, air-popped kind in your pocketbook to snack on.

- One Big Mac and large fries (McDonald's) = the fat content of 1 cup of Crisco (Yuk! Is that what you want to be eating?)

   Most of us would feel repulsed to think about eating a cup of lard or Crisco. But that's what you are doing here: a Big Mac is 590 calories and 34 grams of fat; if you add this to the 26 grams of fat and 540 calories in the fries, you get 60 grams of fat and over 1,130 calories—about the fat equivalent of one cup (2 ounces) of Crisco . . . plus almost your entire day's worth of calories. Stop and think before you pack away all that fat. If you are having a "Big Mac attack," stop and visualize what one cup of Crisco would look like spread on your thighs! Then switch to a grilled chicken *without* the mayo, and just hold the fries—you'll get just as much flavor with a lot fewer calories and fat. And you can feel *so* virtuous.

- 1 pint of Häagen-Dazs ice cream (plain vanilla!) = 2/3 stick of butter

   I know, I like Häagen-Dazs, too . . . and it is all too easy to eat "the whole thing"—after all, it's such a small container, it can't be too bad, right? Wrong. At 1,080 calories and 72 grams of fat, you'll be sorry when you get on the scale again. Not to mention the 82 grams of sugar . . . not exactly a "sweet nothing" for your body. Did you know that one pint of Häagen-Dazs (or any other pint of ice cream for that matter) is meant to make *four* servings? I hear you saying "But I just can't stop, and besides, that's not enough for four people!" But that's really all you should be having—an occasional 270-calorie sweet treat isn't so bad—but 1,080 calories in one sitting is, once again, almost your whole day's supply of calories!

- 1 bagel with cream cheese = 2 1/2 slices of pepperoni pizza

   Bagels have a pretty innocent image—most of us would think the pizza has more calories and fat. But not all bagels are built the same. Bagels from specialty stores, at 4 ounces and 350–500 calories on average, have twice the size and calories of a traditional bagel. A normal serving of cream cheese is about 2 tablespoons or 75 calories. But most bagel specialty stores and delis pile on as much as *half a cup* of cream cheese, bumping the calorie count up to 400! If you just can't go without your morning specialty-shop bagel, then at least try having only half for breakfast, and save the other half for your afternoon snack. At least you won't overdo it in the morning and still hit the afternoon slump at 4 P.M., wanting even more calories! Or, if you just don't have the willpower to save half for later, then scoop out some of the excess bagel dough and scrape off excess cream cheese. The calories you save are worth it for your waist.

Sugars in Soft Drinks and Everywhere Else

It isn't just fat that makes you fatter. So does excess sugar. Moreover, sugars in these soft drinks add further to the neuron damage of excitotoxins by making you fatter and increasing your risk of insulin resistance. Excess intake of sugars leads to a type of cell-damagers called *advanced glycosylation end-products* (AGEs). These AGEs literally *age* your cells while they fill you with empty calories that make you gain weight. A recent scientific study at Boston Children's Hospital confirmed the obvious: Consumption of sugar-sweetened drinks in childhood leads to obesity in children! So ratchet down your sweet tooth a few notches. Be wary of these "no fat" but high-sugar "diet" snacks, cookies, and frozen desserts. Your brain and body will feel better and work better for you . . . and so will your ovaries.

Vegetarian Diets: Benefits to Your Body, Pitfalls for Ovarian Health

I am not against vegetarian diets per se, but I think they have been excessively glorified in the media. Most women don't realize the potential pitfalls of vegetarian diets or how carefully you must plan vegetarian meals in order to make certain you are getting complete proteins, adequate vitamins, and minerals. If a vegetarian diet isn't properly balanced, you end up with subtle deficits of essential amino acids, vitamins, and minerals that can lead to increased problems with infertility, earlier ovarian decline, increased fatigue, muscle pain syndromes, and other "vague" problems.

What are some of the well-documented nutritional deficits of vegetarian diets, especially with a true vegan diet that has no meat, fish, dairy, or eggs? Vegetarians have been found to have low levels of three crucial minerals: iron, zinc, and magnesium, in part because the plant sources provide less than optimal amounts of iron and also a type (non-heme iron) that is not well absorbed. The high fiber and phytate content of a plant-based diet also impairs absorption of these minerals. Magnesium, in particular, is a crucial mineral to help defend against the cell damage from the excitotoxins you read about earlier. Vegetarian diets are also notoriously low in B_{12} because the richest sources of this vitamin are animal foods. Depending on the soil content where vegetables and grains are grown, vegetarian diets may be deficient in iodine as well, which in turn impairs thyroid function, another factor in infertility.

Many vegetarians also have inadequate protein intake, substantiated in studies from many different cultures. This is one of the reasons more vegetarian women have menstrual irregularities. Many grains and vegetables have high levels of estrogenlike compounds (phytoestrogens) that attach to the body's estrogen receptors and impair the ovaries' hormone production. This is another reason for the menstrual irregularities and higher incidence of infertility in vegetarians. Dr. A. Cassidy and co-researchers in Britain analyzed the influence of a soy-based diet on the hormonal status and menstrual cycle of premenopausal women with regular ovulatory cycles. Sixty grams of soy protein containing 45 mg isoflavones were given daily for one month. This caused a significant increase in length of the follicular phase and delayed menstruation. Midcycle bursts of luteinizing hormone and follicle stimulating hormone were significantly suppressed while the women were taking the soy protein. Keep in mind that we see similar responses with tamoxifen, an antiestrogen. These effects are due to nonsteroidal isoflavones and phytoestrogens that sometimes behave as estrogen "boosters" *(agonists)* and sometimes function as estrogen "blockers" *(antagonists)*.

Soy foods in modest amounts may have some potential benefit with respect to later risk factors of breast cancer and high cholesterol. But the flip side is that in younger women, the phytoestrogens in soy can also suppress the menstrual cycle and decrease hormone production, which then impairs fertility. Studies have shown, and the media has reported, that "eating vegetarian" has cardiovascular benefits due to a lower intake of saturated fats. That's true. But for younger women who may be trying to become pregnant, too *little* fat means less of the building blocks to make ovarian hormones, which in turn increases the risk of infertility. You can develop symptoms of low estrogen at unexpectedly early ages.

You can see how important it is to read reputable health articles. It's trendy to eat vegetarian these days. If this is what you want to do, then pay careful attention to getting adequate protein, combining foods properly to get all the essential amino acids, and eating the right balance of foods to have adequate levels of key vitamins and minerals critical for the body's production of hormones and other chemical messengers. Your brain and body deserve it. This is one diet you can't approach haphazardly and expect to stay healthy.

In Summary

Excitatory amino acids. Excitotoxins. Hypothalamic damage. Hormone disruption. These are serious health issues that haven't adequately made it into mainstream medicine. Start now to eliminate as many sources of excitotoxins in your diet as possible. The bottom line is that excitatory amino acids in your foods disrupt the function of the hypothalamus, which oversees the pituitary and in turn regulates ovary cycles and other endocrine organs that produce hormones. It is *your* brain and body that is getting disrupted.

As far as we know with certainty, you only have one life to live. Don't let it—and your health—slide away in a slurp of soda and fat. I hope these shocking facts will make you think twice about what you're eating and drinking when you decide to skip breakfast and have a soft drink. Or grab a Big Mac and fries for lunch. Or have your daily indulgence with one of these ubiquitous "fun foods." When you think about how often the average person may have one or more of these in a day, you can quickly see why we have so many obese children and adults in our country.

When we reflect on all this information and its collective impact on our neuroendocrine system, you can see why premature puberty, PMS, PCOS, and POD are all on the rise. I am not saying you should never eat these things, but be aware of the pitfalls. Watch how often you have them, and control your portion size—you really don't have to eat the whole thing all at once. Don't just unconsciously reach for what's easiest or quickest. Stop and ask yourself: "Do I *really* want this? Will something else satisfy me?" Consider options that are a better use of your daily calorie and fat allowance. Cut out the diet soft drinks and the flavor-enhanced snack foods—the excitotoxin load builds up every day of your life, reaching critical levels of damage. Drink water or seltzer instead of soft drinks . . . they are really *much* better for you! Each positive change you make is a step toward better hormone balance and a healthier body.

5

Ovaries at Risk: "Gender Benders" and Endocrine Disruptors Around You

---

Introduction

For years, I have been exploring the links between environmental chemicals and their effects on our endocrine system. These synthetic, man-made, hormonelike chemicals called *xenoestrogens* interact with the estrogen receptors in our body, sabotage our hormones, and increase our long-term risk of diseases like breast cancer. There are also *xenoandrogens* and *xenoprogestins,* and some of these chemicals have mixed effects, acting at all of our hormone receptors. Since we now know that most chemical pollutants disrupt more hormone pathways and receptors than just our sex hormones, they are more appropriately called *endocrine* or *hormone disruptors.* These synthetic chemicals have been found in the body fat and breast milk of humans throughout the world, as well as mammals on land and in the oceans, fish, birds, reptiles, and amphibians. As you read further and see what they can do, you will see why they are often called *gender benders.* Their damage is found in studies of *all* species tested to date.

Many of these chemicals—such as dioxin, the pesticide DDT and its breakdown product DDE, polychlorinated biphenyls (PCBs), and others—have been linked with increasing rates of breast, prostate, testicular, and bladder cancers and endometriosis. But the issues are even broader. There are ominous indications that they also seriously damage ovarian function. We must look into these issues if we want to have a better understanding of the alarming rise in female infertility, ovarian cysts, PCOS, hormone-triggered depression and anxiety, premature ovarian decline or failure, and immune disorders.

One of the earliest warnings came from Rachel Carson in her classic book *Silent Spring,* first published in 1962, in which she wrote eloquently of the reproductive damage from the pesticide DDT. DDT use was later banned in the United States, but it is still manufactured here for export to countries around the world where it is still in widespread use. DDT then comes back to us on the winds, oceans, rain, and imported foods to continue its dirty work in our bodies. Since *Silent Spring,* the problem has *not* gone away. Quite the contrary, it has gotten far worse and more ominous. Creative chemists have gone on to exponentially increase the problem by creating even more deadly and persistent chemicals in thousands of common products that are used daily. We are the only species with a brain creative enough to make chemicals capable of wiping out our entire race, by insidiously poisoning our hormone and reproductive systems.

Xenos is a Greek word meaning "foreign" or "different." *Xenobiotics* refers to a whole group of chemical compounds that are man-made, foreign to the body, and have generally toxic or damaging biological effects to living organisms. Our bodies do not have the ability to readily metabolize these chemicals, which makes them very long-lasting and more damaging to our bodies. Some are known carcinogens; some don't seem to cause cancer, but all can damage endocrine pathways. Most have never been studied to determine any cancer-causing effects, much less toxicity to reproductive, brain, and hormone function. Keep in mind that although these chemicals may have estrogenic or androgenic effects, their effects are *consistently negative.* They disrupt our body systems because they are not the same as the hormones produced by our bodies.

The headlines scream that "estrogen" increases the risk of breast cancer. The National Toxicology Program recommended adding "estrogen" to the list of human carcinogens. Women are afraid to consider birth control pills or HRT after menopause because of such alarming news. We are made to feel terrified of a hormone our bodies make naturally—in greater or lesser quantities, depending on where we are in our life cycle—our entire life. Why the sudden intense negative focus on our body's natural hormone, as if it is something to fear and loathe? Do we see such headlines about men's testosterone? Are there other pieces of this puzzle being swept under the rug? What is going on here?

Let's look at the way these environmental chemicals put your ovaries, fertility, brain, and long-term health at significant risk. This is a complicated area, but it is critical for you to understand because there are profound implications for you as a woman, and for your daughters and sons.

What Are Endocrine Disruptors and What Do They Do?

These man-made chemicals belong to a group of environmental pollutants that are part of a larger class of both naturally occurring and synthetic molecules that can act like hormones in the body, although they are not really true hormones. Because these man-made compounds, unlike natural ones, persist for decades or even centuries, in the environment without being broken down, they are also called *persistent organic pollutants,* abbreviated POPs. POPs pack a whollop to our endocrine system and hence our bodies: They may *accentuate* or *disrupt,* or completely *alter* or even *block* actions of multiple body hormones, not just estrogen.

These compounds may mimic or block testosterone, thyroid, insulin, or other hormones, so POPs fit under the broader category of "endocrine disruptors" and can affect everything in our body that is governed by our hormones, which means just about our entire body! The number of chemicals with this endocrine-disrupting effect seems to grow almost daily; at this writing we know of several hundred, but these are just the ones that have been studied. There are potentially thousands more. We lack this knowledge because the toxicology stud-

DDT 1970 - 1990's exposure

ies done before these compounds are put on the market focus only on cancer-causing effects. Chemical manufacturers are not required to look into toxic effects on any of the other body systems.

In animal studies and cultures of human ovary cells, many of these chemicals act as *follicular toxicants,* which means they kill ovarian follicles. If your follicles are killed prematurely, it can mean decreased fertility or premature menopause. You then have symptoms like those listed in the introduction that occur when we lose the ovarian hormones our follicles produce. The endocrine disruptors affect the ovarian pathways in another way: Many of them cause profound damage to the thyroid, our master metabolic regulator, which oversees ovarian and many other functions in the body.

Some POPs interfere with iodine metabolism, which can cause hypothyroidism as well as breast and ovarian cysts. Beyond the ovarian and other endocrine pathways, these toxic chemicals are linked to the rising rates of autism, lower IQ, learning disorders, behavioral disorders, lower sperm counts in males, and rising rates of testicular cancer. For example, men in cultures around the world have been found with sperm counts as much as 50 percent lower than men had just thirty years ago, before there was such widespread use of these toxic chemicals. Women's "egg counts" are obviously harder to determine, so we don't have good statistics about the early death of ovarian follicles from these chemicals. But from the increase in young women with symptoms of ovarian failure that I see in my practice, and from the worldwide studies, it is clear women are affected, too.

I do not have the space here to go into all the years of worldwide animal studies that raised the red flags for humans, or the history of how we got in such a mess with chemicals that pollute and sabotage our fertility and survival. If you are interested in the fascinating detective work done by scientists to identify these health effects in animals and humans since Rachel Carson's efforts, I encourage you to read two outstanding and well-researched books: *Our Stolen Future* by scientist Theo Colborn and her team of Dianne Dumanoski and John Peterson Myers, and *Living Downstream* by ecologist Sandra Steingraber. Let their descriptions of the animals' plight and their urgent alarm to humans be *your* health wake-up call.

Why Is This Such a Problem Now?

The short answer is that none of these organic compounds existed before the 1930s. Pre-1930s, people were simply not exposed to such an incredible array of synthetic chemicals. Most have been invented in the "chemical age" that started just prior to World War II. The world was not exposed to these pesticides and industrial chemicals on a wide scale until the 1940s and 1950s. During the period from roughly 1970 through the 1990s, the first human generation ever exposed to DDT and other POPs during fetal life began reaching their own reproductive age. Subtle perturbations and disruptions began to appear.

CHRONOLOGY: DEVELOPMENT OF AND HUMAN EXPOSURE TO SYNTHETIC ENDOCRINE DISRUPTORS (POPS)

1929: Polychlorinated biphenyls (PCBs) developed

1930s: "Nerve gases" developed in Germany, later used by the Nazis in World War II (1939–1945); became basis for pesticides

1938: DDT first synthesized and manufactured and DES synthesized, the first synthetic estrogenic compound

1940–1945: First widespread use of synthetic chemicals worldwide and wide-scale exposure to living organisms

1940s–1950s: First human generation to be exposed in infancy

1940s–1970s: DES in widespread use during pregnancy; first human generations born who were exposed to a potent, synthetic estrogenic chemical in the womb

1950s–1970s: First human generations born who had been exposed to many pesticides and other industrial pollutants (POPs) in the womb

1970s–2000: DES daughters and sons health problems manifest

1970s–1990s: First human generation exposed to POPs in the womb now reaching reproductive age when effect of hormone disruptions become more pronounced and noticeable—for women: infertility, endometriosis, PCOS, premature ovarian decline, thyroid disorders, and others

2000: Second generation DES sons and daughters now old enough for adverse health effects to become manifest

© Elizabeth Lee Vliet, M.D., 2003

Who Are the Players in This Hormone-Disrupting Drama?

These chemicals make up an alphabet soup far less healthy than the food variety. DDT, DDE, DES, TCDD, BHA, PCB, PBB, PAH, and CCA are some common ones. There are hundreds more in this huge group of chemicals not normally found in nature and are potently toxic for living organisms. The man-made ones are consistently damaging, with serious, widespread toxic effects. Many are known carcinogens. Their longer names are all listed in the box on pages 88–90, grouped by categories of where they are found, type of action, and types of damage they cause. I want you to have this information available at home so you can check ingredient labels on foods, cleaning compounds, cosmetics, household "pest" killers, dog and cat flea collars, lawn care products, and so on.

Then there are the naturally occurring compounds, such as the phytoestrogenic isoflavones of soy, grains, and clover. Heavy metals are found in soils and water. Even though all may have significant "endocrine disrupting" effects, a few of the naturally occurring ones have modest positive effects, such as lower cholesterol seen from a diet higher in phytoestrogens. But they may also disrupt the menstrual cycle and impair fertility, as seen in cattle feeding on red clover, which is rich in isoflavones. Others in the naturally occurring group, such as genistein found in soy, have mixed effects: beneficial at some concentrations but showing adverse effects at other concentrations. So let's take a closer look at these chemicals.

Where Are the Chemical Endocrine Disruptors Found?

Simply put, they are now everywhere. Man-made endocrine disruptors, the persistent organic pollutants (POPs) may be found in the water we drink, the food we eat, the air we breathe, and the objects we touch around our homes, workplaces, and recreational areas. They are found in the plastic linings of canned foods and plastic food wrappers. They are found in common chemicals probably sitting under your bathroom and kitchen sinks or in your laundry room and garage. These chemicals are in widespread use in our environment. They are found in cigarette smoke, plastics, detergents, pesticides, herbicides, fungicides, hair dyes, paints, solvents, dry-cleaning solutions, cosmetics, food additives and preservatives, fabric coatings, wall coverings, carpets, playground equipment, and vehicle exhaust—just to name a few of the sources we encounter daily. We also unwittingly add these chemicals into the environment: You may not realize that all the things you flush down the toilet or rinse down the kitchen sink can end up in our water supply, bubbling up in rivers and streams! A U.S. Geological Survey on 140 waterways in 30 states tracked 95 different pollutants, with these surprising results: 74 percent of the samples contained insect repellents; 48 percent contained antibiotics; 40 percent contained reproductive hormones (e.g., birth control pill estrogens and progestins); 32 percent contained other prescription drugs; and 27 percent were found to have chemical compounds used for fragrances. So stop and think before you flush old prescriptions, such as birth control pills and antibiotics, or old perfumes or household cleaners, down the toilet.

Since POPs are fat-soluble, they become concentrated in the fat tissues of fish, animals, and humans. Those animals—and humans—at the top of the food chain accumulate the most POPs in body fat because each step in the series adds a little more of the pollutants to fatty tissues. Birds that eat fish from toxic waters every day build up more concentrated levels than are in each fish. Larger prey that eat the birds get a little more, and so on up the food chain. Polar bears have very high levels of DDT, DDE, PCBs, and other chemicals in their body fat because they eat high-fat seals that have eaten contaminated fish. For human women, the fact that these toxic chemicals build up in fat carries a special risk: We have more overall body fat than men do, and the primarily fatty tissue of our breasts actively store these estrogenic compounds. The breasts and breast milk concentrate these chemicals to a significant degree over a lifetime. Nursing babies get the full brunt of the mother's chemical storehouse, particularly the

CHEMICALS WITH ENDOCRINE-MODULATING ACTIVITY

1. General Categories

Man-Made Chemicals

- Industrial and household products, such as pesticides, cleaners, plasticizers, solvents (e.g., DDT, DDE, PCB, PBB, PAH, TCDD, dioxins, DEHA, toluene, xylene, perchloroethylene, etc.), triazine herbicides
- Pharmaceuticals like DES (diethylstilbestrol), cyclophosphamide (anticancer drug)
- Dietary supplements and food additives, such as MSG, glutamate, aspartate, cysteine, BHT, BHA (butylated hydroxyanisole)

Naturally Occurring Compounds

- Phytoestrogens in plants
- Phthalate esters
- Heavy metals (neurotoxins): lead, mercury, arsenic, cadmium, gallium

2. Examples Based on Types of Actions

Estrogenic

- O,p'-DDT, methoxychlor, Lindane (organochlorine pesticides), Endosulfan, Dieldrin, toxaphene
- Kepone (estrogenic effects in male factory workers)
- Nonylphenols (also weak androgen agonist*)
- Bisphenol-A
- DES
- Benzylbutylphthalate, dibutyl phthalate
- Genistein, other isoflavones found in soy, clover, grains

Estrogen Blockers (Antiestrogenic)

- PCBs (polychlorinated biphenyls) (isomers of DDT)
- Dioxin and related dibenzo-p-dioxins
- Dibenzofurans
- Compounds in cigarette smoke
- Genistein (both agonist and antagonist actions, depending on concentration), other isoflavones

Androgen Blockers (Antiandrogenic)

- P,p'-DDE (metabolite of DDT), also DDT*
- Vinclozolin
- Atrazine
- Bisphenol-A*
- Benzylbutylphthalate*

*Based on recent data from Sohoni (see Appendix II)

Act by Other Mechanisms

- Cyclophosphamide
- Benzo(a)pyrene, anthracenes
- Solvents (toluene, xylene, perchloroethylene)
- Methoxychlor
- Nitrous oxide ("laughing gas" anesthesia)
- Ethylene oxide
- Butadiene
- 4-vinyl cyclohexene
- Alkylphenols
- Phthalate esters
- Triazine herbicides (atrazine, simazine, cyanazine)
- Fungicides (chlorothalonil, Maneb, Metiram, Thiram, Zineb, Ziram)
- Excitatory amino acids (glutamate, MSG, aspartate, etc.)

3. Examples Based on Type of Damage in Women

These are not all of the types of damages caused. I have listed the ones most relevant to the issue of ovaries at risk, the primary subject of this book.

Health Impact	Chemicals Found to Cause†
Breast cancer	DDT, DDE, Lindane, methoxychlor, PCB, TCDD, possibly DES, triazine herbicides (atrazine, simazine, cyanazine), others likely
Ovarian cancer	DES, DDE, PCB, triazine herbicides (most data is on atrazine), possibly many others
Infertility/impaired fertility	Aromatic hydrocarbons in cigarette smoke, isoflavones (soy, red clover), coumestrol, cyclophosphamide, PCB, TCDD, PAH, organochlorine pesticides (DDT, DDE, Lindane, etc.), organic solvents, heavy metals, nitrous oxide, ethylene oxide, 4-vinyl cyclohexene, butadiene, DES, glutamate, aspartate
Menstrual irregularity	DDT, DDE, Lindane, heavy metals, PCB, isoflavones (soy, red clover), coumestrol, PAH, solvents, TCDD, DES, atrazine, glutamate, aspartate
Increased miscarriages	Solvents, nitrous oxide, ethylene oxide, DES, isoflavones (soy, red clover), coumestrol

†Based on studies in animals, humans, or both

DDT pre 1972

Health Impact	Chemicals Found to Cause
Early menopause	PAH, cigarette smoke, butadiene, DES, 4-vinyl cyclohexene, phytoestrogens, isoflavones, possibly many others
Endometriosis	Dioxins (many types), TCDD, PCB, DES
Reduced lactation	DDE, DES, others not well studied
Osteopenia/osteoporosis	Cadmium, lead, cigarette smoke chemicals
Thyroid damage	PCB, organochlorine pesticides (DDT, DDE, Lindane, others), isoflavones (soy, red clover, others), phytates, iodine deficiency (iodine metabolism disrupted by a number of these compounds), MSG, glutamate, aspartate
Immune damage	PCB, dioxins, Dieldrin, may be others. Greater adverse impact on infant with immature immune system when chemicals passed in breast milk
Hypothalamic-pituitary dysfunction	heavy metals, PCB, DES, excitatory amino acids (glutamate, aspartate, cystoic acid, MSG), triazine herbicides (atrazine, etc.)

© Elizabeth Lee Vliet, M.D., 2003

first nursing child. As nursing depletes the mother's breast stores of chemicals, subsequent babies receive smaller amounts.

DDT wasn't banned in the United States until 1972. Everyone born prior to 1972 was exposed to DDT in the diet because the pesticide was commonly found in dairy products and meats as well as on vegetables sprayed with DDT for pest control. If you were born after 1972, you were exposed to DDT from residues in your mother's body fat that flowed across the placenta. As an infant, you were getting DDT residues in either human breast or cows' milk, since cattle that had eaten grains and grasses with DDT residues would have the persistent chemical in their body fat to then leach into their milk, just as in human breast milk. Most Americans alive today carry some DDT residues because it is stored in the environment and the body for decades.

In the body, DDT is metabolized to a compound called DDE. Recent research shows that DDE is an *antiandrogen* that blocks testosterone from activating its receptor complex. This receptor blockade causes undescended testicles in young boys, shorter stature, greater tendency to obesity, and less muscle development. In adult men, DDE causes lowered sperm counts, smaller testicles,

ORGANOHALOGENS

You may frequently see the term *organohalogens* used, and this refers to the following groups of chemicals that have added chlorine (organochlorines) or bromine (organobromines) atoms, which enhances their actions, and their toxicity:

- dichlorodiphenyl dichloroethene (DDE)
- polychlorinated biphenyls (PCBs)
- polybrominated biphenyls (PBBs)

© Elizabeth Lee Vliet, M.D., 2003

and increased testicular cancer. We don't know all the potential adverse reproductive effects DDE has in women because *no research has been done on women.* I suspect we will find that it leads to abnormal testosterone production and action in women.

Even though these chemicals are banned in this country, we are still exposed to them every day because most are still manufactured for export to countries whose laws are less strict. Winds that blow across the ocean to our west coast carry chemical residues from countries where they are still in use. Fish, vegetables, and fruits from other parts of the world are imported and bring POP residues to our tables. Besides, banning their use doesn't help much because these chemicals are so long-lasting. Aldrin, a termite killer, is converted to Dieldrin in body tissues and in the soil, where it remains for years. Dieldrin suppresses the immune system and causes abnormal brain waves in mammals. Although banned in the United States in 1975, Aldrin was allowed as a termite killer until 1987, so people were still exposed to it. Pregnant women exposed to Aldrin would have daughters in their teens and twenties about now, just about the age we start seeing reproductive damage, such as endometriosis, PCOS, severe PMS, irregular cycles, immune problems, and mood-behavioral difficulties. Other chemicals like chlorpyrifos (Dursban or Lorsban), are still infiltrating our lives and health. It is the active ingredient in over a thousand products surrounding us daily, from flea and tick collars for pets and roach and ant sprays under your kitchen counter to the sprays used on crops we eat.

Another group of POPs, called *triazine herbicides* (atrazine, cyanazine, simazine), are water soluble rather than fat soluble. They are widely used across the United States from the cornfields of the Midwest to the fruit groves of Florida and California. When sprayed on vegetable and fruit crops to kill weeds, they are taken up from the soil into *all* plants and leach from the soil into the groundwater as well. We ingest them in produce we eat and in our drinking water. We also get them in meat, poultry, milk, and eggs because POPs contaminate corn feeds for cattle and chickens. All of these compounds are possible carcinogens, and atrazine is a known endocrine disruptor linked to breast and ovarian cancers, as well as other reproductive problems including infertility. Atrazine inhibits the ability to make testosterone and alters pituitary response to the hormones that oversee ovulation. Links between the herbicide triazine and ovarian cancer have been found for women farmers in Italy. These compounds have been in use since the 1950s and yet little has been done to study their link to risk of breast and ovarian cancers, much less investigate the degree of their adverse effects on fertility, reproductive disorders such as endometriosis and PCOS, or hypothalamic-pituitary regulation of our other endocrine systems.

What Are Gender-Bending Endocrine Disruptors Doing to You?

Many of the endocrine disruptors used as pesticides for the last fifty years were actually the chemical descendants, only slightly tamed, of the terrifying organophosphate nerve gases tabun and sarin developed in Germany in the 1930s and used during World War II. Both the early nerve gases and those developed in recent decades for chemical weapons kill by blocking the critical enzyme cholinesterase so that nerve impulses can't be transmitted and the nervous system can't function to regulate the basic functions of life, such as breathing. The slightly tamer organophosphates developed since the 1950s for commercial use as pesticides work the same way: They block cholinesterase and paralyze the nervous systems of insects so they die.

The symptoms people develop when they have been exposed to these chemicals show how they work to interfere with nerve function: blurred vision, nausea, shortness of breath, headaches, dizziness, restlessness, agitation, and even asphyxia. Chemicals like this are involved in the "strange" symptoms experienced by veterans of the Gulf War. And those are only the immediate effects. There are delayed effects on your immune system and nerve function. Death of your developing ovarian follicles leads to delayed effects of loss of your ovarian and thyroid hormones and the resulting damage to body tissues. What about the ways these chemicals work in your body long-term to accomplish their wicked tricks on the estrogen receptors? Or the ways they make breast cancer cells grow faster? They aren't so tame after all.

How Do They Work to Disrupt Our Own Hormones?

I briefly mentioned earlier a few of the types of actions of these compounds, but there are many ways these chemicals disrupt normal body hormone pathways and damage different body systems. POPs and excitotoxins are able to wreak such havoc with the brain's central command centers that direct the function of our entire endocrine system. The chart on page 93 summarizes ways they work to disrupt our endocrine systems.

SUMMARY: MECHANISMS OF ENDOCRINE DISRUPTION

Environmental chemicals that mimic hormones may act in several different ways to disrupt normal body functions. They:

- *Duplicate* normal hormone responses but produce slightly different variations, since their molecules are different from human hormones.
- *Interact* with receptors to *block* normal hormone function (much like the drug tamoxifen does).
- *Interact* with receptors to produce an *abnormal* response. The exaggerated androgen and insulin production in women with PCOS is an example of this type of effect.
- *Interact* with hormones and/or receptors to produce an additive or synergistic response, leading to *exaggerated* hormone effect. We think this is one way that these chemicals increase the risk for ovarian and breast cancers.
- *Interrupt* normal signaling mechanisms that control our body's ability to make proteins, enzymes, and other hormones.
- *Alter genes* that control activation or inactivation of critical pathways. A good example is the Y chromosome I described in Chapter 4, which has to be activated exactly on Day 56 of human gestation to turn on the testicle of a male embryo to make testosterone and convert the "unisex" brain to a male one. If one of these endocrine disruptors blocks that gene from turning on at the right time, a genetic male embryo is destined to live out his life in a hormonal and physical "limbo land," medically called *intersex.* (I'll tell you more about this problem later in the chapter.)
- *Interfere with neurotransmitters* (MAO, ST, NE, DA, ACh, etc.) that oversee the manufacture and release of GnRH, the hormone in the hypothalamus that regulates the pituitary hormones (FSH, LH) governing the ovaries. The result is disruption of the normal menstrual and reproductive cycles.
- *Direct toxic effects* on nerve cells in the pituitary.
- *Direct toxic effects* on the ovaries and testes to disrupt production of sex hormones.
- *Bind* to hormone receptors on sperm and oocytes (cells that become "eggs") to cause abnormal function and impair fertility.

False Reassurances, Hidden Dangers

The really sad part of the women's health story is that researchers and health care professionals have thought, until very recently, that these chemicals were harmless, despite research studies for *forty* years showing serious reproductive damage in multiple animal populations around the world. We were lulled into a false sense of security about POPs because there were a number of misconceptions and misunderstanding floating around scientific circles about how they worked. For example, the estrogenic POPs, and their residues on foods or in water supplies, are present in much lower concentrations in the body than our own body estrogen, so researchers thought there were not enough to do damage. A paper I reviewed in the menopause literature made that statement as recently as 1998. As we are finding out, this has turned out to be seriously wrong.

Researchers also falsely assumed that estrogenic POPs had a chemical structure different enough from our own body estradiol that these molecules could not function as "keys" to unlock or activate the human estrogen receptor (HER) complex. This was another profound mistake, because they *do* activate it. Lab analyses have shown POPs to be less potent than our own body estrogens, in some cases a few thousand times weaker, so researchers thought they didn't have much effect in our bodies. We now know this is also wrong. Many weaker estrogenic compounds, including many plant foods we normally eat (soy is a good example), are loaded with compounds that can interfere with the normal function of our hormone pathways.

The Emerging Truth

The true picture is not as simple or as innocuous and reassuring as researchers once thought. Newer studies reveal a frightening picture far more alarming than many scientists ever realized. POPs have some wicked tricks that turn them into serious, insidious weapons and subtle poisons that affect our bodies in terrible ways, especially our ovaries, breasts, and brain. The following section gives more detail about these deleterious actions. I hope this summary helps you see why I am concerned about all the fear that is focused on HRT when everyone seems to be ignoring the more serious estrogenic threats all around us that wreak such insidious havoc with our bodies. Then, we'll take a look at the POPs and breast cancer connections and explore crucial lessons from the DES experience.

Estrogenic Subverters: POPs' Wicked Tricks

1. The human estrogen receptor (HER) turns out not to be quite as difficult to activate as once thought. HER *works best* with the identical estradiol key our ovary makes, but doesn't *require only* this "identical" key for activation. HER is, unfortunately, rather promiscuous—it will *accept many* molecular "keys" of different sizes and shapes and be activated to some degree by all of them. That doesn't mean, however, that all of these different "keys" will work the same way or have the same effects in the body, as I have described in detail in my earlier books. In addition, different types of estrogenic "keys" may have adverse effects over time, including increased likelihood of cell mutations leading to breast or ovarian cancers.

2. Estrogenic POPs are far more common than researchers realized. Many different compounds and chemicals we use every day at home or in the workplace fall into this category. Many organic compounds such as pesticides, plastics, paints, chemical fragrances, chemical air fresheners, detergents, and many others can trigger estrogenic effects even if their molecules don't look anything at all like estradiol!

3. For even more damage, estrogenic POPs gang up on us, acting *together* to create even worse effects than any one compound alone. In medicine, we refer to this as a *synergistic* effect. In this case, 1+1+1 does *not* equal 3; it may equal 300 or 3,000 instead! Thus, when several estrogenic POPs are present, they may have effects several hundred times, or even several thousand times, *greater* than any one alone. Profound carcinogenic effects have been found when more than one of these compounds is present, even if each one is present in a very low concentration. Dr. Abou-Donia at Duke University showed that the pesticide chlorpyrifos, when combined with the organophosphate propetamphos, caused catastrophic destruction of the nervous system in doses lower than chlorpyrifos would alone.

4. Even though estrogenic POPs are less potent on laboratory measures than the estrogens our bodies make, they make up for their lower potency by sneaking around the body enzymes that break down hormones, and thereby escape the normal metabolism that our bodies use to deactivate our natural hormones. This trick enables the estrogenic POPs to persist in the body much, much longer than our own ovarian hormones do—our natural hormones are broken down in metabolism in a few hours. For example, if you take off an estradiol patch, the blood levels drop within about twelve hours. If you take a tablet of estradiol, it is metabolized to less active or inactive compounds in just a few hours, a very short duration of effect. Premarin, on the other hand, is a mixture of horse estrogens used for menopause estrogen therapy that takes about three months after the last dose to be cleared from the body. Estrogenic POPs may remain for many years after the last exposure. DDT is a good example. Although banned in the United States in 1972, women today, over thirty years later, *still* have measurable DDT residues in their body fat and breast tissue from environmental exposure in infancy and childhood.

5. POPs have another trick to overcome their lower concentration and lower potency. Our own hormones (ovarian, thyroid, and adrenal) are attached to carrier, or transport, proteins in the bloodstream called *sex hormone binding globulin* (SHBG), *thyroid binding globulin, corticotropin binding globulin,* and *albumin.* The binding proteins hold on to the hormones and slow down the rate hormones leave the blood to enter cells. This controls the rate that our hormones activate cell receptors. But POPs are different. They don't attach as tightly to these transport proteins as our own sex hormones do. This means POPs are more easily and quickly released from the carriers,

making POPs *more rapidly* available to activate cellular receptors than are our own hormones. Many pesticides behave like this in the body.

6. POPs don't just *mimic* the actions of our own estrogens; if they did, they wouldn't be so dangerous. POPs compounds can also *intensify* the effects of our own body estrogens to create new, undesirable effects such as increased risk of cell growth and changes that may lead to cancers.

7. Many different POPs actually block the healthy functions of our own estrogens, making us even sicker from the loss of the beneficial effects of our own body's natural 17-beta estradiol. I have seen this clinically in daughters of mothers who took DES in pregnancy.

8. Some POPs stimulate the body to make more estrogen receptors, which means more sites for estrogen actions, but not always in desirable ways. It also means more different types of estrogenic substances can activate all these new receptors. Many researchers think this is one way pesticides increase the growth of breast cancer cells.

9. Estrogenic POPs can change the way our body estrogens are broken down (metabolized). They push the process toward undesirable compounds that new research shows increase the risk for breast cancer.

Our normal healthy direction for estradiol metabolism is the 2-pathway in which it is broken down into "A ring" or catechol estrogens. The undesirable direction for estradiol breakdown is called the 16-pathway, or D-ring metabolites. Current research on breast cancer shows that shifting estradiol metabolism more toward the 2- (A ring) pathway actually *lowers* risk of breast cancer. A shift the other way, into the 16-pathway (D ring) leads to an increased risk of breast cancer.

A number of pesticides like atrazine, benzene, DDT, Endosulfan, and some PCBs all push our bodies to make more of the 16-pathway (D ring) types of estrogens. It is another insidious way that these chemicals turn our natural estradiol into a potent chemical weapon. It is rather like a glitch in a torpedo's program that makes it turn back on the submarine that launched it instead of heading out toward its intended target.

Endocrine Disruptors and Breast Cancer

DDT, Lindane, Chlordane, Dieldrin, Aldrin, heptachlor, chlorpyrifos, toxaphene, Endosulfan, and triazines—all are known or probable carcinogens. For example, toxaphene and Endosulfan cause breast cancer cells in tissue culture to grow faster; DDT converts to DDE in the body, and both have been found in levels 50 to 60 percent higher in breast cancer patients than women without the cancer. In 1993, Dr. Mary Wolff at Mt. Sinai School of Medicine in New York published a study showing that women who developed breast cancer had 35 percent *more* DDE in their blood than women who didn't. Dr. Wolff analyzed the blood specimens of 14,290 women and found that those with the highest DDE levels in their blood were *four times* more likely to have breast cancer than those with the lowest levels of DDE.

In 1990, researchers in Finland found that women with breast cancer had higher concentrations of Lindane-like residues in their breasts. Women with the highest Lindane residues were ten times more likely to have breast cancer than women with lower levels. The combined blood from women with breast cancer was analyzed and had 50 percent *more* of this pesticide residue than the blood from women without breast cancer. An analysis of Connecticut women published in 1992 showed similar trends: Levels of PCB, DDE, and DDT in the breast tissue of women with breast cancer were 50 to 60 percent higher than in women without cancer. So why is it that *all* you hear about in the news is the *slight* increase in risk of breast cancer that may occur with some types of estrogen therapy after menopause? There are many other aspects to this cancer link that are imperative to investigate and take into account in our evaluation of cancer risks.

Similar epidemiological data from Israel links breast cancer rates with the pesticides DDT, Lindane, and BHC. After twenty-five years of *rising* breast cancer rates there, two researchers noted that Israel was the only one of twenty-eight countries showing a significant *decrease* in breast cancer rates over the ten-year period that ended in 1986. Israel had allowed use of DDT, BHC, and Lindane until the mid-1970s, when they were banned. Prior to the ban, all three of these pesticides were found in dramatically high concentrations in dairy milk, other dairy products, and human breast milk. Two years after the ban, studies of human breast milk from residents of Jerusalem showed Lindane levels dropped 90 percent, BHC levels decreased 98 percent, and DDT levels went down 43 percent. Within ten years of the ban, there was a marked drop of 30 percent in breast cancer mortality in women under age forty-four. Researchers could not identify any other significant lifestyle or environmental change to account for these differences except the prohibition against using the three pesticides.

In Sweden, Germany, and Italy, which banned use of DDT in the 1980s, the concentrations of DDE and PCBs in human breast milk have been slowly declining. In addition to all of this damning evidence, epidemiological studies in the United States have clearly shown that certain occupational groups of women have significantly higher risks of breast cancer than the general public. An example is women in the petroleum and chemical industries exposed daily to higher concentrations of these same chemicals.

Breast cancer data from Hawaii suggests that the significant increase in breast cancer rates over the past few decades are related to endocrine disruption by environmental chemicals. Agricultural chemicals, including endocrine disruptors, have been used intensively in Hawaii's island ecosystem over the past forty years, leaching into groundwater and leading to unusually widespread exposures. Hawaiian women have been significantly exposed, in particular, to two endocrine-disrupting chemicals: chlordane-heptachlor and DBCP (1,2-

dibromo-3-chloropropane)—at levels that exceeded federal standards by several thousand times. Specialists there do not think that the increased rates are due solely to improvements in screening and detection; they are concerned that this is the ominous beginning of more serious problems to come as a result of pesticide exposure.

Different mechanisms allow these environmental estrogenic pollutants to act in ways that increase breast cancer risk and spread the disease once it develops. They attach to the estrogen receptors and ramp up the effects of our own body estrogens, stimulating growth of new blood vessels (angiogenesis), altering our DNA, and triggering growth-promoting changes in our body's estrogen target tissues. Yet to date, the American Cancer Society and other U.S. cancer organizations have done little to explore this critical evidence of the role of environmental pollutants in breast and other cancers. Instead, they scare us about our own estrogen, and fuel fear about replenishing hormones after menopause. In my view, this ignores the far more serious issues that we face from insidious exposure to these incredibly damaging, known carcinogens in the environment. We've been steeping in them like a teabag in a teapot for most of our life, perhaps since conception. Why isn't the American Cancer Society focusing on what these estrogenic chemicals do to damage our estrogen receptors and make us more susceptible to female cancers?

The American Cancer Society also spends millions of dollars on ad campaigns exhorting us to clean up our lifestyle, change our diet, and exercise more. The implication is that if we don't do those things and then get cancer, it's our fault. Yes, a healthy diet is important, but this is not the only factor in who gets cancer. A wiser approach would be to use some of the advertising dollars to fund research on cancer links with persistent organic pollutants.

Many of these pesticides also cause earlier onset of puberty. If girls begin menstruating earlier and also delay pregnancy until later, as is common today, there is a longer period of continuous excess estrogen stimulation during critical phases of breast development. Our total estrogen exposure comes not only from natural body estrogens, but also from all the estrogenic chemicals in our environment, including those causing puberty to switch on too early. Although not the only factor in breast cancer risk, current research has found that rapid breast growth in puberty around the time your periods begin is an extremely important factor in your later breast cancer risk. It creates a more serious problem for later life if there is too much stimulation of breast growth around this time, especially if it comes from exposure to non-natural estrogenic chemicals found in POPs. Most breast cancers in later life begin in the breast ducts. These ducts are formed during the phase of rapid breast growth just before your menstrual periods begin. Exposure to these environmental chemicals at this stage of development has the potential to cause much more damage than if such exposure comes later on. The damage that occurs in puberty, however, won't likely appear until several decades later. Many scientists now think that exposure to the estrogenic chemicals in childhood and puberty combines with other known risk factors to increase risk of having breast cancer later in life.

Researchers are looking at these endocrine disruptors' effects on male reproductive function, such as lower sperm counts, but they have not yet systematically looked for similar reproductive effects in *women*. From what studies we *do* have on these environmental contaminants, POPs appear to permanently damage the body's estrogen receptors. Many pesticides *also* interfere with the synthesis of crucial mood-regulating chemical messengers. Dursban (chlorpyrifos) inhibits the conversion of tryptophan to serotonin, a critical neurotransmitter that functions in mood, pain, sleep, appetite, and thirst regulatory pathways. Where do you find Dursban? It is a common ingredient in many pesticides used in homes, schools, and workplaces. And if your ovarian hormones are also too low when you are exposed to Dursban, you have a triple whammy: (1) low estradiol leads to loss of serotonin synthesis and function, (2) decreased absorption of the vitamin and mineral cofactors needed to make more serotonin, and (3) you have the inhibitory, damaging effects from the Dursban. No wonder women with low estrogen get hit especially hard by pesticides and potent synthetic chemicals. It isn't so surprising that many women describe experiencing depression after exposure to pesticides and other POPs.

Synthetic Estrogenic Substances: What Have We Learned from DES?

I have a number of women patients who were "DES babies." It strikes me as more than a coincidence that these women have experienced "strange" hormonal problems since puberty. They also tend to have unusual responses to hormone therapy—either they are exquisitely sensitive to very small doses, or they require doses higher than we would expect. We have decided to do a clinical study of our patients with DES exposure to see if we can discern any consistent patterns in their hormonal challenges. This is a complex problem with many connections. Just what is DES and why is it important in relation to endocrine disruptors?

Diethylstilbestrol, or DES, is a highly potent synthetic, nonsteroidal estrogenic compound first synthesized in Britain in 1938. DES was subsequently used medically for over three decades in more than 5 million women in the United States, the United Kingdom, Europe, and Latin America. Doctors gave it to pregnant women thinking that it would prevent miscarriages. Later, it was more widely used, even in women who had not had prior miscarriages, with the idea that it would create healthier pregnancies and stronger, healthier babies. Its use was further expanded to include emergency "morning after" contraception, to suppress milk production after delivery in women who did not want to nurse, and for treatment of menopausal symptoms such as hot flashes. It even became popular for a while as a way to stop growth if teenage girls were becoming "too tall" to be attractive! Used in animal feed and hormone implants to fatten livestock, DES was even given to chickens to make them develop faster. Even if your mother was not given DES, you could have been exposed to it during your developmental years in foods your mother ate.

During the time DES was used in the 1940s to 1960s, doctors believed the placenta created a "safety barrier" so that drugs given to a pregnant mother did not harm the developing baby. This was seriously flawed thinking. Many substances *do* cross the placenta and have a profound impact on the developing baby, many of which are permanent and irreversible. Some everyday examples are caffeine, alcohol, cigarette smoke, cocaine, and even prescription medicines. You are probably aware that developmental and learning difficulties occur in babies born to mothers using cocaine, tobacco, or alcohol. These drugs tend to produce effects that show up soon after birth. Environmental chemicals, and yes, even hormones like DES, *also* cross the placenta to the baby and typically produce effects that do not show up until many years or even decades later in adolescence or adulthood. This was the case with the rare form of vaginal cancer that developed in young women whose mothers had taken DES. DES has been studied extensively in the decades since this vaginal cancer connection first came to light, and now we know that it causes reproductive tract, immune system, and brain abnormalities in all species studied, including humans, primates, rodents, and birds.

New research has also shown that *amounts* of drugs and other chemicals that don't cause damage or side effects in adult woman can have devastating effects on a developing embryo and fetus. An example is thalidomide, which was safely used in the 1960s as a sleeping pill for women during pregnancy. It turned out that the drug caused profound deformities in the arms and legs of a developing fetus. Thalidomide effects showed up at birth and were obvious to all. But when there are no *visible* defects at birth, doctors tend not to think that a drug will have any long-term adverse effects on the baby. Yet that idea has also turned out to be seriously wrong. An infant's brain and body, especially during key times of organ formation, can be critically and permanently injured in ways that may not show up for decades. This is exactly what occurred with DES. Infant girls and boys *looked* healthy and appeared to develop normally. But the sabotage done by DES within those apparently normal bodies emerged years later.

What were the consequences of being exposed to DES? Daughters of mothers who took DES have high rates of a formerly rare type of vaginal cancer called *adenocarcinoma*. This type of cancer is not only rare, it is usually not seen in women younger than fifty. DES daughters who developed vaginal cancer were hit in their teens and twenties. Some died at very young ages due to the aggressiveness of the DES-induced cancer. DES sons have a greater incidence of malformations of the penis and testicles than in boys not exposed to DES. To cause these effects later in life, the *timing* of DES exposure during the baby's development in the womb is more crucial than the *amount*. For example, female babies exposed before the tenth week of gestation have a higher incidence of the rare vaginal cancer. Those exposed after the twentieth week of gestation, however, did not develop the deformities of the reproductive tract. This pattern of a "critical window" for exposure is seen with other types of endocrine disruptors as well.

Vaginal cancers robbed women of fertility and even their lives. Now we know there are additional insidious ramifications of DES exposure. DES also caused structural deformities of the uterus, fallopian tubes, and ovaries leading to ectopic pregnancies, miscarriages, and infertility. There is also a much higher than normal incidence of endometriosis and other reproductive problems such as PCOS in DES daughters. There is now disturbing evidence that the risks of DES exposure can be passed along to a second generation of children. DES grandchildren—many of you reading this book—will also have to be aware of these risks to your health and fertility.

There are other subtle problems that appear to be related to DES disruption of normal endocrine development and function. I have been suspicious that DES may also have altered brain response to our own body hormones and affected the way in which women responded to birth control pills and hormone therapy at menopause. Many of my patients whose mothers took DES have earlier than usual onset of perimenopause, have more difficulties with severe PMS, atypical depressions, recurrent ovarian cysts, and uterine fibroids. Interestingly, they have often needed higher than usual doses of estrogen to relieve menopausal symptoms. I believe this relates to a higher "set point" of the brain's estrogen receptors in the women exposed during fetal development to this highly potent synthetic estrogen. Often, they do not respond as I would expect to testosterone replacement either. Nor do they experience an improvement in sex drive that I typically see in other women. Another atypical response I see in some of my DES-exposed patients is that they are unusually sensitive to even small amounts of medicines, in particular hormones. It is as if their estrogen receptors have been altered to be overly responsive. All of these adverse effects need to be explored, but to date, there is little research on these subtle types of hormone disruption from exposure to DES and other environmental hormone disruptors.

There are clues in studies on animals, however, to support my concerns. Some of the problems I describe above that I have seen in my patients have also been reported in medical articles. These include increased ovarian inflammation, early depletion of follicles, abnormal follicles, increased number of cysts, absent or decreased number of corpora lutea (normally present from ovulation), thickened interstitial components, abnormal ratios of FSH and LH, elevated production of androgens, and increased number of ovarian, breast, and uterine tumors. Interestingly, the abnormal changes in the ovary after DES exposure are strikingly similar to what is described for PCOS, but you don't see much about this possible connection in the writings on PCOS today.

Animal studies indicate DES acts on other body systems, such as the brain (especially the pituitary), the breast, and the immune system. But these DES effects have not been studied adequately in humans. In mice, DES causes suppression of two important components of the immune system: T-helper cells that oversee our body's total immune response, and the natural killer (NK) cells that patrol the body looking for abnormal cells to eradicate and prevent from spreading. If our NK cells aren't working optimally, we are not able to ward off other carcinogens very well, and we become more likely to develop cancers as we age. Women exposed to DES in the womb have later been found to have permanent, adverse changes in their T-helper and NK cells. I think this explains the clinical observations that women exposed to DES also have higher rates of several autoimmune disorders, such as Hashimoto's thyroiditis, Graves' disease, rheumatoid arthritis, and possibly lupus. DES effects on brain development in the womb are far more difficult to tease out. Research has hardly begun to scratch the surface of potential health effects on brain pathways disrupted during development. You can see from the DES time line below that this is a ticking time bomb.

CHRONOLOGY: THE DES TIME LINE

1938: First synthesized in Britain.

1940s and 1950s: Widespread use for millions of women—to prevent miscarriages, to help "support" a healthy pregnancy, for a "morning after" contraceptive, to treat menopausal symptoms, etc.

1952: Dr. William Dieckmann and colleagues at the University of Chicago published their study of two thousand pregnant women, half given DES and half given placebo, to see the effect on miscarriage rate. Their conclusions were unequivocal: DES did not decrease *either* the number of miscarriages or the number of premature births. Later analysis of their data showed that there was an *increase* in miscarriages, an increase in premature births, and an increase in deaths of newborns in women given DES. *In spite of these terrible findings, the FDA did not take any action to curb its use.*

1952–1970s: Some doctors begin to cut back on DES use after the University of Chicago study is published, but hundreds of thousands of pregnant women are still given DES in the belief that it would reduce miscarriages and lead to healthier babies.

1966–1969: Specialists at Massachusetts General Hospital, affiliated with Harvard Medical School, had seven cases of clear cell adenocarcinoma, all in the unusually young age range of fifteen to twenty-two. Normally this cancer isn't seen until after age fifty, and even then it is very rare.

April 22, 1971: The MGH-Harvard researchers publish an article in the *New England Journal of Medicine* reporting that seven of the eight young women with the rare vaginal cancer had mothers who took DES in the first three months of pregnancy.

1970s, 1980s, 1990s: Researchers found other abnormalities in children of DES mothers:

DES Daughters
- Deformed uteruses that could not sustain pregnancy
- Deformed fallopian tubes and ovaries
- Higher than normal rates of infertility
- Increased rates of ectopic pregnancies and miscarriages
- Increased rates of premature babies
- Increased rates of endometriosis
- Increased rates of uterine tumors, both benign (fibroids) and malignant (sarcomas and endometrial cancer)
- Increased rates of both benign and malignant breast tumors
- Increased frequency of ovarian cysts and abnormal follicles (also seen in PCOS)
- Diminished formation of corpora lutea ("eggs")
- Abnormal progesterone and estrogen production, abnormal receptor function
- Increased incidence of prolactinomas (a benign pituitary tumor) and elevated blood levels of prolactin (also seen in PCOS)
- Immune system problems
- Abnormal glucose tolerance and decreased glucose utilization (also seen in PCOS)
- Abnormal development of gender-specific sexual behavior in DES offspring (males feminized, females masculinized), suggesting that DES caused abnormal sex differentiation of the hypothalamus during fetal development

DES Sons
- Increased genital defects
- Undescended testicles
- Stunted testicles and penises
- Cysts in the epididymis
- Low sperm counts
- Abnormal sperm
- Reduced fertility
- Hypospadius (deformity of the penis)
- Increased rates of testicular cancer at earlier ages than expected
- Immune system problems
- Abnormal glucose tolerance and glucose utilization
- Abnormal development of male sexual behavior

1980s–present: Second generation of DES children reaching puberty and early adulthood showing similar problems as above.

Beyond the Ovary: Endocrine Disruptors' Effects on the Thyroid

The endocrine disruptors I have been describing, especially polychlorinated biphenyls (PCBs) and dioxins, also seriously interfere with thyroid hormone action in addition to our ovarian hormones. PCBs bear a striking structural resemblance to our body's active thyroid hormones and appear to fool the body's thyroid receptors, acting as agonists, antagonists, or partial agonists to thyroid hormones. They may also increase the number of thyroid hormone receptors, which then means the brain and body will need even more hormones to function properly. Our thyroid hormones play a major role in regulating metabolism of the body and brain, as well as in modulating reproductive functions, including our ovarian cycles. Exposure to synthetic chemicals that interfere with thyroid function as we develop in the womb has profound effects on brain function for the rest of our lives. Human brain development occurs at very specific windows of time throughout our time in the womb, and it is essential to have the proper levels of thyroid hormones during these critical windows. If we don't have the thyroid hormones and iodine present in the proper amounts and balance during brain development, permanent brain damage occurs. The type of brain damage, and the symptoms that occur in childhood or later life, will depend on *when* and *how much* disruption occurs in the thyroid hormones. Thyroid hormone deficiency during brain development is one of the leading causes worldwide of learning and attention deficit disorders and other subtle types of neurological/cognitive dysfunction, as well as a severe form of mental retardation.

POPs may interfere with normal thyroid metabolism and hormone synthesis by a number of different mechanisms. The simplified flow chart on page 105 shows how POPs interfere with thyroid activity and how this cascade effect impacts the ovaries. Healthy thyroid function is crucial for normal fertility and healthy ovarian hormone production, so POPs' disruption of thyroid activity is another way that they disrupt fertility, as well as lead to premature menopause. If you suspect you may have a thyroid disorder in addition to problems with your ovaries, see the discussion in Chapter 7.

Heavy Metals and Menstrual Disturbances

Naturally occurring heavy metals—lead, mercury, arsenic, cadmium, and gallium—have long been known to cause nervous system damage, including producing severe psychosis. I am sure you have heard the phrase "mad as a hatter." This refers to a mental illness caused by mercury that manifested with hallucinations, delusions, and disordered thinking. This type of illness occurred in hatmakers (hatters) in the seventeenth century, when mercury was used to tan animal hides. The symptoms of psychosis were identical to what we see in the psychiatric disorder schizophrenia, but here they were produced by toxic brain damage from the hatters' chronic exposure to a physical agent, mercury.

These metals can produce multiple neurological symptoms, even from exposure to low levels. I had a patient recently who presented with a bizarre cluster of

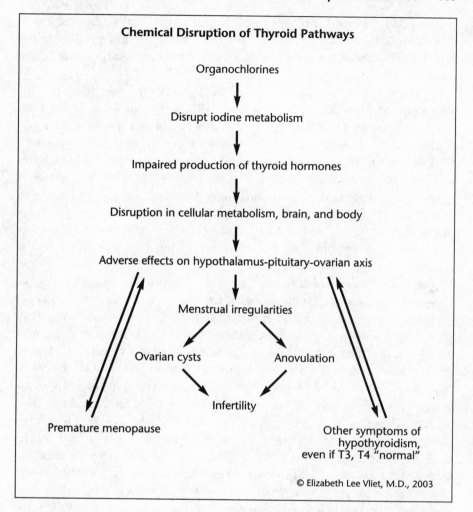

neurological symptoms that was quite a challenge to unravel. After a lot of detective work, we were able to determine that she was unknowingly poisoned with low levels of arsenic, in addition to her other serious problems, including bone loss from her low estradiol and testosterone. What were her symptoms? Severe exhaustion, dizziness, light-headedness, marked difficulty with word recall, concentration problems, dull headaches, vomiting, and weight loss, among others. The difficulty with arsenic and other heavy-metal toxicity is that symptoms are so nonspecific they can be caused by a hundred different things. She had seen two neurologists, but all the neurological studies and brain imaging studies were normal. But I had several clues that her symptoms were not all due to her ovarian hormones. First, her symptoms did not improve with estradiol the way I would have expected, and second, she was much sicker than I usually see in women who just have low estradiol. I decided to order a blood test for heavy metals, and it showed the elevated arsenic levels. As with other chronic heavy-metal intoxication, arsenic exposure had caused damage to brain pathways, and it had also disrupted her menstrual cycle, leading to diminished production of ovarian hormones.

In younger women, chronic heavy-metal exposure can cause infertility. One group of researchers found that low levels of lead exposure over several years disrupted menstrual cycles in Rhesus monkeys. The monkeys were given drinking water that contained lead acetate daily for three one-year exposures over a five-year period. The monkeys had further lead intake for three additional consecutive years, providing additional time to observe the effects on menstrual cycles. The lead acetate in the drinking water produced average circulating lead concentrations in the blood between 44 and 89 mcg/100 ml and zinc protoporphyrin concentrations between 87 and 105 mcg/100 ml. These are not unusually high concentrations, but menstrual cycles were significantly impaired even at these levels.

Even though the lead-treated monkeys had completely normal menstrual cycles prior to the study, for the entire last two years of lead exposure their cycles decreased in frequency (called *oligomenorrhea*), and their cycles were longer with greater variability in intervals between bleeding. The number of bleeding days also decreased compared to the monkeys who did not receive any lead (control group), which indicates a hormone imbalance. These changes were not due to differences in exposure to environmental influences such as light or diet, because when the monkeys were no longer getting lead in their drinking water, their menstrual bleeding returned to normal duration. The other effects of lead exposure, however, remained *for over a year* after they stopped getting lead in their drinking water. This was troubling. It indicates that adverse effects on fertility can remain even after lead exposure is eliminated. Even more worrisome was that the monkeys had none of the usual observable signs of lead toxicity, such as loss of appetite, weight loss, or a change in blood counts such as hematocrit. For a woman, this means it could be difficult to recognize exposure to lead or some other heavy metal.

Menstrual cycle disruptions due to prolonged lead or other heavy-metal exposure may also lead to premature menopause. It may be difficult to know whether you are getting excess lead or other metals from environmental sources because the level that disrupts the menstrual cycle may not produce any obvious or classic signs or symptoms of heavy-metal toxicities. I wanted you to be aware of the subtle effects of these metals so that if your menstrual cycle changes and you have symptoms like fatigue, low energy, "blah" mood, fuzzy thinking or other "vague" symptoms without apparent cause, or symptoms that don't respond to the usual treatments for more common problems, you may want to consider asking for a screening blood test for heavy-metal exposure.

In Summary

Silent Spring was an early warning that what happened in animal populations could affect all of us. Over forty years have passed since Rachel Carson published her alarm, yet we have even more reason for concern now. More endocrine-disrupting chemicals have been created. These chemicals are more potent than ever, and more persistent. We know that they cause significant perturbations in our exquisitely sensitive endocrine system. Everything in this chapter should help you see how sensitive you are to the harmful effects of endocrine-disruptor chemicals. Pay attention to your menstrual cycles. Know what is normal and what is not. Pay attention *when* in the menstrual cycle symptoms occur. Follow the action plan in Section IV and clean up the way you eat, eliminating as many of these toxic chemical products as possible. Check around your home, and eliminate products with chemicals included in the list in this chapter. Speak out for better information and regulation of substances that wreak havoc with our health and the health of children yet to be born. You can make a difference.

6

Ovaries at Risk: Toxic Effects of Cigarettes, Alcohol, Marijuana, and Other Drugs

Cigarette Smoking

You have heard a thousand times or more that smoking cigarettes is bad for you, and that it increases your risk of lung cancer, heart disease, and stroke. Although smoking is down overall about 40 percent since 1965, lung cancer deaths in women have increased more than 600 percent since 1950. At the same time, rates have been dropping in men as more have stopped smoking. Twenty-two million women now smoke; as a result, women now make up over half of all the new cases of lung cancer each year. At least 1.5 million adolescent girls in the United States smoke cigarettes, and nearly 3,000 teenagers a day become regular smokers. The younger you start, the greater the risk of severe nicotine addiction as you get older. If you are like many young women in their teens, twenties, and thirties who smoke, you probably aren't all that concerned about lung cancer or heart attacks. I can hear you saying to yourself right now, "I'm young, so it really isn't a problem. It won't hurt *me* because I can stop any time I want to." If that's the case, why don't you? Could it be that you are more addicted than you think?

Even though you may still be young, you should look at some new research that has serious implications for all women who smoke or live with someone who does. Cigarette smoke, whether from your own or secondhand from others, increases your risk of having one of several defective genes recently much in the news, called *K-ras, GSTM1,* and *GRPR.* Each of these genes create a much higher than average risk of developing lung cancer. For example, the K-ras gene mutation, three times more common in women, enhances the growth of cancerous tumors. The GSTM1 gene normally functions to deactivate carcinogens in tobacco smoke; secondhand (environmental) smoke alters this gene so that it cannot detoxify the carcinogens. The more secondhand smoke you live and work with, the more likely you are to have this defective gene, and the greater your risk of lung cancer. The GRPR gene, fueled by exposure to nicotine, helps lung cancers grow. This gene is more common in the airways of women than men, which is another reason that smoking is a greater cancer risk for women than men.

Okay, so maybe you are too young to be worried about lung cancer. But did you know that cigarette smoking can damage your ovaries, even if you are "only" a teenager or in your twenties? And what about when you want to have a child? Did you know that smoking cigarettes can lead to infertility? Did you know that women who smoke have more risk of endometriosis and ovarian cysts? Did you know that cigarette smoking may lead to premature menopause in women as young as thirty?

Many components of cigarette smoke not only cause cancer, but are also *directly toxic* to the follicles in your ovaries. The more you smoke, the more follicles you kill off. And remember, unlike men who make more sperm throughout their lives, women are born with all the follicles we will ever have. When follicles are gone, they are permanently gone. Without follicles, you lose your hormone-producing factories; that means lower estradiol levels, lower testosterone levels, and abnormal menstrual cycles. Lower hormone levels also mean less energy, loss of sex drive, loss of mental sharpness, poor sleep, an immune system that doesn't work as well, and a host of other problems described earlier.

Multiple studies from many different countries over the past forty years have shown the relationship between smoking cigarettes and impaired fertility. Getting pregnant is more difficult for smokers, and smokers have much higher rates of infertility than nonsmokers. In one 1985 study, women who smoked cigarettes, compared to nonsmokers, were 57 to 75 percent *less likely* to conceive, depending on how much they smoked. For those smokers who finally did get pregnant, it took over a year longer to conceive than it did for the nonsmokers. Women smokers who go through in vitro fertilization and other assisted reproduction techniques have lower success rates than nonsmokers. In addition, smokers are more likely to have significant fetal growth retardation, creating smaller babies, more likely to be born prematurely. And the problems don't stop there. Female children born to women who smoked during pregnancy can have problems conceiving their own children, even if they do not smoke. Specialists think this occurs because smoking during pregnancy actually kills some of the primordial follicles in the developing female baby. Since she isn't born with the normal number of follicles, she has a harder time getting pregnant later.

Most patients and many physicians still do not know that cigarette smoking causes earlier menopause, and this includes exposure to secondhand smoke. Women who smoke regularly may go through menopause five to seven years sooner than nonsmokers. Many of my patients tell me that when they ask other physicians about a relationship between smoking and early menopause, their doctors say, "There isn't one. I never heard of this problem." Yet medical studies showing this connection were published over *twenty-five years ago!* Even before their periods completely stop, women who smoke cigarettes have significant declines in their levels of estradiol for years prior to menopause.

There are many mechanisms by which the chemicals in cigarette smoke can cause earlier menopause:

- *Death of cells in the ovary that become eggs (oocytes)*
- *Reduction in the ovaries' ability to make estradiol*
- *Increased metabolic breakdown of estradiol by liver enzymes that are induced (i.e., made overactive) by cigarette smoking*

- *Disruption by nicotine of the hypothalamus and pituitary, which regulate the secretion of hormones that oversee the proper cycling of the ovaries*
- *Suppression of the GnRH pulse generator that maintains normal cycles*
- *The carcinogenic effects of the compounds in cigarette smoke**

In my practice, I see smokers with multiple hormone-related health problems, and most of them also have muscle and joint pain syndromes. What are some of these connections that might explain why smokers have more of these muscle and joint problems as well? Pain regulation is one of estradiol's many functions. Estradiol also helps muscle metabolism and repair. Healthy levels of estradiol help prevent pain from occurring, reduce pain when it strikes, and also help (along with testosterone) to build healthy muscle tissue. So, if cigarette smoking has lowered your estradiol, you lose some pain-relieving benefits. Other adverse effects of cigarette smoking on pain pathways include:

- *Diminished serotonin production.*
- *Constriction of small arteries that serve muscles and nerves, which leads to diminished blood flow and diminished supply of vital nutrients to body tissues, nutrients needed for building, repairing, and healing microtrauma from daily use.*
- *Reduced oxygen-carrying capacity of the red blood cells, since smoking replaces oxygen with carbon monoxide. The loss of oxygen supply not only leads to fatigue but also to a build-up of metabolic waste products in muscle tissues, causing more muscle pain.*
- *Decreased blood flow and nutrients to cells, along with a reduction in vitamin C from smoking, causes an increase in oxidative (free-radical) damage to nerve and muscle cells, and release of inflammatory prostaglandins and other body chemicals that intensify pain.*
- *Diminished stomach acidity and decreased absorption of many vitamins, especially the B group, needed for the brain and body to make pain-relieving neurotransmitters.*
- *Nicotine also increases pain perception by several mechanisms and, as a stimulant, leads to increased anxiety and irritability, both of which are already present from the "stimulant" effect of pain itself.*
- *Nicotine withdrawal while you are asleep leads to more frequent awakenings and loss of Stage 4 deep sleep that is crucial for muscle repair, growth hormone secretion, and keeping the brain healthy, among other restorative functions.*

---

*Cigarette smoke is a complex "witches' brew" of chemicals, many of which are known carcinogens: alkaloids (nicotine), polycyclic aromatic hydrocarbons (PAH), nitroso compounds, aromatic amines, and protein pyrolysates). For example, PAH causes ovarian tumors and ooycte death in animals.

So when you put all the pieces together, the picture for women who smoke is not pretty. Take a look at this young woman, who started smoking at age twelve. Like hundreds of young women I have seen in my practice over the years, she thought she "wouldn't have any problems" from smoking cigarettes.

Bev is now thirty-eight years old and has smoked at least a pack of cigarettes a day since she was twelve. Her periods also began about age twelve, and over the next ten years, she had a wide range of troubling symptoms she called "weird." She said at her initial visit, "No one could tell me what was happening to me. I had this dizziness, swimming in my head; I felt like my brain was in a fog; my body would shake at times, and I felt more and more anxious/depressed/foggy, and just never felt quite right. I felt like something chemical was happening in my body, but none of the doctors could ever explain what was going on. Then, in my early twenties, I was getting worse and could barely function. I would wake up with numb arms every night, feeling disconnected in my motor movements, and would have split-second moments of memory glitches and not know where I was. I thought I was losing my mind. Then all of a sudden my period came three times in one month, and I had intense panic attacks. I also had this weird muscle tension where I would realize my muscles would be tense and I would have to consciously try to relax them. My libido totally disappeared and has never returned.

"In desperation, I went to a psychiatrist and an OB/GYN. The psychiatrist put me on an antidepressant and said I was dysthymic. The GYN just thought I was under stress. I had watched my body, and I realized that these weird things were happening at certain times of my cycle. I also saw that my cycles were changing. I put two and two together and figured that something must be affecting my hormones.

"I demanded that my GYN do hormone tests, but he just said I was too young and it wasn't necessary. I demanded that he humor me and do them. When he called me with the results, I almost cried, I was so relieved and validated. I had high prolactin and really low estrogen, so he sent me to an endocrinologist who started me on Parlodel (bromocriptine). I felt a lot better, especially considering the state I was coming from, but I never felt a hundred percent. I still felt there was more to it than just taking Parlodel, but I decided to settle for what relief I had at that point.

"I tried for over two years to become pregnant and never could, so I finally went on Clomid and got pregnant. I stopped smoking during my pregnancy until after my son was born, and I figured there wasn't a problem if I went back to smoking. But then I had postpartum depression and went on Paxil, which helped, but I felt really tired all day and my sex drive was totally gone. About six months after the baby was born, I went back on Parlodel, which only made me feel worse. I felt like I had a hangover—fatigue, brain fog, just no sense of clarity in my thinking. It really has such a dramatic effect on me.

"For the next two years I was on a hormonal roller coaster with anxiety, mood swings, a quaking feeling, intermittent brain fog, et cetera. Then I had a miscarriage that they said was a blighted ovum, and I had to have a D and C. I just didn't feel well all this time, so I finally decided I wanted to have this consult with you. I feel like there is something else going on hormonally that causes my severe fatigue, brain fog, and makes it hard to concentrate. It isn't all month long, but seems to come for a few days in a row and then lifts some, then later comes back. I just don't have a good sense of well-being. It always feels like there is something chemical going on and my body isn't quite adjusted. I find that my body is tensing all over, even if I am not stressed. My muscles hurt, my joints ache, and I feel like an old woman before my time."

When Bev and I reviewed her lab tests, I could see why she was still having so many problems. Clearly the cigarette smoking had damaged her ovaries over all these years, and she was having the problems that occur in smokers due to loss of estradiol. She had a really low Day 1 estradiol of only 30 pg/ml (optimal is 80–90 pg/ml), and her Day 20 (luteal phase) estradiol level was only 105 pg/ml, which is only about *half* the healthy level at this time of the cycle. Her low levels went right along with what research studies show for hormone levels in smokers. Her low estradiol also decreased sex hormone binding globulin (SHBG) and pushed more testosterone into the free fraction. Too much testosterone in the free fraction can cause irritability, insomnia, anxiety, agitation, tense muscles, to name a few symptoms, because the testosterone is more available to overstimulate the receptors. If estradiol is too low, it makes the symptoms of excess available testosterone even worse, so this helps explain why she would feel worse during her periods, the time of her cycle when the estradiol was the lowest.

You may recall that she said her libido had vanished. How can she have excess free testosterone *and* a loss of libido? This happens when estradiol levels are too low to properly "prime" the testosterone receptors in the brain so that the testosterone can work optimally for women, unlike the way it works in men. Her low libido was aggravated by the high progesterone relative to her low estradiol in the second half of her cycle. Progesterone blocks testosterone from acting at its receptor sites. Progesterone breakdown products (metabolites) act as central nervous system depressants much like Valium, Ativan, Xanax, or Klonopin. All drugs or hormones that bind at these brain sites can cause low libido. In addition, higher levels of progesterone relative to the estradiol in the luteal phase of her cycle added to her brain fog, much as she would experience from taking Valium or Klonopin.

There is no question Bev had perimenopausal levels of estradiol, even though she was still having periods. In addition, her bone density test (DEXA) showed early bone loss (osteopenia) at the hip, giving further support to my conclusion that her estradiol level was too low. Early bone loss is also common in women who smoke, primarily due to the lower level of estradiol. Most of her brain symptoms— fuzzy thinking, brain fog, memory loss, and problems concentrating—occurred because her estradiol was too low. I explained to her that the cigarette smoking was a direct cause of her low estradiol, and had also probably contributed to her high prolactin found by the other physician. High prolactin adds to the smoking-induced suppression of her ovaries and decrease in hormone production.

Bev had already had saliva hormone tests done before I saw her. The report of that test said she had "estrogen dominance and low progesterone." This is exactly the same description I have seen on every single saliva test report I have ever reviewed, so I suspect it is given all the time and has little relevance to what is actually happening in *your* body. When we tested the more reliable blood hormone levels, the results showed a clear decrease in estradiol throughout her cycle, and a normal rise in progesterone in the luteal phase of her cycle. The blood tests fit exactly with what we would expect based on her symptoms and on the known consequences of cigarette smoking, including bone loss.

Low levels of estradiol and cigarette smoking also cause changes in the pH of the stomach and intestine, affecting the body's ability to absorb nutrients, such as calcium, magnesium, iron, B vitamins, and others. Loss of these important vitamins and minerals made her brain fog and memory problems even worse.

All of Bev's problems were directly related to her twenty-five years of smoking cigarettes. Smoking had profoundly damaged her ovaries and brain pathways, including the pituitary, in several different ways:

1. *Nicotine disrupts chemical messengers that regulate the pituitary and prolactin release.*
2. *Nicotine and the other chemicals in cigarette smoke kill off follicles, causing early ovarian decline and lower estradiol levels.*
3. *Smoking increases activity of liver enzymes that metabolize hormones, which means hormones are broken down or inactivated faster.*
4. *Nicotine interferes with normal production of mood- and sleep-regulating chemical messengers.*
5. *Smoking contributes to impaired absorption of vitamins and minerals from the gut at the same time it increases the body's need for these same vitamins and minerals.*

This shows you how damaging smoking can be for young women's fertility. And then in 1986, lung cancer became the leading cause of cancer death in women. Every year since, lung cancer deaths in women exceed deaths due to breast cancer. Most women still think breast cancer is the leading cause of death. The reality is starkly different: Lung cancer and heart disease, both increased by smoking, together kill more than *10 times* as many women as breast cancer.

Cigarette smoking itself increases your risk of breast cancer. This risk is more pronounced for young, premenopausal women than for postmenopausal women. Tobacco smoke in the body contains many direct carcinogens and adversely affects immune system function, as well as the metabolism of estrogens and other important hormones. Two recent studies found that premenopausal women who have ever smoked daily have approximately a twofold increased risk of breast cancer compared to women who *never* smoked. Women who are currently heavy smokers have *four* times the risk of breast cancer compared to the risk for nonsmokers.

These are much bigger increases in risk than any that have been attributed to taking estrogen. With smoking, it is a "dose-dependent" relationship. *The more you smoke, the higher the risk.*

If you are still smoking cigarettes, give it up now. Take steps to prevent any more damage to your ovaries that can cause infertility and lead to even more serious problems later.

Alcohol

Alcohol is a socially acceptable, legal drug available everywhere. Drinking among young people has risen dramatically in recent years, and more ominously, *binge* drinking is on the rise in adolescent and college-age girls. Alcohol is widely touted as a sexual enhancer. It's legal, so it must be safe, right? But this legal drug takes an insidious toll on our health, especially for women. Compared to men, women don't have as much of the enzyme that breaks down alcohol, so alcohol is far more damaging, even if the amount consumed is similar to what a man drinks. Let's look at all the ways alcohol is an endocrine disruptor that affects your hormones, sexual responsiveness, fertility, and your total health.

Folk wisdom has always said that alcohol increased sexual desire but took away the ability to perform! It decreases men's testosterone, causing impotence. It also acts as a depressant drug on the brain and nerves, so nerve endings in the clitoris and penis are less sensitive to sexual stimulation, leading to difficulties having an orgasm. The brain's sexual circuits are also dulled, another negative effect on arousal and orgasm. Even women who are "just social drinkers" report more disruption of their sexual responsiveness.

How does alcohol affect the menstrual cycle and fertility? Over many years, studies from a variety of countries have consistently shown that regular use of alcohol disrupts the normal menstrual cycle and causes problems with ovulation and the ability to get pregnant. Alcohol also lowers production of estradiol and testosterone, leading to earlier onset of menopause. The box on page 115 shows how alcohol affects women more severely than men.

Now what about the ways that your menstrual cycle hormone changes may actually increase your alcohol cravings? This gets scant attention in most alcohol treatment programs, but it is an enormous factor that perpetuates alcohol abuse in a large percentage of women. One twenty-eight-year-old woman started binge drinking at age twelve, soon after her periods began. She had several hospital admissions for alcohol abuse complications and was struggling to maintain her sobriety. She described the premenstrual cravings quite graphically: "*I do fine staying off alcohol from the end of my period until I ovulate, and then all hell breaks loose. I feel like I have an uncontrollable demon inside me that won't let me alone and demands that I go get a drink! I have an awful time resisting these cravings when they start after ovulation and become especially intense the week before my period starts. That's the time I had my relapses and had to go back to the hospital. I*

GENDER MATTERS:
ALCOHOL EFFECTS ON FERTILITY, MENSTRUAL CYCLES, AND HORMONE PRODUCTION

- Alcohol impairs the brain's GnRH pulse generator that triggers proper release of FSH and LH. This in turn causes low estradiol and reduced ovarian function in women.
- Cycle length shows greater variability in women drinkers than in non-drinkers—some cycles are long, some are short, and there are more skipped cycles.
- Estradiol and testosterone levels decline earlier in women who drink alcohol regularly, which lead to a rise in FSH at younger ages. All of these changes lead to decreased fertility.
- Women drinkers have more cycles in which they do not ovulate, another way that fertility is impaired. They are also more likely to suffer amenorrhea, or unpredictable loss of regular menses.
- Women who drink alcohol regularly have heavier menstrual flow and more painful menstruation (dysmenorrhea). In one study, this effect was seen in women who had just one six-drink "binge" a week; these effects are also seen in women who average three or more drinks a day.
- Alcohol use leads to markedly higher rates of premenstrual distress and severe PMS, regardless of age, income, educational level, or occupation.
- Women have greater sensitivity to brain damage and neurotoxicity from alcohol than men do. In a 2001 study, Dr. D. W. Hommer found that women alcoholics had significantly smaller volumes of gray and white matter as well as greater volumes of cerebrospinal fluid in the brain than nonalcoholic women; alcoholic women also had smaller volumes of gray matter than alcoholic men.
- Alcohol (a depressant drug) causes more problems with decrease in sexual desire, arousal, and orgasm in women than in men. Studies show that 70 to 75 percent of women drinkers had these problems.
- In addition to alcohol causing early loss of ovarian hormones, it also causes early bone loss by decreasing absorption of calcium, increasing calcium loss in urine, and decreasing the action of bone-building osteoblasts.
- Regular alcohol use causes an increase in early abortions and miscarriages.
- Alcohol causes birth defects by acting as a teratogen: Fetal alcohol syndrome consists of growth retardation; small head circumference; mild to moderate mental retardation; plus a variety of skeletal, joint, genital, heart, kidney, and skin effects.
- Women who overuse alcohol have higher rates of stillbirths, premature births, and babies with birth defects.

feel like it is something chemical, like a switch is flipped in my brain, and I have to have that alcohol. It's a horrible feeling."

What chemical change with her cycle could explain this? Many women don't realize that the rise in progesterone in the second half of the cycle causes more difficulty handling simple sugars. Especially if the estradiol is lower than optimal as progesterone rises, your body has even more difficulty responding normally to glucose. You have more glucose fluctuations and drops in blood glucose, which we call *reactive hypoglycemia*. The drop in blood sugar is a powerful trigger for alcohol cravings because alcohol behaves in the digestive process like sugars and it will quickly raise blood glucose. All the symptoms from falling or low blood sugar—anxiety, restlessness, low energy, etc.—are relieved quickly by alcohol, and you feel better for a short while. Then, as alcohol levels drop, blood sugar falls, the symptoms return, and you crave alcohol again. The drop in estradiol and progesterone just before your bleeding begins also causes a fall in brain endorphins and serotonin. These are your "feel good" brain chemicals, and when they fall quickly, it causes more anxiety, insomnia, blue moods, irritability, and low energy. Many women then "treat" these problems with a glass of wine, beer, or liquor, and the cycle continues. Alcohol also affects metabolism of the hormones you take in birth control pills or for menopause, adding another factor to the potential for alcohol cravings. Breaking free of this vicious cycle means taking steps to stop alcohol use *and* to stabilize the hormone fluctuations at the same time.

There is another health risk for women to consider. Alcohol use is an *independent* risk factor for breast cancer. This means that the increased risk is not due to other variables, such as total calories, fat, fiber, vitamins, or whether you take hormones. The *age* at which you begin drinking is important; the earlier you start drinking, the greater your risk, regardless of how much you drink later in life. Risk of breast cancer is greatest if regular drinking begins during the vulnerable time of breast development in your teens.

The first study to link alcohol consumption to breast cancer risk was published in 1977. Since then, we have many studies from a variety of countries showing similar results: Even moderate alcohol consumption—*three or more drinks per week*—increases breast cancer risk anywhere from 20 to 70 percent. Your risk is increased even more if you drink more than nine drinks. The more you drink, the more upper body fat you gain, and this further adds to breast cancer risk, as well as risk of diabetes and heart disease.

The mechanism for alcohol effect on cancer risk is not yet fully known. There is speculation that it may alter hormonal balance by increasing estrone and the androgens in fat tissue. Alcohol causes a rise in the blood level of estrone by several pathways: It stimulates the liver to make more estrone, and it also stimulates fat tissues to convert more androgen (androstenedione) to estrone. As you read earlier, estrone is the form of estrogen associated with a higher risk of breast and endometrial cancer. You can minimize the "estrone factor" in risk for both cancers by reducing or eliminating alcohol use, and by losing excess body fat.

In women taking hormones, alcohol raises the blood levels of estrone significantly. In women taking Premarin, estrone and estradiol levels increased more than threefold after drinking alcohol; this same effect also occurred in women taking micronized estradiol tablets. Among current hormone users in the Nurses Health Study and the Iowa Women's Health Study, the risk of breast cancer was increased *only* among those women who also drank alcohol. In both of these studies, the excess risk of breast cancer was *not* seen in all estrogen users, just those who also drank alcohol. Yet all you hear in the news is that "estrogen" increases breast cancer risk! A study from Italy published in 2000 found that alcohol use accounted for about 12 percent of the risk for breast cancer, making alcohol a highly significant, and avoidable, risk factor. In addition to effects on hormone metabolism, alcohol also interferes with normal immune function and stimulates excessively high levels of insulin, another newly identified independent risk factor for breast cancer.

You may have heard that alcohol lowers the risk of heart disease. It turns out that this effect was primarily seen in men, not women. For men, the risk of heart disease decreased significantly even in the higher ranges of alcohol intake. In women, there was a slight decrease in heart disease risk at the lowest levels of alcohol use each week, but a marked increase in deaths from heart disease at higher levels of alcohol use per week. Women's bodies simply show more of the damaging effects from alcohol than do men's. Given all the negative effects on your ovaries, fertility, mood, sleep, memory, and body weight, I encourage you to minimize alcohol use.

Marijuana

Few people today haven't heard of marijuana, a mixture of dried, shredded leaves, stems, seeds, and flowers of the hemp plant. You may have even tried smoking it, and may already know its many mind-altering properties. Women who smoke marijuana regularly also have disturbances in ovulation that make it hard to become pregnant; marijuana also causes more frequent early miscarriages. Marijuana causes abnormalities in the baby, such as abnormal brain function, small head size, shorter height, and lower birth weight, even if the baby is carried full term.

THC, or tetrahydrocannabinol, is the primary brain-active chemical in marijuana that makes you high. The amount of THC varies greatly depending on the type of marijuana and where it is grown. All forms of marijuana affect brain pathways directly. It causes impaired memory, attention, and concentration, as well as difficulty thinking, diminished problem-solving, loss of coordination, and distorted perception. For women athletes, marijuana interferes with timing, causing slower movements and impaired coordination, so you don't perform your best. It also impairs judgment, perception, ability to judge distances, and the ability to react quickly. These same marijuana effects also interfere with your ability to drive a car, causing similar incoordination and slowed reactions as alcohol does in standard drunk-driver tests.

What many young people, and even doctors, overlook is that marijuana disrupts brain centers that regulate hormone production in both males and females. Luteinizing hormone (LH) is suppressed by marijuana so that it doesn't rise at midcycle to trigger ovulation. This is one way it can impair your fertility if used regularly. Extracts of marijuana plants contain two chemicals—*cannabidiol* and *apigenin* (a flavinoid phytoestrogen)—that compete with estradiol for binding at the estrogen receptor. Marijuana also can elevate prolactin, a pituitary hormone that in turn suppresses the normal menstrual cycle and ovarian hormone production. So marijuana can decrease ovarian estradiol production, as well as compete with what estradiol you do produce for binding at the estrogen receptor. If you and your partner are having trouble getting pregnant, keep in mind that marijuana also leads to abnormal sperm development and significantly decreased testosterone in men. The hormone effects of marijuana can even cause men to develop enlarged breasts (gynecomastia) and to have difficulty having an erection. Endocrine effects of marijuana can damage sexual function and fertility in both sexes.

If all this weren't enough, a study published in June of 2001 found that the risk of a heart attack jumps nearly fivefold during the first hour after smoking marijuana, posing a particular threat to anyone with other risk factors for heart disease. Researchers at Beth Israel Deaconess Medical Center in Boston found that heart rate can double after smoking a single marijuana cigarette. Marijuana may initiate a heart attack by causing a piece of plaque inside a coronary artery to rupture and form a clot, which then blocks the flow of blood to the heart muscle. Marijuana also decreases blood flow to the heart by increasing blood pressure. This means that active chemicals in marijuana increase the heart's demand for oxygen, while at the same time decreasing the supply of oxygen in the blood. The likelihood of suffering a heart attack was 4.8 times greater in the first hour after smoking marijuana when compared to periods of not smoking the drug.

The fact that marijuana causes earlier loss of estradiol and its immune-enhancing functions makes women even more vulnerable to marijuana's other adverse effects, such as on the lungs. Marijuana contains cancer-causing compounds similar to those found in cigarette smoke, although the ones in marijuana are even more damaging to the lungs than tobacco smoke. For example, someone who smokes five joints a week is getting as many cancer-causing chemicals as a cigarette smoker who smokes a whole pack of cigarettes a day. Chemicals in marijuana are also irritating to the lungs and can lead to immediate problems with chronic coughs, wheezing, and even asthma in susceptible people. Women who regularly smoke marijuana, like cigarette smokers, have more frequent respiratory infections and pneumonias both from the suppression of their ovarian hormones and from the direct toxic effects of the drug itself.

Although some people say they use marijuana because it "calms" them, it can also increase heart rate and actually cause anxiety. And it leads to palpitations and anxiety as it wears off. Either way, you may find that you are *more* anxious if you are using marijuana regularly. Since it also reduces the hormones of the ovary, such as estradiol and progesterone, you may also experience more anxiety as a result of lower levels of these hormones. THC and other chemicals in marijuana also disrupt normal immune function, leading to more episodes of chronic illness. Obviously, this "recreational" drug is much more damaging than you may have realized.

CNS Stimulants: Cocaine and Others

Cocaine and other brain stimulants such as ecstasy have the potential to disrupt the hormone-regulating pathways of the hypothalamus and pituitary that govern ovarian cycles. Women who abuse these drugs often have changes in their menstrual cycles, particularly if there is significant weight loss due to the appetite-suppressing effects of regular use. Cocaine also changes how fallopian tubes function, interfering with your ability to get pregnant. We don't yet know exactly how this tubal abnormality occurs in cocaine users, but it is important if you have trouble conceiving.

Brain effects of these drugs can be profound. In 2001, Dutch scientists reported that women are more likely than men to suffer brain cell damage from regular use of the party drug ecstasy. The damage appears to selectively hit nerve endings that release serotonin, but may also damage brain cells that oversee nerve signal transmission. Using sophisticated PET scans of brain function, recent studies in the United States have shown that a single "hit" of cocaine causes permanent changes in the brain that set you up for addiction and the vicious cycle of highs followed by severe crashes into profound, sometimes suicidal, depression. Cocaine also causes constriction of the arteries serving the heart and can increase the risk of heart attack up to twenty-five-fold during the first hour after use. This is one of the reasons for the "sudden death" that occurs in cocaine users. For women at certain low estrogen stages of the menstrual cycle, the risk of coronary artery spasm and low blood flow to the heart is even greater with cocaine use. Besides contributing to infertility and ovarian hormone problems, "coke" can permanently scramble your brain, send your blood pressure soaring, or kill your heart.

In Summary

I see women every day having problems with menstrually triggered mood swings, headaches, body aches, low energy, loss of sex drive, changes in menstrual cycle, trouble getting pregnant, or a number of other bothersome symptoms related to hormone changes. Many of my patients haven't even considered that something that seems socially accepted like smoking, drinking, or "recreational" drug use could be directly linked to problems with their ovaries and hormones. These are not simple pleasures or harmless ways to relax. For all the many reasons I have described, just say *no* to these chemicals that mess up your hormones!

LIFESTYLE HABIT	ACTIONS	OVARY EFFECT
Cigarette smoking	↓ serotonin production ↓ blood flow ↑ norepinephrine (Nicotine is a stimulant.)	Toxic to follicles; increases liver breakdown of E2; causes premature menopause

Caffeine	Diuretic—depletes minerals
	Stimulant effects on brain
	Disrupts normal sleep
	    (↓ Stage 4)
	Alters serotonin-
	    norepinephrine balance
		May disrupt normal
		menstrual cycles if used
		to excess

Alcohol	Depresses CNS
	Adrenaline rebound
	    (when wears off)
	Interferes with ovarian
	    function
	Damages muscle fibers
	↓ absorption of B vitamins
	↓ Stage 4 sleep
	Damage to nerve endings
		Even moderate use
		increases estrone levels,
		disrupts normal
		menstrual cycle;
		associated with
		infertility if used
		heavily; increases risk of
		breast cancer

Marijuana	Alters serotonin-
	    norepinephrine balance
	Suppresses LH
	Elevates prolactin
	Competes with estrogen
	    at receptors
		Disrupts ovarian cycles;
		decreases hormone
		levels; kills follicles;
		impairs fertility

7

Ovary Shutdown: The Toxic Role of Stress Overload and Sleep Deprivation

———

Long Days, Short Nights, Overloaded Lives!

Many of my patients tell me they think they have chronic fatigue syndrome (CFS), but when I ask them to describe a typical day, I'm not so sure a medical syndrome is the source of their fatigue! Let's look at a typical weekday schedule for one of my patients, *Harriet,* a thirty-six-year-old married school administrator and mother of three. Harriet sought a consult for "fatigue, insomnia, low energy, headaches, loss of libido, and difficulty concentrating." This is a snapshot of her usual routine:

Harriet

5:00 A.M.: *Alarm goes off. She gets up, takes a shower, and then starts the family going.*

5:15–6:30 A.M.: *Rousts her husband, three sons, finishes fixing school lunches, prepares quick breakfast (cereal and milk), does quick "tidy up" housework, gets dressed for work while watching the morning news, makes sure the kids have homework, books, and lunches.*

6:30 A.M.: *Husband leaves, taking one son to wrestling practice; arrives at his office between 7:15 and 7:30 A.M.*

6:45 A.M.: *Harriet takes the other two children to school, then drives another forty-five minutes to her office at a large urban junior high school.*

8:00 A.M.: *Her workday "officially" starts and includes dealing with discipline problems, supervising teachers, preparing meeting agendas for teachers and PTA, reviewing school policy and curriculum issues with central-office administrators, monitoring bus lines, meetings with local law enforcement officials about drug and alcohol problems among students, meetings with parents, troubleshooting other administrative problems. Since teachers and principals patrol the cafeteria during lunch, she rarely has time to eat lunch, and usually grabs a soft drink two to three times through the day so the sugar and caffeine keep her going.*

5:30 P.M.: *Leaves work to pick up two of the children at sports practices. Runs errands, picks up a few groceries on her way home.*

6:45–7:00 P.M.: *Arrives home, fixes dinner, oversees the kids' homework (or takes kids to soccer or baseball practice or church youth meetings three nights a week); while waiting for the kids at practices, she pays bills, reads, and sorts mail.*

7:30 P.M.: Husband arrives home; dinner.

8:00–10:30 P.M.: Helps kids with homework, does housework, does several loads of wash, and reviews her own work memos.

10:30 P.M.: Gets the kids to bed, helps lay out clothes and books for the morning, prepares kids' lunches for the next day.

11:45 P.M.: Goes to bed herself, but it often takes her a half hour or more to "unwind" and fall asleep, exhausted after another grueling day.

These are her weekdays. Saturdays are spent cleaning house, doing laundry, planning dinners, buying groceries, paying bills, balancing the checkbook, driving kids to various games, and running errands. Her husband often works at his office on Saturday or takes the kids to events if he is available. On Sundays, they sleep "late," usually getting up about 8:30 or 9:00 A.M. to get ready for Sunday school and church. Sunday afternoons, Dad and the boys typically watch whatever sports events are on television. Mom calls family, tries to get a few "odds and ends" done, and begins getting ready for the week ahead. Sunday dinner is the one meal of the week the entire family is usually together.

Not only is Harriet getting very little sleep, but take a look at what she eats each day. She is nowhere close to a balanced, steady intake of "fuel" for her brain and body. She has a small bowl of cereal and skim milk for breakfast—carbohydrates with little protein or fat to sustain energy and blood sugar over the morning, let alone the rest of the day. This breakfast will sustain blood glucose for about two hours. She doesn't eat lunch; instead, she has a high-sugar soft drink with a jolt of caffeine for an energy boost. The sugar boost lasts about thirty to forty-five minutes before the "crash" of low blood sugar. She has another soft drink, and the cycle repeats. She doesn't eat again until dinner. By then, her body has determined that it's in a famine and has increased its level of the stress hormone cortisol, holding on to every last calorie to store as fat. No wonder she is eating less and gaining weight.

Harriet has a caring, stable marriage; she loves her kids and enjoys her job. She does not perceive her life as overly stressful, just "busy." She had no clue she was reaching perimenopausal levels of her ovarian hormones, and no one she had seen for her health problems considered that issue. Her primary care doctor and gynecologist simply told her to slow down, take some stress-management classes, and "relax more."

In spite of her healthy outlook on life, Harriet's overloaded schedule, poor nutrition, and fragmented sleep were *physiological stressors* that had suppressed her ovaries. Her cycles were now longer with shorter, lighter bleeding days. She was only thirty-six, but she was in premature ovarian decline (POD). Her hormone levels really told the story: her Day 1 estradiol was only 20 pg/ml, and her Day 20 estradiol was only 61 pg/ml (about one fourth an optimal E2 level for this cycle day), progesterone was 8.0 (the lower end of the ovulatory range), and her testosterone was only 10 ng/dl (100 pg/ml).

No wonder she was tired, had headaches, trouble concentrating, no libido, and couldn't sleep. She didn't eat enough *food* fuel, and she certainly didn't have enough *hormone* fuel to sustain her schedule, or enough *sleep* to recharge her body. The three primary solutions were straightforward: I gave her a low-progestin, steady-dose birth control pill to restore her cycles and provide hormone stability. We designed a balanced plan of quick, healthy, simple meals and snacks to sustain energy at work and give her body nutrients. I recommended appropriate doses of vitamins and minerals and encouraged her to take some time for herself and get some exercise!

June was forty-one when I treated her. Her POD symptoms—fatigue, insomnia, headaches, difficulty concentrating, and lack of interest in sex—had an entirely different cause from Harriet's. She had recently lost her parents, both deaths completely unexpected and three months apart. She owned and operated a demanding restaurant business where she put in long hours. After her father died, she took over and ran her father's automobile dealership—clearly a stressful, male-dominated world—in addition to her own business. She was a single mom with two children, and she cared for a younger sister with a serious chronic illness. She had also just broken an engagement. Her losses of significant people were catastrophic, particularly occurring so close together. Although she ate well and exercised several times a week, these overwhelming life stresses affected her health and her ovaries. Her ovarian hormone levels were similar to Harriet's, except her stress hormone, cortisol, was significantly higher. She certainly benefited from hormone management, but I also recommended a therapist for help with her grief, as well as prioritizing her goals for family and businesses.

These women are typical of the ones I see in my office every day. They lead more complex lives with multiple demands—at work, at home, and with extended family. Jobs that were once "men's work" have been added to traditional female roles. Our lives may not be as *physically* demanding as the workloads of our foremothers, but our roles are certainly more stress-filled and mentally demanding. Society pushes us to operate at a higher level. We want and need to function at higher levels of physical and emotional energy as well as cognitive performance. We expect much of ourselves, and feel devastated when we can't achieve all that we want. These combined stresses take their toll.

Stress and What It Does to Your Health

Stress is a constant, inevitable, even *necessary* part of life itself. We live with stress, all of the time. In its broadest sense, stress simply means a stimulus that causes change and adaptation to maintain *homeostasis,* or balance, of our body systems. The stimuli that alter homeostasis are called *stressors.* They come from changes inside the body, like rising or falling blood sugar, or from outside the body, like a hot day that makes you sweat. The stimulus, or stressor, may be an event in your life or a thought or image that comes into your mind. We are constantly bombarded with millions of such stimuli every day. You can't be alive and have *no* stress, because the body itself is undergoing the stimulation (stress) of constant change every moment of every day. The brain monitors and modulates all incoming stimuli, and constantly guides the responses of body systems.

So if stress is constant, and our body always deals with it, how does it cause problems with our health? You read about stress and its body-wrecking effects: cancer, heart attacks, high blood pressure, infertility, allergies, and so on. Is there a balance between the stress that allows the body to survive and thrive, and the stress that slowly destroys us? Why do some people thrive on the stress levels others find overwhelming? Why do some people cope with catastrophic stress and others cave in over trivial events? Physicians and scientists have pondered these observations through the ages.

Viruses, bacteria, and carcinogens alone do not cause illness in every exposed individual. After decades of stress research, we now have a better understanding of the role that individual vulnerability plays in who becomes ill. Most diseases we "moderns" develop are greatly influenced by the physical and psychological environment of our bodies. We now know that many factors play a role in determining who gets sick, how sick they get, and how quickly they recover. Our attitudes, the foods we eat, the vitamins we take, our hormone balance, our energy, our feelings of control and choice, our degree of social support, our faith—all these things matter. The balance between risk factors and our "resistance," or hardiness, helps determine whether we stay healthy or develop acute or chronic illness.

Think about it. Have you unwittingly made your body a compromised host, a fertile "soil" for viral, bacterial, and carcinogenic invaders by the way you live, like Harriet? Or have you developed lifestyle habits and thought patterns that serve as an "inoculation" against disease, such as the way June paid attention to her diet and exercise? Although it isn't a guarantee against "out of nowhere" deaths from cancer, circulatory diseases, and other serious illnesses, there is a lot we can do that will improve our ability to resist the ravages of stress.

What Exactly Is Stress?

Remember, your body faces daily external situational and environmental stressors as well as internal body changes (physiological stressors), and the body itself is the "final common pathway" through which all of these changes act and operate to produce the necessary responses. The body has a set range of responses, regardless of the particular stressor that triggers a response. Our brain constantly perceives and processes information from the world and from moment-to-moment changes within the body. Our brain is a *physiological* organ, as well as the *psychological* organ expressing personality, thoughts, moods, and guiding behavior. Thoughts, moods, and behaviors governed by the brain are a result of both physical and psychological causes.

Many times, patients are diagnosed with a psychological or psychiatric disorder because of changes in mood or behavior. Doctors are *taught* that such symptoms have psychological causes that can be either internal thoughts or external situations. But the brain is a physical organ, so it is just as susceptible to biochemical changes that can trigger the same "psychological"—mood or behavior—symptoms. Anxious or depressed moods may have physical as well as psychological causes. It is a fact of basic biology that falling or low estradiol causes brain changes in chemical messengers (physical changes) that cause anxiety episodes, depressed moods, or difficulty sleeping (psychological symptoms). Likewise, psychological stressors lead to profound physical changes in every cell in the body: blood, arteries, veins, intestinal tract, ovaries, thyroid, immune cells, pain-regulating neurotransmitters, nerve endings, blood sugar levels, brain chemistry, and so on. The equation runs both ways:

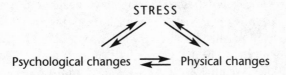

STRESS

Psychological changes ⇌ Physical changes

© Elizabeth Lee Vliet, M.D., 2003

This critical two-way street is often overlooked in health care today, especially when related to women and hormone imbalances.

The Fight-or-Flight Response

The body's "stress response" is sometimes called the *fight-or-flight* pathway. When change hits, it activates the brain's alarm center in the locus ceruleus, setting off a burst of norepinephrine and other chemical messengers that notify the rest of the body within milliseconds to respond. The body reacts to the fight-or-flight signals in hundreds of ways: The adrenal glands rev up production of cortisol, another hormone that oversees stress response. The heart rate goes up to pump more blood. Eyes dilate so we can see better. Blood vessels dilate to deliver more blood to the critical organs—especially the brain and heart and big muscle groups—and blood vessels constrict to decrease blood flow to less critical areas—intestines, hands, feet, scalp. The liver makes more glucose and releases it into the bloodstream to maintain energy. Muscles tense for action. Platelets are put on alert in case they are needed to stop bleeding. All over the body, cells and organs are put on ready alert, all in a split second.

When the "emergency" is over, the body slowly settles back to its normal pace and functions. Everything calms down . . . or does it? What about the way we live today? Rushing around, going long hours without food, staying up late, getting up early, feeling angry, short-tempered, frustrated, overloaded . . . These are all signals that continually activate the fight-or-flight emergency responses. Instead of a short-lived emergency like running from a wild animal as our Stone Age ancestors did, we now keep our bodies in a perpetual state of hyperalert. It's like asking your body to run a marathon every day, with no rest and recovery in between, and not much food for fuel along the way. No smart runner does that! Yet that's what is happening when you live a daily schedule like Harriet's. What does this do to our health over the long haul?

Prolonged stress of any kind disrupts the body's balance, or homeostasis, and causes symptoms related to the constant overactivity of the fight-or-flight stress response pathways—headaches, muscle spasms, fatigue, fuzzy thinking, high blood pressure, irritable bowel, colitis, angina, eczema, frequent infections, irregular periods, acne, weight gain, allergies, hives, herpes outbreaks, anxious/panicky feelings, insomnia, depression, angry/irritable moods, heart disease, cancer.

So you shouldn't be surprised that prolonged stress can lead to suppression of the ovaries. It is part of Mother Nature's protective effects to prevent pregnancy if we are too physiologically "stressed" for our own health and not in optimal shape to sustain a healthy pregnancy. The same biological principle occurs in all species. Mice lose fertility when kept in crowded cages with inadequate food and water and not enough room for their normal "territory." Our biology operates in a similar way to prevent further drain on the body's resources when it is already "running on empty." Look at the consequences of stress on the body in the diagram on page 127. It is no surprise that a doctor's pat on the back and direction to "relax more" or "take an antidepressant" simply won't cut it. You need ways to reduce the damaging effects of toxic stress, which in turn helps all your body systems work better.

Stress, Estrogen, and Coping

Constant stress also suppresses ovarian cycles and decreases estradiol, testosterone, progesterone, and DHEA production. Many studies show a connection, often overlooked, between stress and lower levels of ovarian estrogen, testosterone, and the cyclic production of progesterone. A stress-induced decrease in estradiol then contributes to an imbalance in norepinephrine, serotonin, dopamine, acetylcholine, and other brain-body messengers that regulate pain pathways, sleep, muscle repair, appetite, metabolism, memory, mood, energy, sex drive, and other functions. Women describe being able to cope successfully at other times of their lives, when their hormones were more optimal. Decreased estradiol also negatively affects the brain's chemical messengers, causing a direct impact on women's ability to function optimally when their hormones are out of kilter. Forty-five-year-old *Janie* said it well: "I raised six kids as a single mom, worked full-time, took college classes at night, and I coped just fine with all that stress when I was younger. Now I hit perimenopause and I can't seem to deal with even the smallest stresses without falling apart!"

Women's observations about coping better during times of optimal estradiol fits with what science now shows about the protective effects of this powerful hormone. For example, estradiol acts as an antioxidant, much like vitamins E and C,

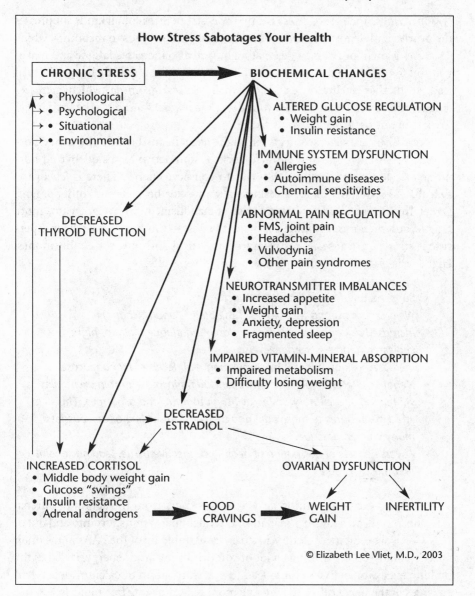

How Stress Sabotages Your Health

CHRONIC STRESS → BIOCHEMICAL CHANGES

- Physiological
- Psychological
- Situational
- Environmental

ALTERED GLUCOSE REGULATION
- Weight gain
- Insulin resistance

IMMUNE SYSTEM DYSFUNCTION
- Allergies
- Autoimmune diseases
- Chemical sensitivities

DECREASED
THYROID FUNCTION

ABNORMAL PAIN REGULATION
- FMS, joint pain
- Headaches
- Vulvodynia
- Other pain syndromes

NEUROTRANSMITTER IMBALANCES
- Increased appetite
- Weight gain
- Anxiety, depression
- Fragmented sleep

IMPAIRED VITAMIN-MINERAL ABSORPTION
- Impaired metabolism
- Difficulty losing weight

DECREASED
ESTRADIOL

INCREASED CORTISOL
- Middle body weight gain
- Glucose "swings"
- Insulin resistance
- Adrenal androgens

OVARIAN DYSFUNCTION

FOOD CRAVINGS → WEIGHT GAIN   INFERTILITY

© Elizabeth Lee Vliet, M.D., 2003

to scavenge "free radicals" made constantly during metabolic processes. Free-radical production increases under stress, contributing to more cell damage. Antioxidants inactivate these free radicals and prevent their damage. Estradiol also helps dilate arteries, including those that serve the heart. When you are under stress, adequate estradiol improves blood flow. All your organs work better with more oxygen, especially your brain! The combined effects of estrogenic hormones help improve our physiological reaction to stress and also regulate vascular metabolic, cognitive, and immune functions critical for us to cope with stress.

Once again, the role of stress is a two-way street: Stress of all kinds suppresses the ovaries and decreases production of estradiol. This leads to insomnia, which decreases growth hormone release at night, and also increases fatigue and makes you feel foggy-brained. The stress of all these negative physical changes in turn leads to further decline in estradiol, which causes insomnia, which increases fatigue, and so on. It can feel like you're stuck in a quicksand pit—the harder you work to get out, the deeper you sink.

Stress also has adverse effects through mechanisms beyond the ovary hormones. Persistent stress and elevated cortisol shift active forms of thyroid hormone into less active, or bound, forms to conserve energy. There is *less* of the available T3 so important for metabolism in muscle, the brain, and other organs. Lower free T3 results in more sluggish metabolism, more weight gain, more fatigue, and then more trouble coping with stress—another stress! Chronic persistent stress also causes excessive adrenal cortisol and other stress hormones. High levels of cortisol over time have many adverse effects:

- *Suppression of normal immune function*
- *Weight gain around the middle of the body ("apple" shape)*
- *Increased risk of heart disease by promoting plaque buildup, higher cholesterol and triglyceride levels*
- *Increased risk of diabetes by stimulating high levels of blood glucose*
- *Negative effects on pain pathways, including increased brain excitability, via release of excitatory amino acids, glutamate, and aspartate. This effect contributes to more pain and the constant feeling of anxiousness many women describe.*
- *Adverse effects on formation of healthy connective tissue, leading to joint and muscle problems*

Release of excitatory amino acids (EAAs) occurs from the action of adrenal stress hormones on sodium, potassium, and calcium ion transport into and out of cells. Cortisol overactivity alone leads to excessive build up of the EAAs in the brain and nerves. If you are drinking a lot of soft drinks for quick energy, it makes the buildup even worse. Excess EAAs lead to overstimulation of calcium-dependent enzymes in the nerve cells and generate more cell-damaging free radicals.

The result is nerve cells die, leading to impaired conduction, abnormal pain regulation, and impaired memory, attention, and concentration. As stress persists, cortisol effects continue to build up over time, further damaging nerve cells in the brain's memory centers. This whole sequence is thought to be one way that memory, thinking, concentration, and focus all diminish when we are under prolonged stress, or have the stress of illness or chronic pain. Women often euphemistically call it "brain fog." Fibromyalgia sufferers call this "fibro-fog."

Besides a toxic effect on brain cells, excess cortisol impairs normal metabolism of collagen, which is the basis of healthy connective tissue, or fascia. You then have more muscle and joint injuries and pain. Wound healing becomes impaired. Overproduction of cortisol also disrupts the sleep cycle, which in turn means more fatigue, less growth hormone release, and less muscle repair at night. These negative changes further compound the sleep problems and muscle-damaging effects already occurring from the declining estradiol. High cortisol levels and prolonged stress also increase the body's need for antioxidants, vitamins, minerals, and all the macronutrients. But lower than optimal estradiol means these aren't as well absorbed from the stomach and intestinal tract. Plus, when we are stressed and don't feel well, we don't take the time to eat nutritionally balanced meals—we may eat too much junk food, or overeat or undereat. Poor nutrition then becomes another stress on our body. It is all intertwined.

Prenatal Stress: Does It Set Up Problems for Life?

We have discussed the effects of stress, mostly after puberty. But what about its impact on a developing baby? This is another adverse consequence of our high-stress lives. The damaging effects of prenatal stress have been found in studies of both humans and animals. These effects in offspring include attentional deficits, learning disorders, hyperanxiety, disturbed social behavior, and impaired coping skills. Many are similar to those of a biological depression, which suggests that stress on mothers during pregnancy can increase the possibility for children to develop depression later in life.

The specific mechanisms of this are not fully known. High levels of the mother's stress hormones during pregnancy appear to cause long-lasting changes in the brain of the developing baby. These brain changes include disturbance in the regulation of the hypothalamic-pituitary-adrenal pathways, decreased feed-back inhibition of corticotropin-releasing hormone (CRH), higher overall levels of CRH in parts of the brain, elevated cortisol production in response to stress, ✗ fewer cortisol receptors in the brain's memory center, reduced effectiveness of the inhibitory activity of the brain's GABA (benzodiazepine) and endorphin (opioid) chemical messenger systems. If there is less effective function of the GABA and endorphin systems, there are more anxiety, pain, and sleep problems.

Children of mothers overly stressed during pregnancy can experience delayed puberty because of alterations in the normal patterns of FSH and LH that over-see the ovaries and regulate menstrual cycles. Stress increases release of the brain hormone corticotropin-releasing factor (CRF), which in turn inhibits release of the hormone GnRH, which governs our menstrual cycles. If GnRH isn't released properly, the ovarian cycles don't occur normally, resulting in low hormone production, which in turn affects all the multiple body pathways we have been discussing.

Stress: It is complicated and has profound implications for all aspects of women's health. The cumulative effects of persistent high cortisol levels and chronic stress adversely affect practically every pathway in the human body, especially women's ovarian hormone balance. If you want more information, read *Why Zebras Don't Get Ulcers* by Robert M. Sapolsky, an excellent, humorous review of the damaging effects of excess corticosteroids over time.

Sleep Deprivation: Toxic to Your Ovaries and Your Health

Tossing and turning, waking up wide-eyed, looking at the clock, going back to sleep, waking up, looking at the clock. I have experienced episodes of disturbed sleep and thought I'd go nuts. I had always been a good sleeper until I hit age thirty-seven or thirty-eight. I couldn't figure out what was happening. My doctors thought it was the stress of a medical practice (made sense, given how busy I was), and I acquiesced to that idea. Premature menopause never entered my head. Later, it dawned on me that I had been under a lot of stress at other times in my life and did not have the same problems. What was going on? It turned out, probably from all the running I was doing at the time, my estradiol levels were actually quite low even though I had not yet hit forty. The loss of estradiol caused the frequent waking up. Within two weeks of starting on the estradiol patch, I was back to my normal sound sleep again.

A good night's sleep is more crucial to our health and well-being than most women realize. The quality of sleep is a major determinant of whether we are healthy, have an enjoyable life, and function optimally on a daily basis. Women are 50 percent more likely than men to suffer chronic insomnia. About 75 percent of women in this country get less than eight hours of sleep a night. Close to one in five women get less than six hours of sleep each night during the workweek. Women are also prescribed far more sleeping pills than men, but common hormonal causes of insomnia are rarely ever checked. Persistent sleep disruption and loss of sleep over time leads to drowsiness and fatigue, feeling "foggy"-brained, memory loss, difficulties with concentration and focus, impaired judgment, depression, agitated-anxious moods, suppression of optimal ovarian hormone production, muscle pain syndromes, disruption of the immune system, and even loss of libido. A recent study even found that reaction times slow down when we are sleep-deprived: up to 50 percent slower after seventeen to nineteen hours awake than they are if you are legally drunk. This study of people in their thirties and forties looked at several measures: mental and physical reaction times, accuracy, coordination, and attention span. The more hours without sleep, the worse they performed. And I haven't even listed *all* the negative effects of sleep loss.

Based on the above, you see how lack of sleep costs society billions of dollars in lost productivity, and leads to over 100,000 car and truck accidents a year. And if sleep deprivation is prolonged, it can lead to acute psychosis with full-blown hallucinations and delusions. Sleep deprivation is regularly used in POW camps as a form of torture, and can lead to sudden death syndromes. If laboratory rats are robbed of sleep, they die within a few weeks. Sleep deprivation is too critical to ignore. Insomnia has many causes. I list some common ones on page 131.

SOME COMMON CAUSES OF INSOMNIA

- Hormonal changes (ovary, thyroid, adrenal, pituitary, etc.)
- Pregnancy—physical and hormonal changes
- Drug and alcohol abuse (acute effects and withdrawal)
- Tobacco (nicotine) use, nicotine patches
- Excess caffeine (sodas, coffee, tea, chocolate)
- Stimulants in "metabolic" or "energy" boosters (examples include herbs with ephedra, also called *ma huang,* phenylpropanolamine [PPA])
- Use of OTC weight-loss products (many contain gotu kola and other herbal stimulants)
- Medical disorders, such as asthma, allergies, other types of breathing disorders, congestive heart failure, diabetes, fibromyalgia, sleep apnea, narcolepsy, restless legs syndrome, myoclonus, and many others
- Medications, such as decongestants in allergy and cold medicines, theophylline (asthma), some antidepressants, testosterone or DHEA (if taken at night), corticosteroids (e.g., Prednisone), beta-blockers, and many others
- Jet lag, or shift work that disrupts normal sleep-wake cycles
- Working late after the evening meal
- Sensitivity to environmental chemicals, perfumes, cleaning products
- Clinical depression, generalized anxiety disorders
- Life stress, persistent worries, bereavement, post-traumatic stress disorders
- Poor sleep habits (Making your bed a home office doesn't help you relax!)

© Elizabeth Lee Vliet, M.D., 2003

Sleep 101

We take sleep for granted, although it seems rather mysterious. We breathe, yet it is as if we are unconscious. We dream of action and movement, but our muscles are completely paralyzed. What is sleep, really? What are the normal stages we go through each night? What does sleep actually do? Let's review some basics, since it is so critical to our well-being.

Sleep architecture is the medical term used to describe the normal pattern of sleep stages (shown in the table on page 132). Each is characterized by different electrical activity, or "brain wave" patterns, measured on electroencephalogram (EEG) tracings, eye movement measures (EOM), and muscle activity (EMG). Non-REM sleep (NREM) are the four stages in which dreaming does not occur. REM sleep is the stage in which dreaming occurs, along with other physiological responses like penile erections or clitoral engorgement. Problems with sleep (apnea, narcolepsy, and others) are evaluated in sleep laboratories to determine the specific type of disorder, which helps determine proper treatment.

Normal Sleep Architecture

	TYPES OF BRAIN WAVE PATTERNS (EEG)	EYE MOVEMENTS	MUSCLE ACTION, VITAL SIGNS
Awake	Mainly alpha waves, some beta	Depends on task	Normal tone; able to have directed, voluntary movement
NREM— Stage 1	Mixed theta, beta waves; alpha less than 50 percent	Slow, rolling	Relaxed; less tone; slower heart and breathing rates; lower blood pressure (BP)
NREM— Stage 2 etc.	Theta, bursts of sleep spindles,	Slow, rolling	Relaxed; less tone; slow heart and breathing rate; lower BP
NREM— Stage 3 (deep sleep)	Delta waves ("slow wave sleep") 20 to 50 percent	Slow	Relaxed, limp; slow heart and breathing rate, low BP; release of growth hormone
NREM— Stage 4 (deep sleep)	Delta waves now more than 50 percent on EEG	Slow	Relaxed, limp; slow heart and breathing rate, low BP; blood flow directed toward muscles, less to brain; GH released
REM (dreaming)	Similar to waking	Symmetrical, rapid, jerky	None (muscles are in effect "paralyzed"); penile erections, clitoral engorgement occur

© Elizabeth Lee Vliet, M.D., 2003

You experience seventy- to one-hundred-minute cycles of all stages each night. You have more non-REM sleep in the first half of the night, and more REM (dreaming) sleep in the second half. NREM Stages 3 and 4, called *deep sleep*, are the stages where the physical body's "wear and tear" are repaired and restored. Most Stage 3 and 4 deep sleep occurs in the first half of the night. Toward morning, REM sleep stages get longer and alternate with Stage 2 sleep. REM accounts for about 20 percent of our total sleep time, and on average, you enter REM sleep about every ninety minutes throughout the night. Just as non-REM deep sleep restores the body, REM, or dreaming, sleep is thought to restore the brain-mind and helps maintain normal learning and memory during the day.

As an example of a way that deep sleep restores the body, most of our daily amount of growth hormone (GH) is secreted in Stages 3 and 4 each night. GH oversees muscle growth and repair as one of its many functions. If these sleep stages are disrupted, such as by declining estradiol, then you lose the benefits of optimal GH to build new muscle tissue and repair the minor tears in muscle fibers. Loss of optimal GH means you are likely to gain weight, because new muscle isn't made. Leptin is another hormone decreased by sleep deprivation. When leptin is present in normal amounts and cells respond to it properly, it tells us when we are full after eating. If sleep loss persists, leptin decreases and you crave carbohydrates, even though you may actually have had enough total calories for the day. This is another reason we gain fat. Most of us really need eight hours of sleep each night, yet the overwhelming majority of Americans average between six and seven hours. It is not true that we need less sleep as we get older, but sleep *quality* declines for both men and women for a number of reasons, even in healthy individuals. Poor-quality sleep can be caused by many factors, such as hormone declines with age, obesity, alcohol use, cigarette smoking, use of decongestants, drinking coffee late in the evening, plus a number of medical disorders.

People often turn to sleeping pills to treat insomnia, but this causes problems if you use them for more than a couple of weeks. They interrupt normal sleep stages and alter the normal balance and progression of sleep stages so that it is actually harder to get good-quality sleep. Many people who take longer-acting sleeping pills, such as Klonopin, Restoril, or Dalmane, wake up feeling groggy and tired in the morning. Shorter-acting ones, such as Halcion or Ambien, may wake you up too early because they wear off in about 3 hours. Eventually, sleeping pills make it harder for the body and brain to function normally and further impair energy, mood, and memory. These are some of the reasons I do not like women to use sleeping pills without first looking for the underlying causes of sleep problems, *including* hormone changes. If insomnia persists after your hormone levels are optimal and other simple causes corrected, I think the next step should be a sleep study to check for more serious disorders. Sleep apnea, for example, can be dangerous in combination with sleeping pills and causes many other health problems.

Your Hormones and Sleep

Estradiol produced in the ovary is one of the primary hormones regulating the brain's sleep center. When estradiol declines, whether from menopause or other causes, we experience difficulty falling asleep and disruption of our normal stages of sleep, especially Stage 4, our deep, restorative sleep. This is a common scenario I see in my patients. It doesn't matter what age you are; if you have a hormone imbalance and too little estradiol, it can lead to insomnia, whether it occurs from PCOS making too much testosterone and DHEA and not enough estradiol, a postpartum hormone crash, having a hysterectomy with removal of the ovaries and not enough estradiol replacement, or hitting perimenopause.

Low estradiol makes it hard to fall asleep in several ways, such as by decreased serotonin activity and changes in the balance of other chemical messengers in the brain. You lay there, your mind obsessively stuck in worries from the day, unable to drift off to sleep. As estradiol levels drop—whether before a menstrual period, after ovulation, after a baby is born, from too much dieting or exercise, or at menopause—it triggers the "alarm" centers in the brain. These centers then discharge a burst of an adrenaline-type chemical messengers that "alert" you and you wake up. The burst of adrenaline also hits the brain's heat-regulating center, short-circuits those pathways, and triggers a "hot flash" or "flush," followed by sweating that also wakes you up. These awakening episodes may be just a few, or may be many times a night. They leave you tired, groggy, and often grumpy. Women must have adequate estradiol for normal deep, restful sleep.

Progesterone also has effects on sleep, but acts on different pathways from those regulated by estradiol. Taking progesterone doesn't *eliminate* the need for estradiol to restore sleep, as some books claim. A number of progesterone metabolites act at the same brain receptors as barbiturates and benzodiazepines, medications such as Klonopin, Ativan, Valium, Xanax, and Ambien. The result is progesterone breakdown products that can have potent sedative effects.

During the first few days of bleeding each month, many women report restless sleep. Some blame headaches or cramps, but falling estradiol and progesterone are more likely triggers for difficulty falling asleep, restless sleep, and early morning wakening. Falling estradiol disrupts the sleep regulatory cycle, and falling progesterone takes the lid off the GABA inhibitory pathways—much like stopping Valium suddenly. Both of these effects cause increased release of norepinephrine, which acts like little jolts of electric current stimulating brain and body, keeping you awake or waking you up throughout the night.

How you take progesterone makes a significant difference in the sedative effects it produces. The liver "first pass" metabolism makes most of these sedative breakdown compounds from progesterone, which means you have a much greater sedative effect if you take progesterone orally. A non-oral form—vaginal gel, rectal suppository, sublingual troche, or an injection—is directly absorbed into the bloodstream and bypasses the first step in the liver, so it means less sedative effects. Since progesterone can make you sleepy, there are occasionally times when it is a useful addition to hormone therapy, even if you've had a hysterectomy and don't need progesterone to prevent uterine cancer. For progesterone to be effective in helping you sleep, however, estradiol also needs to be restored to optimal levels. Taking progesterone every night for sleep must be balanced against its unwanted, potentially negative metabolic effects such as weight gain. If progesterone is used just to improve sleep for a woman who has had a hysterectomy, it can be effective in a lower dose (such as 25–50 mg) than what is needed to prevent excess buildup of the uterine lining.

When Sleep Isn't Normal: Sleep Disorders and Your Health

Fragmented sleep, multiple awakenings, jerky movements, and abnormal breathing during sleep can all be triggered by loss of our optimal estradiol. Young women with PCOS, women with excessive weight gain as result of hormone imbalance, young women whose diet/intense exercise or stress suppressed their ovaries, postpartum women whose estradiol has plummeted, perimenopausal or menopausal women with low hormone levels—all have the potential for sleep disruption. Disordered sleep can progress to more severe forms, such as restless legs syndrome (RLS) or sleep apnea syndrome (SAS), a potentially serious disorder. RLS can occur in women with thyroid abnormalities or low iron stores (ferritin). While RLS is not potentially life-threatening in the way sleep apnea is, it does cause frequent awakenings. And because it interferes with deep Stage 4 sleep that restores the mind and body, it is a cause of daytime fatigue, mood problems, and even weight gain.

If the sleep disturbance is severe, prolonged, and includes significant apnea (stopped breathing) spells that cause oxygen loss, the consequences can be more severe. Sleep apnea is a significant contributing risk factor for high blood pressure, cardiovascular disease, heart attacks, early morning sudden death, major depression, and sexual dysfunction. Such serious consequences occur from the dangerous drops in oxygen (O_2 saturation) in the blood when you stop breathing.

Sleep apnea combined with a drop in estradiol from perimenopause, menopause, or POD results in *combined* effects, causing women to have a greater vulnerability to sudden death or heart attack than men. Oxygen saturation drops when you stop breathing. Low oxygen is made worse by the drop in estradiol, which causes a burst of catecholamines that trigger pounding heartbeats, palpitations, and unstable heart rate and blood pressure. This fall in estradiol and the burst of catecholamines is the same trigger for hot flashes and night sweats. The result is that lower oxygen content in the blood creates less effective blood delivery to the heart due to both high blood pressure and too rapid a heartbeat . . . all of which increase the possibility of a sudden heart attack.

Current therapeutic options for sleep apnea are limited to weight loss, surgery, and/or continuous positive airway pressure (CPAP), so it would be helpful to know whether hormone changes (as in PCOS, postpartum, perimenopause, or menopause) play a role in the development of sleep apnea, and whether the use of hormone therapies to restore optimal balance can alleviate sleep disorder symptoms. Recent studies from several countries show positive benefits of estrogen on sleep apnea. Earlier studies found no effect on sleep apnea from progestin without estrogen. Both estradiol alone and estradiol with medroxyprogesterone acetate (MPA) regimens decreased sleep apnea significantly. Researchers concluded that hormone therapy has a potential role in reducing sleep apnea syndrome and its many associated health risks.

Doctors previously thought fragmented sleep and the multiple awakenings women commonly experience in postpartum, perimenopause, or menopause were due solely to nighttime hot flashes. This sleep apnea study, however, showed this assumption is not correct: 40 percent of the waking episodes in the study were *not* associated with hot flashes. Waking episodes and hot flashes are each separate and *independent* ways the brain responds to falling or low estradiol. This explains why so many younger women with hormone problems report waking up frequently at night, without classic hot flashes.

Since sleep apnea is a more serious sleep problem, such positive findings about hormone therapy effects on sleep are promising for women with milder forms of insomnia. There are many mechanisms by which estradiol, alone or with progesterone/progestins, interacts with neurotransmitters and regulates brain centers involved in sleep pathways. Women have told doctors all along that our ovarian hormones *do* play a significant role in normal sleep, and when our hormones are out of kilter we don't sleep well. It doesn't matter how old or young we are, because this is a *hormone* effect, not an *age* effect. I have adolescent patients with low estradiol who have exactly the same fragmented sleep as my menopausal patients with low estradiol. My patients consistently say their sleep is better when hormone therapy includes estradiol.

I think it is important for physicians not to dismiss sleep problems in women as "just stress," and prescribe sleeping pills, if they haven't checked hormone levels. If women actually have sleep apnea, sleeping pills can cause more episodes of not breathing, making a bad situation even worse. If your bed partner says your legs move all night, or you snore, or that you seem to stop breathing and then "jerk" back into a loud breathing, talk with a physician about sleep studies and insist on getting your estradiol level checked.

Anger and Our Hormones: Toxic Effects of Negativity

One of our nurse practitioners is a wise woman and astute clinician who cares deeply about her work in women's health and who often has "pithy" insights. She and I, both sufferers of hormone-related problems of varying degrees, were talking about some of the difficult situations we encounter with our patients. She said: "You know, a lot of these women are really *angry* about all they have been through. They are angry at doctors who have dismissed these hormone connections."

Click. Something fell into place in my mind. Yes. I have felt the anger from many patients during consults, although I may not have verbalized it. These women have both expressed and suppressed anger for many reasons: anger at losing significant relationships when sexual interest dies from lack of hormone catalysts; anger at having headaches; anger at feeling betrayed by the body and not having the energy to do what they want; anger at not feeling listened to or validated when they sought help; anger about not getting answers as to how to feel better; and anger at losing quality of life. As one woman said, "I think these hormone problems *robbed* me of my life and career!"

People cannot be separated into emotions or body. We are both. If the mind is tortured with angry, negative feelings, the body responds with an outpouring of cortisol, a stress response that blocks healthy function of both ovaries and thyroid. If your emotions are "out of control," the stress feeds back to the body and leads to a physical shutdown. The anger—whatever the source or cause—must be resolved for healing to take place.

You have likely experienced the way anger causes physical symptoms: neck muscles tighten up and spasm, or you get a headache or diarrhea. Maybe you have hives, or your herpes breaks out again. There are a hundred ways anger is felt physically. Muscles bound by the threads of anger tension are *going* to hurt. Do a check right now. Think of something that makes you really angry, concentrate on it, and notice what happens to your neck and shoulder muscles. What happens to your gut? What happens to your heartbeat? You can't avoid the physiological responses anger produces.

Recently, a patient shared a story that graphically demonstrated this anger-hormone connection. This young woman, in her mid-thirties, had a problem with cyclic acne and mood changes, along with memory problems that grew worse at the time of her menstrual period—pretty typical POD "low estrogen"–type symptoms. At her appointment, she seemed to lack full range of motion of her neck and held her head rigidly. It was obvious she was in pain. When I asked her about it, she said, "I really don't know what happened—my neck just started getting tighter and tighter. I'm having trouble turning my head and it really hurts. I can't think of any injury. I skipped my period this month, but that's the only thing I noticed that was different."

After we had talked about her hormone lab results, and therapy with the estradiol patch, I decided to revisit the neck pain and muscle spasms. She casually observed, "You know, my patch seems to be wearing off sooner lately. . . . It seems related to all the stress at my house. . . . My sister-in-law and her three children came to live with us until her husband is transferred back here, and it has really been a zoo at home with my three kids and her three kids. And we don't see eye-to-eye on the way we discipline the kids, so it makes it really hard. I find myself feeling angry with her a lot of the time now. I can't say anything because she's my husband's sister. I get angry that she doesn't seem to appreciate what we are doing for them, and I get angry that she lets her kids do things I don't let mine do. Then I feel bad about myself for being so angry."

Another *click*. I realized the connection between her neck muscle spasms and pain, her missed period, and the estradiol patches wearing off sooner. Her stress hormones were working overtime. By holding her anger, she unconsciously tensed her neck as she literally, and figuratively, "clenched" her jaw to keep from saying something she would regret.

The undercurrent of anger affected her physical body, her menstrual cycle, and how she metabolized the estradiol in the patches. But she didn't appreciate the connection and said, "Oh, I'm really not that angry, we'll get through it; it's really no big deal." I adjusted her estradiol patch dose, and suggested massage therapy sessions for her neck. A month later, the pain pattern had affected her sleep, making her more tired and tense, and less able to "go with the flow" at home. She said at one point, "I can't remember what it feels like to feel normal anymore."

One day I received a letter from her. With big exclamation points she wrote that her neck pain was completely gone, and her menstrual cycles were more regular. "It's amazing. Just as suddenly as all this had come, it dissipated. My sister-in-law and I had finally reached a point where we weren't speaking to one another and she moved out. My symptoms got worse over the next few weeks, and I realized how much anger and resentment I was harboring toward her. One day, just before Christmas, I called her, we apologized to each other, and I ended the conversation with 'take care.' I meant it. That night at dinner I noticed, with complete surprise, that the pain in my neck was completely gone. When I thought back over things, I could see how the simple act of being pleasant to my sister-in-law released the intense anger that was keeping my jaws clenched and my neck muscles so tight. I was amazed at the difference in my body. There are still a lot of hurt feelings in this situation, but I feel I had a big breakthrough in making a choice that helps me feel better, both physically and emotionally."

Her story illustrates a further point. Part of her body tension and hormone disruption was a result of anger, and part was a result of her negative judgments that she was "bad" because she felt angry. In our culture, women are taught that it is "ugly" or "bad" to express anger. We grow up with the message "If you can't say something nice, don't say anything at all." This gets translated into "If you can't be nice, don't be at all." So we clam up, tense up, jam the anger down deep inside where we hope no one will see it. We smile to cover up the anger, trying to pretend all is well.

No matter how bad we feel, we are taught to look pretty and be nice. We wear makeup. We dress nicely. Above all, we smile. If we look pretty and smile, people—including doctors—then say, "How can you be having any problems? You look healthy, you look like you feel fine." This is an important issue, since *hormone imbalance tends not to be a very visible problem*—unless, of course, you are noticeably pale, gaunt, and have lost your hair. For women, showing you don't feel well is often a two-edged sword. If you convey how bad you actually feel, you may be accused of trying to "manipulate" others, or you may be labeled a hypochondriac. It's a catch-22. My staff is often surprised when women come in for their appointments looking so good, after they have talked to them on the phone. In the front office, our patients are wearing their "public face." It is only in the privacy of the consult room that the facade is dropped and their face shows pain, often with tears. But this happens only *if* they feel safe, listened to, and cared about.

When you see many doctors and still don't feel any better, you may feel angry. The anger is built on disappointment and frustration that may be understandable, but it leads you to the next physician carrying the baggage of negative emotions that can alienate the physician and staff from the start. If you are labeled difficult, complaining, or demanding, you become more alienated, feel devalued and discounted, and get angrier. The downward spiral perpetuates itself.

Your conscious mind may pretend the anger doesn't exist, but your body carries the anger. After all, it isn't "acceptable" for a *woman* to feel and show her anger. You're afraid people won't love you if you show your anger, or you may drive away those who could help you. You can fool me, you can fool your other doctors, and you can fool your family. But you cannot fool your body. Your body *knows*.

Like an undertow at the beach sweeping you away, anger can drag you down and drown you if you don't learn effective ways to feel it, flow with it, and release it.

Anger is often a mask for fear. Take a time-out, look inward honestly, and ask yourself, "If I am feeling angry, what am I afraid of? Is there fear hiding under the anger?" You know. Your soul knows. Your body knows. Ask, and then listen. With answers, you can focus on ways of releasing the pent-up corrosive feelings.

"Anger hormones" disrupt the balance of all the others in your body. Anger and fear can be resolved, but you must first admit they are there. Then commit yourself to release the negativity. None of the other medical approaches will work optimally unless you add this one, too. Create an environment where it is safe to express and release your anger—it is essential to getting well. You don't have to do it alone—it's okay to ask for help. There are friends, family, therapists, and others who can guide you. A healthy balance in all aspects of your life is necessary for healing and to keep all your hormones in balance and functioning well.

8

Lifestyle Habits and Cultural Issues—
Unexpected Stress for Our Ovaries

Introduction

Many factors affect ovaries and cause changes in your menstrual cycles. Some result in subtle decreases in frequency of periods, while others cause extreme changes or stop your cycles altogether. Many times we are too busy to notice these changes, or we may actually feel relieved to be rid of the inconvenience. After all, not many of us like the bother of bleeding every month. A lot of young women, particularly athletes, have told me that they were pleased when their periods came less often or stopped. Other patients tell me that even their doctors dismiss the concern, saying things like, "Oh, don't worry about it. You probably don't miss the nuisance anyway." But there are hidden consequences. The "convenience" of no periods can have adverse effects on your body and your future fertility.

The rhythmical nature of our menstrual cycles is governed by the brain's gonadotrophin releasing hormone (GnRH), or "pulse generator," that integrates all the hormonal, metabolic, and neural signals for the normal workings of the ovaries and reproductive function. Before puberty, the brain has mechanisms to keep the GnRH pulse generator in check and prevent menstruation from beginning too soon. After puberty, there are a variety of lifestyle factors, such as frequent use of cigarettes, alcohol, marijuana, cocaine, ecstasy, and other drugs, chronic dieting, as well as the many chemicals, illnesses, and environmental influences that can interfere with the brain's ability to properly regulate the menstrual cycle. Excess stress (both physical and psychological), being significantly underweight (such as anorexia nervosa), obesity, other metabolic disorders, and emotional losses can all disrupt or even stop your normal menstrual cycle.

Lessons from the Track: A Young Woman's Wake-Up Call

Exercise is good, right? We have all heard that it is one of the best "medicines" of all and we should exercise more. Certainly, a balanced program, designed for your needs and limitations, is an essential part of your health plan. But what about the amount of exercise? We all know that *too little* exercise is detrimental, but can you exercise *too much*? Absolutely. Exercise puts a physical demand, or stress, on the body. Too much can lead to injuries and shut down your ovaries, as this young athlete found out.

Tobra was twenty-one. She started running track in high school and had a successful college career. Just before her college graduation, however, she had stress fractures in her spine and was diagnosed with significant bone loss. Her trainer suggested she see me to discuss hormone options, and the possibility of adding other medication to preserve and rebuild bone. Her menstrual periods had begun at about age eleven. She began running competitively at age fourteen, and by fifteen, her periods stopped completely. At nineteen she stopped running for a year because of injury. During this time her menstrual periods returned, although the flow was light. When she resumed competitive running, she again lost her menses. By the time I saw her, she had not had any periods for three years.

In addition to the bone loss and lack of menstrual periods, she was having difficulty sleeping and would wake up feeling tired and slow. She was up multiple times during the night to urinate, and had been embarrassed recently by urinary leakage, especially at the end of races. She had trouble concentrating on her schoolwork, and said, "My short-term memory seems shot. I feel irritable a lot of the time, I cry over little things for no real reason, I don't have any interest in sex, and I have this awful fatigue much of the time now. I just don't feel like myself anymore."

Tobra didn't have any of the usual risk factors for bone loss, such as alcohol use, too many soft drinks, cigarette smoking, stimulant abuse, poor diet, or too little calcium. The extensive training schedule, running five to ten miles a day every day was her only risk factor. Even though running is a weight-bearing activity, her intensive training suppressed her ovaries so that she no longer menstruated. This also meant she didn't have adequate estradiol; her level was less than 20 pg/ml instead of being well over 100 pg/ml, as it should have been at that time in the cycle. Her physical exam showed typical effects of low estrogen such as excess downy facial hair and decreased breast mass. Her DEXA test for bone mineral density (BMD) was far too low for her age at both the spine and the hip. Exercise can only give full benefit to build bone if your estradiol is at a healthy level.

Her doctor had tried to restore her periods with Ortho Tri-Cyclen birth control pills, but she had intolerable side effects and stopped. "I was very emotional, sad, had mood swings, water retention and swelling, especially in my face and legs, along with weight gain and fatigue. I felt horrible and I could hardly run at all." Since she did poorly on that particular balance of estrogen and progestin and the varying hormone doses, I suggested she try Ovcon 35, a steady dose pill with less progestin and more estrogen. I also recommended Actonel, a medicine that prevents bone breakdown and helps build new, healthy bone mass. She also needed to increase her food intake to provide better nutrition for her workouts and recovery, and she had to cut back her training to give her body more time to recover.

After a couple of months, she was sleeping better and had a higher energy level. At six months, the markers of bone breakdown had improved, and she was feeling better, with none of the mood problems she had with Ortho Tri-Cyclen. A year later, Tobra had stopped the birth control pill, thinking she didn't need the hormones if she increased soy in her diet. She was drinking soy shakes, eating tofu instead of meat, and taking soy isoflavone capsules daily. "I thought these were healthy things to do," she said.

But when I repeated her BMD, she had quite a shock: She had lost another 5 percent of her bone mass. I explained to her that soy alone would not restore lost bone, and could inhibit the positive effects of her own body estradiol. I recommended she restart Ovcon 35 and Actonel and stay on both for several years until her bone mineral density built up to a normal range. She continues to do well on this regimen without any adverse side effects. Her bone density improves steadily each year. She now exercises for pleasure and fitness, keeping to a more realistic level that doesn't overstress her body.

Athletic Training and Your Ovaries

The medical term for exercise-induced ovarian suppression is *hypogonadotrophic hypogonadism,* or *hypothalamic amenorrhea.* This condition has been recognized and researched for decades. It has only come to the forefront in recent years with the emergence of competitors in "women's" events who are still prepubescent girls, particularly in such highly publicized events as the Olympics. It is well known that eating disorders and loss of regular menses are common among gymnasts, figure skaters, divers, and swimmers, to name a few. Girls in these sports deal with demanding, incredibly rigorous, training schedules, spending hours every day in practice sessions and weight workouts. They are also under tremendous pressure to have a "perfect body," at least that is true for the skaters, divers, and gymnasts, since judges also evaluate their "artistic presentation" (i.e., appearance).

Two major reasons make these issues of great concern: First, many young nonathletic women are compulsively overexercising, trying to live up to the current images of beauty in our culture. Second, with greater acceptance and encouragement of women athletes, we now have millions of school-age girls, teenagers, and college-age women participating in competitive athletics. Female athletes are pushing the envelope to optimize performance, to win. Competitive levels are now similar to their male counterparts. While these are wonderful opportunities for girls of all ages, we must pay attention to the effect of athletic training on ovarian cycles.

There is a lot more at stake today for elite women athletes: scholarships, multimillion-dollar sport and advertising contracts, endorsements, and cereal-box covers await the best. The underlying message is that skill is not enough; *image* is everything. Female athletes often feel pressured by agents and others to present the "complete package" of top performance and a "perfect"-looking body. In addition to training schedules that keep them quite lean, they often diet to keep perceived excess weight in check. The combination of intensive athletic training and dieting can be devastating: Ovaries shut down, menstrual cycles stop, bone breakdown increases, sleep goes haywire, muscle declines, energy fades. Many athletes encounter declining performance, but don't have a clear picture of why.

Research supports this relationship between exercise intensity and ovary effects. Both gymnasts and long-distance runners have lost menstrual periods at a higher rate and for longer periods than control groups. The findings also show that women who did not have regular periods had a much higher incidence of running-related fractures and lower bone density of the lumbar spine than did women who still had their periods. The women runners who had ceased menstrual periods also had lower thyroid levels, so another important hormone was out of balance and wreaking havoc on body function.

Even relatively mild exercise can disrupt the normal menstrual cycle phases. Studies by researchers at Boston University, published in 1999, found that short-term exercise can cause "egg" (corpus luteum) dysfunction even when exercise is limited to just one half of the cycle, either the follicular or luteal phase. Luteal phase defect was found in 40 percent of women who exercised during the first half (follicular phase) of the cycle, and in 50 percent of women who exercised during the second half, or premenstrual (luteal), phase. This meant there were fewer ovulatory cycles, which could affect fertility. In the control group that didn't exercise, none of the women developed any corpus luteum dysfunction. The researchers concluded the abrupt onset of training altered proper ovulatory function in the second (luteal) phase of the cycle, regardless of which phase of the menstrual cycle the exercise occurred. This is why you should start slowly with a new exercise program and increase intensity gradually. It is also a reason that many fertility specialists recommend women cut back on exercise when they are trying to get pregnant.

We are not certain of all the mechanisms by which exercise suppresses the ovaries, but we do know there are abnormal patterns of hormone secretion in women athletes. Athletic training alters the GnRH pulse generator in the hypothalamus so that it fails to trigger the normal cyclic activity of hypothalamic-pituitary-ovarian pathways. German research found that athletes with menstrual disorders also had significantly lower resting metabolic rates (RMR), even though daily caloric intake did not differ from athletes without menstrual disorders. Estradiol plays an important role in our metabolism, so this study suggests that overtraining and low estradiol decreased metabolic rate. That's the opposite of what we want: We exercise to increase our metabolism, not decrease it!

Chronic Dieting, Anorexia, and Bulimia—Risks to Your Ovaries

By the fourth grade, 80 percent of girls in the United States are already unhappy with their bodies. They think they are too fat, so they start a diet. Dieting slows your metabolism, and makes it harder to maintain healthy weight as you age. More important, dieting damages normal ovarian and thyroid function, which has wide-ranging effects on your entire body and health. The severest forms of dieting—anorexia and bulimia—are devastating to young women's fertility, and set them up for a lifetime struggle with weight. Chronic dieting is often the precursor to obesity, insulin resistance, and diabetes because metabolism is severely disrupted. Why are so many young girls, adolescents, and young adults so obsessed with weight and body size?

One explanation lies in the way we are brainwashed to believe we must be *thin* to be successful, happy, and to attract a man. The distinct message is that if we are not thin, we are not worthwhile. In 2002, the women in fashion magazines and advertisements are thinner than ever, despite years of concern about sending the wrong message about healthy female body size. These images begin in early childhood and continue our entire lives. Most of the time, we are not conscious of how such images profoundly influence us and shape our sense of self and self-worth.

Think about it. What is the image of *"woman"* we are conditioned to believe is desirable? The ideal "woman" in ads is thin, young, muscular, usually white, beautifully groomed, with long legs, sexy feet, perfect white teeth, flawless skin, long thick hair. Most of all, this woman is extremely thin. Size 2 or size 4 thin. She has no body fat; her bones protrude at the shoulder, clavicle, and hip. We think that is how we are supposed to look. Then we berate ourselves if we don't. Pushing ourselves to reach this "ideal" thin body profoundly perturbs all our body systems, in particular the normal healthy function of ovaries and thyroid glands.

Thinness, which usually occurs from undernutrition, is one of the most frequent "suppressors" of normal menstrual cycles and healthy hormone production in young women. Women with full-blown anorexia nervosa lose their menstrual periods completely. But even women without the full-blown disorder push themselves to degrees of thinness that cause irregular cycles, low estradiol production, difficulty getting pregnant, and early bone loss. A 1985 study of women ages twenty to twenty-nine found that dieting for only six weeks (approximately 800–1000 kcal/day) caused plasma estradiol levels to decrease to *menopausal* concentrations during the final two weeks of dieting. In two out of every three women, menstrual cycles were disrupted. It took three to six months for regular cycles to resume after dieting ended. The authors concluded that even *mild* dieting interferes with ovarian hormone production, and causes disturbances of the menstrual cycle.

Ask women to choose thinness or health. Thin wins ninety-nine times out of a hundred. We feel that, at all costs, we must look thinner and younger. Women are affected by these societal images far more than men. Culturally, our identity is tied up with our appearance rather than our career. Women restrict calories, restrict fat (and count every single dirty little fat gram), cut meat, cut dairy, and so on, until nutrition is so imbalanced, the body shuts down and metabolism slows to conserve fuel. That's when you feel cold, tired, and irritable, have dry skin and lifeless hair. You worry you have "chronic fatigue" and spend thousands of dollars on medical consultations, tests, and supplements. But still, you persist with the dieting, always focused on a thinner body, obsessed with wearing a size smaller. I commented to a patient that she was killing herself with dieting and food restriction. I was shocked when she said, "Then at least I will die thin!"

Low ferritin is one dieting-induced physiologic stress that causes fatigue and the likelihood of menstrual cycle disruption. Dietary intake of iron is often insufficient for girls, particularly those who cut out red meat to lose weight or decrease dietary fat. The average American girl today gets 40 to 45 percent of the recommended daily iron. Losing iron in your menstrual blood, coupled with dietary deficits, is likely to cause low ferritin, which stresses the body because it impairs optimal delivery of oxygen, particularly during intensive exercise. Low ferritin also leads to "restless leg" syndrome that disrupts sleep, another physical stress. A study of competitive swimmers found low ferritin levels in 46.8 percent of the girls tested, compared to *none* of the boys. These women did not have full-blown anemia evident on their red–blood cell counts, but they nevertheless had iron depletion with serum ferritin (iron stores) levels less than 12 mcg/L. The researchers did not find that ferritin levels became lower over the course of the swimming season, so they concluded the training had not caused the low ferritin. The cause was low dietary intake along with loss of iron during menstruation. Menstruating girls and women should supplement with iron because of monthly blood loss. Men don't have this monthly source of iron loss and usually get plenty of iron from red meat and other dietary sources.

Dieting ultimately makes you sick, in addition to disrupting your ovaries and their critical hormones. A truly healthy female body cannot coexist with such extreme degrees of thinness. The ovaries simply won't tolerate it. Much like a petulant child pouting in the corner, they shut down and refuse to make the hormones we need. Dieting-induced ovarian suppression and loss of estradiol and testosterone means you push yourself into premature menopause, even though you may only be in your twenties.

We have earlier ovarian decline than our mothers did and are entering perimenopause at younger and younger ages. I am convinced this constant dieting is a factor, and also contributes to infertility. Dieting to reach such impossible goals pushes the body to skip or stop menstruation, sending estradiol production lower than normal, and ovulation occurs less and less often. Thyroid hormones are affected because the active, free hormone converts to the inactive bound portion as a protective response to low food intake in order to conserve energy. Pushing our bodies to such thinness thwarts Mother Nature's plan to keep us fertile. Female hormones are designed to help store fat so we can sustain pregnancies and nourish a growing baby. You won't get pregnant without a minimum percent of body fat because it is the signal to our regulatory systems that there is enough food for mother and baby.

Sadly, I can't fight Hollywood and the media machines that perpetuate these images, but I hope this gives you perspective on the choice between health and thinness. If you are tired and run down, cold, losing hair and sex drive, and your periods are barely there or don't come at all, you need a thorough nutrition evaluation and complete hormone tests, including both ovarian and thyroid hormones, not just a TSH check.

Another Diet Pitfall: The Low-Fat Diet and Your Ovaries

Extremely low-fat diets may not be all the hype people would have us believe, especially for women. It was through studies done primarily on men that researchers Dean Ornish and Nathan Pritikin found a reduced risk of cardiovascular disease with diets having less than about 15 percent fat. Women, though, have different biological needs. Optimal production of ovarian and adrenal steroid hormones that support fertility and pregnancy require a minimum level of fat in the diet so that the liver can make cholesterol, which then becomes the building block for estradiol, progesterone, testosterone, DHEA, cortisol, and aldosterone. When women do not eat enough fat in the diet, the body cannot make hormones and the metabolism slows down, along with other effects such as mood changes, sleep problems, loss of libido, joint and muscle aches, dry skin and hair, brittle nails, and other problems. Without adequate fat, several crucial vitamins cannot be absorbed. These fat-soluble vitamins—A, D, E, and K—help the body with a variety of functions, including the synthesis of important enzymes and proteins and the prevention of cell-damaging free-radical buildup. How much fat is enough? For women, 20 to 30 percent of calories as fat is a healthy range for optimal hormone production, as well as optimal energy levels.

Women often restrict dietary fat. Since many sources of fat are also sources of protein, a very low-fat diet is often low in protein, especially high-quality animal protein. Too little protein causes an increased production of sex hormone binding globulin (SHBG), which in turn means that a higher percentage of ovarian hormones present in the bloodstream are now attached to this carrier protein, and are *less* available in the free, active form to make cells function properly. Higher SHBG levels mean even less of your hormones are free to do their critical metabolic jobs throughout the brain and body. As a result, a low-protein diet makes you tired, listless, lethargic, and "dull." These symptoms are easy to confuse with hypothyroidism, yet due to an entirely different cause.

A twenty-seven-year-old patient found out about these issues when she reduced her fat intake to 8 to 10 percent of her total calories. It almost cost her the ability to become pregnant. She saw me because of joint pain, extreme fatigue, hair loss, daily headaches, dry skin and premature wrinkling, and waistline weight gain despite her rigorous diet. She only had three or four periods a year, with the flow scant and short cycles. Her gynecologist said not to worry, since there couldn't be hormone problems at her age. She had not been able to get pregnant even though she and her husband had not used contraception for two years. I ordered a bone density test, and it showed she had significant bone loss (osteopenia), even though she was still in her twenties.

During her evaluation she admitted being on an extremely low-fat diet. Our analysis showed inadequate protein and an excess intake of simple carbohydrates and sweets. My detailed hormone analysis identified markedly low estradiol, progesterone, testosterone, and DHEA. She also had a very low free T3 even though her TSH of 1.45 was optimal. Low free T3 is a compensatory, protective reaction to inadequate nutrition. I recommended she increase her fat and protein intake to desirable ranges. Eight weeks later, she said, "Adding more fat and protein really seemed strange at first, after all the years of feeling brainwashed by the no-fat gurus. But I had more energy and my sweet cravings disappeared . . . like someone turned off a switch! Pretty soon, my hair even started to get fuller and thicker again. I felt like I had my body back."

Her new eating plan provided balance that gradually restored her ovarian and adrenal hormones, and her free T3 returned to the desirable level as well. Until the diet changes took effect, I also suggested that she take a low dose of bioidentical 17-beta estradiol, testosterone, and cyclic natural progesterone to help restore hormone balance. After six months her hormone levels had returned to healthy levels, and her cycles were now regular. She was able to go off the supplemental hormones. A year after that, she called back to report she had a healthy baby girl.

Occupational Hazards—Forewarned Is Forearmed

There are many occupational groups with increased risk of certain diseases and/or injuries because of exposure to industrial hazards and/or chemicals. Flight attendants, a group that has been predominantly female, get overlooked. I spend a fair amount of time in airplanes, and I talk with a lot of the flight attendants, particularly after they find out what I do. I see in their faces, based on years observing women with hormonal problems, changes in skin and hair. I hear about their problems—insomnia, headaches, fatigue, no libido, allergies, memory problems, PMS getting worse, gaining weight for no reason, and the list goes on. My observations and conversations with a limited "sample" of flight attendants does not make a scientific study, but I see patterns that are similar to what I see in women who come to our offices for hormone evaluations. These connections need to be explored.

Why are flight attendants any different from other groups of women in their age group? There are some unique aspects to this career that may contribute to women having earlier than usual "perimenopausal"-type hormone changes. The role of flight attendant combines a number of risk factors that are already known to contribute to early ovarian decline or suppression:

- *Hours at high* altitude
- *Exposure to* ionizing radiation
- *Loss of normal* sleep
- *Frequent changes in* sleep *schedules*
- *Frequent* time zone changes *that affect circadian rhythms*
- Dehydration
- Erratic nutrition
- *Exposure to* secondhand cigarette smoke *(for those who have been in this career longer, since smoking on planes was only banned on all planes in the United States within the last few years)*

Each of these elements are found to *independently* cause early menopause, or at least a decline in ovarian hormones, especially estradiol. We have already discussed the many adverse effects from poor nutrition, cigarette smoking, and sleep deprivation. Practically every flight attendant I have ever talked with has commented about their poor eating habits while traveling. When they do get to their destination and grab a meal, it's often airport fast food—high in saturated fat, sugar, salt, and preservatives. This isn't the way to a healthy body or healthy ovaries.

A number of studies around the world have found that women living at high altitudes, above 7,000 feet, commonly have earlier menopause than women at lower elevations. Since most planes are pressurized to an approximate elevation of 8,000 to 10,000 feet, flight attendants are spending a lot of time in an environment equivalent of living on a mountaintop. The air is drier at these elevations, contributing to dehydration, and exposure to ionizing radiation is more intense. Ionizing radiation causes many different types of damage to the body, depending upon the exposure.

If you have been in this career for a number of years and have begun experiencing changes in your menstrual cycles or having other symptoms I describe, I encourage you to pursue having a comprehensive hormone evaluation and bone density testing, as described in Section IV.

Negative Self-Talk, Self-Image

I am talking about the impact of our "inner tapes," those thoughts and feelings that go around and around our minds, some good, some critical, some self-doubting, and some chastising. Some are there from childhood scars; others are there from present-day disappointments or wounds from careless comments by the people around us. Whatever their source, all of these are "stresses" that over-stimulate the body's physiological reactions and affect our hormone balance.

An example of negative "inner talk" many of us share is summed up well in this ad from the 1990s, written for Nike by *women* writers:

> *Fear of Failure*
> *Fear of Success*
> *Fear of Losing Your Health*
> *Fear of Losing Your Mind*
> *Fear of Being Taken Too Seriously*
> *Fear of Not Being Taken Seriously Enough*
> *Fear That You Worry Too Much*
> *Fear That You Don't Worry Enough*
> *Your Mother's Fear You'll Never Marry*
> *Your Father's Fear That You Will*
> *. . . it's not so surprising that there are a lot of conflicts*
> *and a lot of fears.*

This ad poignantly describe the double bind in which women often find themselves. We struggle with the burden of our perceived inadequacies alone. All of us have these doubts and worries due in large measure to the culture in which we live. The psychological pressure creates more physical stress in our bodies, which in turn affects our hormone balance and leads to physical and psychological symptoms.

We are also bombarded with psychological messages that say *someone else* will take care of us. That "someone else" is often a husband, a doctor, an attorney, or a businessperson. The weight of the entire culture supports this message. This gives us the unconscious impression that there will be an outside authority to tell us what to do. As a result, we may not feel confident in our own decisions. It is not surprising that health care is another paternalistic system, one in which women are "told" what is best by authority figures. It is also not surprising that in this system, women are labeled as worriers, hypochondriacs, neurotic, anxious, hysterical, and overutilizers of medical care when we go in as patients, trying to explain unusual or puzzling symptoms that fall outside the organized, medical specialty "boxes."

In addition, women are the usual caregivers for everyone else, far more than men. Many women tell me they feel overloaded with the responsibilities of caring for everyone around them and hardly have a moment to call their own. They feel "selfish" for taking time out to take care of themselves. Some of my patients tell me they feel guilty taking time to read, saying, "I found myself constantly justifying the value of the information for the amount of time I spent on myself reading this!" Most of my patients constantly struggle with this issue of finding time and space for themselves in their lives.

I thought about this overload of caregiving responsibilities as I read the tragic headlines about Andrea Yates, the young mother with postpartum psychosis who killed her five children. Even with her own catastrophic illness, she had been caring for an invalid father with Alzheimer's and her five very young children, even home-schooling them. We see the disastrous, horrifying consequences that can occur when a woman reaches her breaking point. The tragedy is how she, and the children in her care, were failed by all those around her—the family who didn't "see" that she was drowning in illness and overload, medical professionals who didn't evaluate the hormone connection in her postpartum depression, the doctors who didn't "see" her psychosis was still there and stopped critical medication prematurely. Ultimately, she was failed by a legal system woefully unprepared to comprehend the enormity of a psychotic mental illness and "see" that it is more than simply knowing right from wrong.

In Summary

The collective impact of all these stressors, both psychological and physiological, produce profound changes in the body, whether they are lifestyle choices or societal stereotypes and cultural biases. Over time, the cumulative effect plays out in our body and disrupts our ovaries' ability to make critical hormones. The health of our ovaries as well as the rest of our body is affected. The consequences vary from woman to woman, but overall, there are similar patterns to the symptoms women experience regardless of age. Recognize these factors and their very real consequences on your health. Make appropriate lifestyle changes to improve your health. And, if you have any of the symptoms or body changes described, see someone knowledgeable and have your hormones checked properly. Don't compromise your needs. *You are worth some caretaking, too!*

9

Ovaries at Risk: Unusual Effects of Viruses and Medical Illnesses

––––––

Introduction

Mysterious, puzzling, and *bizarre* are words that often run through my mind as I listen to the experiences of my patients as they describe the time their hormone symptoms began. Tick bite? Black widow spider bite? Viral illness? Chlamydia infection? Hemorrhage following delivery? All of these unusual triggers have led to sudden and premature menopause in patients I have evaluated. Perhaps our ovaries are more at risk, and more sensitive, than doctors appreciate. My patients and I are on a journey, rather like detective work, to understand the causes and triggers of their problems and find solutions to help regain their health. While sometimes we may never know for certain what triggered the premature ovarian decline, we are usually able to identify clues in women's experiences that correlate with good science. The science can help validate women's own observations, which encourages trust in body experiences and intuition.

Women often ask me which type of specialist they should see for these problems—is an internist or endocrinologist or a gynecologist better. My short answer: whichever specialist listens, will do complete testing, and helps you improve your health. Many of these problems cause symptoms that cross the "specialty" boxes of our current health care system. Don't get caught up in doctors' "turf" issues over who is "supposed" to check your hormones. The point is to get the problem *correctly* identified and *properly* treated.

Toxins from Ticks, Spiders, and Viruses

Lyme Disease, transmitted by the deer tick, has gotten a great deal of attention in recent years. Just one tick bite can cause peculiar problems. You may be familiar with the symptoms—bull's-eye rash, diffuse joint pain, muscle aches, and persistent fatigue. But I doubt you have read much about tick bites triggering premature ovarian decline, or premature menopause. In fact, the doctors with whom I have discussed this have usually said, "Impossible." There usually isn't much conversation or discussion. Most doctors simply dismiss the idea with the comment, "It can't be," and move on. I have to say, however, I have learned that with the human body, very few things are "impossible."

I have a number of patients for whom I could find no other trigger in their medical, lifestyle, or family history to account for the sudden onset of menopause-like symptoms *except* the tick bite, or a spider bite, or severe viral illness such as "mono" (infectious mononucleosis). These types of illnesses can trigger an inflammation of the ovary that we call *oophoritis*. But since we don't have good tests to measure oophoritis, it often goes undiagnosed. Oophoritis is a nonspecific term; you can have a viral, bacterial, toxic, or autoimmune oophoritis. The symptoms are similar to low estradiol that occurs in PMS, menopause, or is due to other causes, so the connection with the bacteria, virus, or "bug" is usually missed. Sometimes this isn't critical, because the treatments may be the same, regardless of cause. But other times, such as with Lyme disease or chlamydia, it is important to ferret out the cause because you may need antibiotic therapy to prevent long-term complications.

So if you have a bug bite or viral illness and then notice changes in your menstrual cycle, or you start having hot flashes, night sweats, or other menopauselike symptoms, make sure that you insist on a thorough hormone evaluation. In patients I have seen, these unusual triggers have caused such significant loss of ovarian hormones that they developed osteoporosis in their thirties. You, and your doctors, need to take these issues seriously. Examples of my patients show what can happen when these types of oophoritis are missed.

Linda had a sudden, full-blown menopause at thirty, in spite of excellent health and *no* risk factors for early menopause. I first saw her about ten years after her symptoms began because she was "tired of being so tired all the time and just not feeling well." She said that all her symptoms—hot flashes, night sweats, restless sleep, joint and muscle pain, fatigue, and abrupt loss of her periods—began shortly after she had been bitten by a black widow spider, which made her quite ill. She was certain the toxins in the spider venom triggered her menopause, but "My doctors just blew me off and pooh-poohed that idea. They said I was too young for this to be menopause!" She was treated for many years with antidepressants for a low-grade, depressed mood, loss of energy, and problems sleeping. There was not a great deal of improvement. She also tried many different herbs and vitamin supplements, but nothing seemed to restore her former sense of well-being. By the time I checked both her hormone levels and her bone density, she had developed osteoporosis even though she was only forty years old. The character and pattern of her symptoms, the obvious sign of losing her periods, and the bone loss, convinced me that she had been thrown into menopause by the toxins in that spider bite. There simply were no other risk factors and no history of early menopause in her family. Now that we have found a hormone combination that works well for her, she has regained much of her former vitality and is also rebuilding bone to replace what she lost. Today, she feels angry, and sad, too, that her insights were discounted and she spent so many years not feeling well.

I've had quite a number of patients, mainly from the East Coast where deer ticks are widespread, who had clearly documented Lyme disease followed soon after by the usual symptoms of ovarian failure, including loss of periods. *Coleen* was in her twenties when diagnosed with Lyme disease. This was followed by severe, intractable PMS with marked mood swings, joint aches, muscle pain, chronic fatigue. She also gained thirty pounds she couldn't lose, no matter how diligently she followed a diet and exercise program. Her periods didn't stop completely, but her menstrual cycles and bleeding pattern changed dramatically—her cycles were now closer to thirty-five days with heavy bleeding and severe cramps. Even though she, too, had no other risk factors for early ovarian decline, her hormone profile told the story. Thyroid and adrenal tests were excellent, but she had lost bone density and had a Day 20 estradiol of 98 pg/ml even though her progesterone was excellent at 18.5 ng/dl, showing she still ovulated. After we found a steady dose birth control pill (Orthocyclen) that worked well, her symptoms improved markedly, and she no longer had the monthly "crazies" with her mood swings.

Both of these women, as well as most of those I have seen with similar stories, had seen multiple doctors and spent thousands of dollars on sophisticated medical tests. Of course, no one checked the basic ovarian hormone levels that might have confirmed what the women suspected all along.

Chlamydia and Other Sexually Transmitted Diseases

Sexual transmission of viruses and bacteria may lead to similar oophoritis syndromes and loss of healthy hormone production. *Chlamydia* is one of the most common sexually transmitted bacterial infections in the United States, but it is notoriously difficult to diagnose. In the early stages, it often causes such subtle, vague, and indolent symptoms that women don't know they have been infected and mistake symptoms for "stress." One woman began in her late twenties having painful bladder problems and recurring vaginal infections that were increasingly difficult to treat. Then, in her early thirties, she started having menopauselike symptoms. After twenty-five years of suffering bladder pain, chronic vaginal infections, debilitating fatigue, loss of sex drive, and unexplained infertility, she was finally diagnosed by an infertility specialist in New York with chlamydia, who said this had been the cause of her problems all along. I saw her for a consult a few months after she had begun treatment for the chlamydia. She said:

"I went to the top doctors in New York. They never checked for it, and I certainly didn't know I might have been exposed to it. I started trying to get pregnant in my thirties, but I never was able to. I finally went to a fertility specialist who was the first doctor that checked me for chlamydia. He put my husband and me on antibiotics, and finally it resolved. After the chlamydia was treated, my ovaries started working again, and I could feel my ovulation—but here I am now at forty-eight, and it is really too late for me to try and have a child. It affected me terribly for so long. I had very painful periods, really bad PMS with terrible hormone swings, and I was told I needed estrogen and was put on Premarin years ago, even though I had it all over my medical charts that I had severe allergic reactions whenever I got around horses! I was so angry that I suffered all that time, now knowing what was wrong with me, and not knowing why I never could get pregnant."

Once she had been successfully treated for chlamydia, her ovaries began to cycle again, the bladder problems gradually resolved, the recurring vaginal infections stopped, and her PMS improved. She had already scheduled the consultation with me, and decided to see what additional suggestions I had for her hormone management, even though she could see that the antibiotic treatment for chlamydia had dramatically improved her cycle function and symptoms. At our meeting, I found that her estradiol was still low at 30 pg/ml, and her testosterone was also low at 17 ng/dl. This fit with her residual symptoms of insomnia, hot flashes, difficulty with short-term memory, and loss of interest in sex. I recommended increasing the dose of her estradiol patch and adding a low dose of natural testosterone. Since she had such an excellent response from her antibiotic treatment for the chlamydia, I did not make any further changes to her therapy. The unrecognized chlamydia caused her ovarian dysfunction and inability to become pregnant. She will never recover her lost potential to have her own child.

Chlamydia organisms must live inside cells of the body to survive. We call this type of organism an *obligate* intracellular parasite. It is difficult to diagnose because it hides in white blood cells (macrophages and monocytes) that travel throughout the body in the blood. Camouflaged in our own cells, chlamydia organisms can be carried from the vagina via the bloodstream to other parts of the body, including the ovaries and joints. Chlamydia has long been known to cause pelvic inflammatory disease (PID) as well as infertility. Chlamydia infections, however, can cause additional problems that may surprise you.

Both chlamydia and the sexually transmitted bacteria that cause gonorrhea can also lead to *inflammatory arthritis* and are one of the most common causes of arthritis in young women. There is another type of joint inflammation, however, that is far more common in women, at a ratio of about eight women sufferers to every one male: temporomandibular joint pain-dysfunction syndrome (TMJ). It causes significant pain, debilitating quality of life, lost productivity, and costs sufferers thousands of dollars for evaluation and treatment. There is now evidence that a hidden chlamydia infection can play a role in the enormous female preponderance of TMJ, and also contribute to decline in ovarian hormones.

United States dentists Drs. C. H. Henry, A. P. Hudson, and H. C. Gerard examined the synovial fluid of TMJ sufferers for the presence of chlamydia, thinking that it could be an example of an inflammatory arthritis from infection with this organism. This study, published in 1999, was the first to show that, in fact, chlamydia organisms are present in large numbers in the synovial tissue lining the jaw joint of patients with TMJ. Most surprising was that *all* the patients with both chlamydia and TMJ were *women*, with an average age of thirty-four to thirty-seven years. *None* of the males in their study tested positive for the chlamydia organism in the synovial tissue. After finding that so many women with TMJ also had the chlamydia organism present in the jaw joint, these dentists concluded that TMJ dysfunction and pain can be an unrecognized inflammatory, infectious arthritis. If TMJ is caused in some women by chlamydia, then early treatment with the right antibiotics may help prevent this debilitating syndrome.

If chlamydia can be disseminated through the bloodstream to infect the jaw joint, it can also travel to infiltrate the ovary. Since chlamydial infections often go undetected, particularly in women, there is a strong possibility that this organism may be a trigger for an infectious oophoritis that can lead to early loss of the ovarian hormones, as well as cause arthritis. Early disruption in healthy function of your ovaries can lead to the whole gamut of symptoms described throughout this book.

Don't let this happen to you. Practice safe sex, and ask your doctor to test for the sexually transmitted infections at your annual pelvic exam.

Thyroid Disorders and Your Ovaries

The statistics are eye-opening: Thyroid disease affects more than 10 million women, and is *eight to twenty* times more common in women than men. According to the Thyroid Foundation of America, more than half of the people with thyroid disorders are undiagnosed. Why is this in a book about ovaries? Because the thyroid gland is a critical regulator of ovarian function and fertility. It turns out there are thyroid hormone receptors on the ovary, and ovarian hormone receptors on the thyroid, so they are in constant direct hormone communication with each other, as well as with the brain through the hypothalamus and pituitary, the two glands that oversee ovarian function.

By the age of fifty, at least 10 percent of women will have a clearly diagnosable thyroid disorder. By age sixty, this number jumps to 17 percent, which means *millions* of women. But younger women today have a high incidence of subtle thyroid dysfunction that we call *subclinical,* and it can affect the ovaries as well as leave you feeling sluggish and moody. PMS symptoms intensify, and you may have difficulty getting pregnant. I have evaluated hundreds of women over the years with undiagnosed thyroid disorders that caused ovarian problems. In younger women, thyroid disorders are more damaging to reproductive function than in men. The specific effects depend on which type of thyroid problem you have—*hypo*thyroidism (low thyroid) or *hyper*thyroidism (excess thyroid)—and at what age it occurs.

Thyroid imbalances also cause a wide range of both physical and emotional symptoms, from anxiety, agitation, depression, and mania to rapid-cycling "bipolar"-type syndromes. Thyroid disease is "the great imitator," causing just about every physical, mood, or cognitive symptom ever described! Many of the same symptoms can be caused by loss of the ovarian estradiol, which makes it even more critical to check all of these hormones carefully when symptoms appear.

As you get older, and *hypo*thyroidism goes untreated, it can lead to high cholesterol by impairing the body's ability to remove "bad" LDL and VLDL cholesterol particles from circulation. Untreated hypothyroidism also leads to high blood pressure, early heart attacks, stroke, marked weight gain, clinical depression, and dementia. If overactive thyroid (*hyper*thyroidism) goes untreated, serious health problems result, including atrial fibrillation, congestive heart failure, osteoporosis, muscle wasting and weakness, anxiety, agitated depressive syndromes, persistent insomnia, and cognitive difficulties similar to attention deficit disorder.

These multiple effects are not surprising when you consider that thyroid hormones help translate our DNA codes that guide cells to make and use nutrients, vitamins, hormones, and the other various building blocks used by the body and brain. Let's look at the thyroid hormones and how they are regulated, since they are intimately involved with the normal function of our ovaries and fertility.

A Guide to Your Thyroid Hormones

The thyroid system is controlled by the brain's master control center in the hypothalamus. The hypothalamus produces *thyrotropin releasing hormone* (TRH), which stimulates the pituitary to produce and release *thyroid stimulating hormone* (TSH). TSH circulates in the blood and directs the thyroid gland to make T4 *(thyroxine)*. T4 made in the thyroid gland is converted in the gland and in body tissues to the more active form, T3 *(triiodothyronine)—if* all the pathways are working properly. The thyroid gland has several important enzymes, such as thyroid peroxidase (TPO), that are essential for converting T4 to T3. If the body doesn't make enough T3 from T4, the result may be symptoms of a thyroid disorder even when standard thyroid function blood tests fall within the "normal" laboratory range.

T4 and T3 circulate in the bloodstream to serve the entire body and also report to the pituitary and hypothalamus about the thyroid gland's production—not enough, too much, or just right. This feedback determines how much TRH and TSH to make, which in turn directs T4 and T3 production. Very little T3 and T4 occur in the free, active form in the blood; over 99 percent of the T3 and T4 is attached, or "bound," to three carrier proteins: *thyroid binding globulin* (TBG), *transthyretin* (TTR), and *albumin.* For example, only about 0.2 percent of T3 is in the free, unattached form. This means that anything in your diet or medications that changes the balance of the carrier proteins can have a huge impact on how your thyroid hormones work.

The whole process of thyroid regulation is similar to your house thermostat that registers hot or cold relative to where you set the temperature. If it's too hot, signals go back to the cooling system and directs it to turn on—and vice versa. As you read this chapter, keep in mind that if the thyroid gland is not making *enough* T4 and T3, then the pituitary puts out *more* of the stimulating hormone, TSH. This means an underactive thyroid gland shows up with a *high* TSH, usually greater than 5. Many patients think a low TSH means hypothyroidism. It is the opposite. A *low* TSH means the pituitary senses *too much* thyroid hormone in the bloodstream and shuts *off* the stimulating hormone. If TSH is too low (less than 0.5), this indicates an *overactive* thyroid gland. Just remember, it's the reverse of what you expect: low TSH = *hyper*thyroid, high TSH = *hypo*thyroid.

Thyroid hormones are essential for normal body metabolism, brain development, and normal reproductive function in most species, especially humans. T3 and T4 regulate our ovarian cycles along with many aspects of brain and nerve function, from growth of neurons to the movement of nerve cells to the proper areas for their function. They oversee the formation of normal nerve cell junctions (synapses), and formation of the protective fatty sheath (myelin) around nerve cell extensions (axons) that connect one cell to another. Thyroid hormones are also crucial for fetal brain development during pregnancy. Human brain development occurs at specific windows throughout our time in the womb. Proper levels of thyroid hormones are critical during these times. If we don't have thyroid hormones and iodine in the right amount, at the right time, and in the right balance, permanent brain damage occurs, leading to neurological and learning disorders. This type of brain damage, and the symptoms that occur later, depends on *when* in the pregnancy and *how severe* the disruption was.

Worldwide, low thyroid hormone during brain development is one of the leading causes of learning disorders, attention deficit disorders, and other subtle types of neurological/cognitive dysfunction. Learning disorders and mental retardation are common in areas of the world where iodine is deficient in the diet. Although iodine is added to salt in the United States, chemicals in our environment can interfere with adequate dietary iodine so that it cannot be used normally by the thyroid gland to make thyroid hormones. This is another way that exposure to synthetic chemicals during pregnancy can have damaging effects. By interfering with normal thyroid hormone action when the baby's brain is developing in the womb, these chemicals profoundly affect the brain's ability to function normally the rest of your child's life.

How do *your* thyroid hormones affect your baby? Some cross the placenta, primarily as thyroxine (T4). If you are exposed to chemicals such as pesticides while pregnant, they can interfere with your ability to make enough T4 and so less T4 is available for your baby's developing brain. I described above that T3 is the most active form of our thyroid hormones, especially in the brain. Most of the T3 for our brain is actually made there from T4 and by the action of the enzyme, *thyroid peroxidase* (TPO). Pesticides may also damage this enzyme, making it incapable of helping to make enough T3. High soy intake also blocks the action of this enzyme. This type of enzyme deficiency could explain why, even though serum T4 and T3 levels are normal, an infant or young child can have hypothyroidism causing learning and neurological deficits.

A study, published in April 2001, of 182 Swedish fishermen's wives found that the women who ate more fish had higher blood and body fat levels of persistent organochlorines and PCBs and also lower levels of thyroid hormones than did women who ate very little fish. This suggests that the chemical contamination of foods can affect thyroid hormone levels in adult women. These findings are especially important for women during pregnancy because of potential long-term damage to the baby.

The Role of Iodine and Iodine Deficiency

Iodine is a critical element needed by the thyroid gland to make its thyroid hormones in the process called *iodination*. There are three iodine molecules added to make T3, and four to make T4. You can see how the balance of iodine available to the thyroid gland is important for optimal thyroid hormone synthesis. *Excess* iodine intake over time may lead to hyperthyroidism, more so in older people. Iodine *deficiency* can produce hypothyroidism and increasing likelihood of goiter. Long-term, both iodine deficiency and goiter are risk factors for one type of thyroid cancer. Likewise, too much iodine intake over a long time may disrupt thyroid hormone actions and also cause hypothyroidism and goiter, as we see with the high incidence of goiter in certain areas of Japan where seaweed is eaten regularly. Most of the time, however, people who get too much iodine will remain normal because our thyroid gland has several ways to regulate its iodine metabolism to maintain balance.

Many areas of the world have soils deficient in iodine, and that includes major areas of the midwestern United States, the so-called goiter belt. Adding iodine to salt in this country helped decrease the incidence of goiter, but there has been a rise in recent years, in part because so many people (women especially) have cut down on salt. A recent study from Switzerland showed a similar pattern. High goiter rates in iodine-deficient areas were virtually eliminated with the introduction of iodized salt. Then, in 1991–1992, researchers saw a rise in goiter rates, for several reasons: reduced intake of salt, increased use of foods prepared with noniodized salt, and more diverse diets. The Swiss health officials recommended people use iodized salt again. I think we should follow this recommendation as well.

There is another reason for iodine deficiency to reappear: Many chemicals in the environmental POP endocrine-disruptor group can interfere with our ability to use the iodine in our diet. This is caused by a number of mechanisms. POPs interfere with the function of the enzymes needed to manufacture T4 and T3, and interfere with thyroid hormone action at receptor sites in the hypothalamus and at other body receptors. There may be other ways that our sensitive thyroid pathway can be disrupted by POPs in our environment. For example, PCBs, nitrates, organochlorine insecticides, thiocyanate, and possibly many other compounds may cause impaired iodine utilization. Thus, you may have adequate iodine in your diet but be unable to use it due to exposure to such chemicals. This is how gradual symptoms of hypothyroidism can develop over time.

If the iodine content of your diet is low, your thyroid gland will initially adapt by increasing iodine concentration from the bloodstream, by enhancing iodination to make T4 and T3, by decreasing iodine storage in the gland, and by better recycling of iodine from a breakdown of thyroid hormones. TSH will also stimulate the thyroid gland tissue to grow (hyperplasia), which adds more hormone-producing tissue. People respond in a variety of ways to iodine deficiency, depending on genetic makeup, diet, medications, and environmental chemical exposure. Some people develop an enlarged gland goiter, others have only a mild increase in TSH, and still others have marked symptoms of hypothyroidism even when measures of T3 and T4 are normal. But over the long haul, low iodine intake dramatically decreases levels of T3 and T4 in several areas of the brain by 30 to 50 percent. This leads to subtle brain symptoms of hypothyroidism such as depressed mood, memory loss, scattered thinking, a feeling of "fuzzy brain." As hypothyroidism progresses, there is disruption in the brain pathways that regulate the ovaries and other endocrine systems, leading to a decrease in these other hormones. Later, the hypothyroidism may become overt and obvious as it affects more body systems. Another reason for young women to be aware of iodine deficiency is that there is an increased risk of cancer in later life. Iodine deficiency, chemical goiter-inducers (*goitrogens*), and thyroid toxins promote tumor growth in the thyroid gland and have also been linked to breast cancer.

The diagram on page 105 shows how exposure to environmental chemicals may affect iodine metabolism and lead to thyroid and other health problems.

Hypothyroidism

Hypothyroidism is more common than hyperthyroidism and is more likely to go unrecognized because the symptoms are subtle. Its manifestations can be so varied that they are easily confused with other problems. Gynecologists may miss thyroid dysfunction because it so closely mimics other, more common gynecological disorders that also cause breast discharge (galactorrhea), excess facial and body hair (hirsutism), loss of menses (amenorrhea), infrequent menses (oligomenorrhea), and even infertility. A thyroid connection to infertility can easily be missed if thyroid antibodies are not checked, even if TSH is checked and found "normal" (see Chapter 14 for hypothyroidism and fertility). When hypothyroidism first occurs has some bearing on the symptoms you may experience. Let's look at the differences.

Hypothyroidism Before Puberty

Girls who become hypothyroid before they reach puberty will typically be shorter than if thyroid function had remained normal. They may also have either *delayed* puberty, or a different syndrome called *precocious puberty,* which leads to premature menstrual bleeding, breast enlargement, a milky discharge (galactorrhea) from the breasts due to a parallel rise in the brain hormone prolactin, which causes normal pubic hair growth. So if a girl has breast development and vaginal bleeding but no pubic hair, it is an important clue to check the thyroid carefully.

If premature puberty is caused by low thyroid function, these changes generally reverse when treated with thyroid hormones. It is important to identify and treat hypothyroidism quickly before puberty so that girls reach their normal height and have healthy ovarian and cognitive function. Loss of memory and concentration from hypothyroidism can also severely affect school performance.

A ten-year-old girl I saw recently illustrates how important this can be. *Sandie* is an active soccer player who gets plenty of daily exercise, eats a healthy diet, and

COMPARISON

Normal Puberty	Precocious Puberty of Hypothyroidism
• Pubic hair growth	Delayed pubic hair growth
• Normal bone growth	Delayed bone development
• Breast enlargement	Breast enlargement
• Vagina plus estrogen effects	Vagina plus estrogen effects
• Vaginal bleeding	Vaginal bleeding
• TSH normal	TSH elevated*
• FSH, LH normal	FSH, LH may be consistently elevated
• Normal prolactin	Prolactin elevated,* often proportional to rise in TSH
• Normal SHBG	SHBG decreased,* with elevated free E1, E2, and elevated free androgens (hirsutism, acne, truncal weight gain)
• Normal menses	Amenorrhea or menorrhagia
• No breast discharge	May have galactorrhea

*These three laboratory findings are not seen in normal puberty. If they are abnormal, it can help point to an underlying hypothyroid condition.

© Elizabeth Lee Vliet, M.D., 2003

doesn't have more than an occasional soft drink. But she keeps gaining weight, feels sluggish, has trouble concentrating at school, and her grades have been slipping. She feels so tired that she comes home from school and takes a nap. Her mother was worried about these changes. Because so many people in the family have thyroid problems, she thought this might be happening to Sandie. They had consulted a pediatric endocrinologist at a local Children's Hospital, and had been told that Sandie's thyroid and ovarian hormones were "just fine." Her mother wasn't satisfied with this answer as she watched her daughter change from a vibrant, energetic, athletic girl into a tired, chubby, lethargic person.

At her consult, I discussed with Sandie and her mother all the changes they had noticed, particularly the decline in school performance. Earlier doctors had not asked about this, and her mother had not realized it might be important to mention. Her first evaluation had not checked thyroid antibodies, free T3, free T4, or the glucose and insulin responses after eating. I reviewed our findings, which showed a TSH of 3.8, low free T3, low free T4, and markedly elevated thyroid antibodies. Normally, I might not start thyroid hormones when the TSH isn't any higher, but I was very concerned about Sandie's change in cognitive performance at school, and the amount of weight she had gained even with all her exercise. She also had findings of insulin resistance that went along with this weight gain, which put her a greater risk of diabetes later in adolescence.

My clinical judgment was that she had an early thyroiditis that was negatively affecting brain function, metabolism, and weight even though the TSH was still in the "normal" range. Her mother was very eager for Sandie to try thyroid medication, and I decided this was reasonable, as long as her TSH wasn't pushed too low. I started Sandie on just 12.5 mcg of T4 the first two weeks to see how she did on a very low dose, then increased to 25 mcg daily. After four weeks, her mother reported: "It was like a miracle! She has more energy to play soccer, she doesn't take naps in the afternoon, she has lost seven pounds, and best of all, she's alert and able to concentrate again at school. She is so happy about how much better she feels on this little bit of thyroid. I can't believe the difference in my daughter!" This was a time when carefully evaluating the patient and her needs, rather than just focusing rigidly on lab tests alone, tipped the balance toward cautious use of thyroid hormone. This young girl will likely have much better health in the years ahead because her mother was persistent in seeking answers that made sense to her from her observations of her daughter. Likewise, I found it very meaningful to see this delightful ten-year-old get her energy and enthusiasm back, and improve her performance at school, too.

Hypothyroidism Occurring in Adolescence

Adolescent girls normally have some degree of menstrual irregularity until their cycles develop their particular rhythm. But significant menstrual irregularity is common if hypothyroidism occurs in adolescence because low thyroid hormones cause lack of ovulation. There may also be heavy bleeding, which is unusual. There may also be a rise in prolactin from the increase in brain TRH that stimulates TSH and prolactin release, or from thyroid effects on dopamine pathways that regulate prolactin. If prolactin is too high, it can cause breast enlargement, milky discharge, weight gain, depression, headaches, more cycles with no ovulation, and decreased levels of estradiol and progesterone.

Hypothyroidism also leads to a decreased breakdown of the *androstenedione* (an androgen made in the ovary) as well as *estrone,* an estrogen produced in body fat from androstenedione. Higher levels of androstenedione cause more acne and excess body hair. Higher levels of both hormones add to the gain in fat around the waist. The increase in fat around the middle (called *central* or *truncal fat*) doesn't respond well to the usual weight-loss efforts and causes more likelihood of insulin resistance. In fact, the more you diet, the more your thyroid hormones don't work properly and the higher the increase in cortisol (your stress hormone), which stores more fat. You get fatter and fatter!

Hypothyroidism also converts more estradiol (E2) to estriol (E3), which causes abnormal feedback to the pituitary, so it releases more FSH and LH that disrupt ovulation and increase the ovary production of androgens (androstenedione, DHEA, and testosterone). Increased production plus decreased breakdown means girls with this problem have serious middle-body weight gain, acne, and excess body hair. These same symptoms occur with other disorders, such as

PCOS. Treatments for each are different, so you need a careful evaluation of the thyroid as well as the ovary hormones to determine the problem.

Hypothyroidism Occurring in Adult Women or During Pregnancy

Besides robbing your energy, mental clarity, and mood, hypothyroidism can have a profound impact on the health and function of your ovaries. Depression is sometimes the first clue to a subtle thyroid disorder that can cause serious disruptions if untreated. This has been known for a long time, yet it is not often taken into account when evaluating women for depression. For example, one study published almost twenty years ago showed that 20 percent of a series of psychiatric inpatients with depression had elevated thyroid antibodies (*antimicrosomal* antibody and *antithyroglobulin* antibody). This rate was much higher than the 5 to 10 percent observed in people without depression. These patients had subtle thyroid dysfunction contributing to the depression, but they *all* had "normal" standard thyroid tests, which is why the hormone connection was missed. Except for the depression, they had no apparent symptoms of a thyroid disorder. Because thyroid hormones play such a big role in the brain, mood changes may be one of the earliest clues that something is amiss with the thyroid gland. As the thyroiditis and hypothyroidism progress, disruption of the menstrual cycle is often the next thing that occurs. This illustrates again why I think it is so important to check thyroid antibodies in women with symptoms like depression or fatigue, even if their TSH is normal.

If you have normal, regular menstrual cycles, and then become hypothyroid, it typically causes longer or shorter cycles. Bleeding patterns also commonly change, becoming much heavier, often with severe menstrual pain and cramping. Hypothyroidism also leads to loss of normal ovulation, which makes it difficult to get pregnant. Even milder forms of thyroid decline, especially early stages of autoimmune disorders like Hashimoto's or Graves' disease, may also cause a defect in the luteal (ovulatory) phase of progesterone and estradiol production, also contributing to infertility.

Although hypothyroidism normally reduces fertility, women who do become pregnant when they have unrecognized hypothyroidism have an increase in spontaneous abortions ("miscarriages") in the first three months. Untreated hypothyroidism during pregnancy also causes higher incidence of pregnancy-related high blood pressure, which in turn increases the risk of toxemia (also called *preeclampsia*) before delivery. Various studies also indicate untreated hypothyroidism *doubles* the risk of early spontaneous abortions, stillbirths, and premature births, while it *triples* the risk of congenital abnormalities in the baby. You can reduce these risks if the thyroid problem is corrected. Even with thyroid hormone supplementation, however, women who have had hypothyroidism still have a higher than normal risk of having a baby with a congenital malformation.

You see why it is critical to know about thyroid function before you try to get pregnant. Later in this chapter I will recommend tests that can be done by your gynecologist or primary care physician. If you were treated in the past for hypothyroidism and then become pregnant, you should have your OB doctor or an endocrinologist monitor your thyroid medicine carefully, because you will often need higher doses to keep within the optimal range as the ovarian hormones change rapidly during pregnancy. The high levels of ovarian hormones increase the binding proteins that carry T4 and T3 in the bloodstream during pregnancy, and lead to a decrease in the amount of free, active thyroid hormones present. Because of these changes, TSH should be checked *at least* once every trimester so that the dose remains correct as the hormones change. If your thyroid condition is particularly unstable, your doctor should check the TSH and other levels more often.

If you are on thyroid medication when you become pregnant, it is wise not to stop your medicine abruptly. If you just stop thyroid hormones instead of slowly tapering down, your own thyroid gland can't immediately start to make all it needs. This means you can be hypothyroid until the gland fully takes over again, which could cause problems for the pregnancy as I described above. Only small amounts of the mother's T4 and T3 cross the placenta, so it isn't likely that your replacement dose of thyroid hormone will harm the baby unless you are taking so much that you are *hyper*thyroid (TSH lower than 0.5). Just be sure your doctors check this regularly during pregnancy.

Hyperthyroidism

Problems from excess thyroid hormone activity are also quite varied, and hit most organ systems in our body. Symptoms range from mood effects and heart palpitations to bone loss, hair loss, muscle weakness, and, yes, even weight gain and fatigue, which many do not associate with excess thyroid hormones. Hyperthyroidism in the early stages may also be overlooked and misdiagnosed as an anxiety or panic disorder, or even as a "bipolar" illness because of the mood changes it can produce. The specific effects will depend on how severe the excess, when it happens, and how long it has been present, just as I described for hypothyroidism.

Hyperthyroidism Before Puberty

If a prepubescent girl becomes hyperthyroid, she may have delayed sexual development and begin menstrual periods later than usual. This appears to be caused by lower body fat in hyperthyroid individuals, since we know that a certain threshold, or set point, of body fat is needed before menstruation begins. Physical development in other areas is generally normal, although a girl who is hyperthyroid may be thinner and taller than her peers. Excess thyroid increases bone growth, making bones of the legs and arms longer, but bones are often less dense than normal because excess thyroid causes too much bone breakdown. Excess thyroid activity also causes scattered thinking, hyperactivity, and difficulty with focus that can be mistaken for an attention-deficit hyperactivity disorder (ADHD). If you have hyperthyroidism and you are put on the stimulant Ritalin with the thinking that the problem is ADHD, it can worsen the learning disorder and cause serious heart rhythm problems. Demand a careful medical evaluation and ask to be checked for thyroid problems instead of starting medicines like Ritalin or Adderall based only on evaluations of learning and behavior.

Hyperthyroidism Occurring in Adolescents and Adult Women

Hyperthyroidism may also cause infertility, although it has effects on menstrual function and fertility that are different from hypothyroidism. Excess thyroid can make the cycle longer or shorter so that the luteal phase doesn't develop properly. This elevates FSH and LH, which often causes loss of ovulation and diminished menstrual flow. The decreased menstrual flow results when too little endometrial lining is built up, which makes it harder for a fertilized egg to implant properly. But sometimes hyperthyroid women still ovulate normally, unlike those with hypothyroidism. So if you miss menstrual periods, you could be pregnant and should have a pregnancy test.

Excess thyroid activity causes an *increase* in sex hormone binding globulin (SHBG), an opposite effect from hypothyroidism. This means that less testosterone is in the free, available form even though the total amount of testosterone is often increased. Hyperthyroidism also increases the conversion of androgens to estrogens and shifts estrogen metabolism preferentially to estradiol and estrone. The higher estradiol and estrone, along with a lower *free* testosterone, helps to explain why your skin is softer, with fine downy hair, when you have too much thyroid hormone.

Since hyperthyroidism suppresses appetite, in addition to being a major metabolic "stressor," it often leads to nutritional deficiencies that aggravate the menstrual disturbances and contribute to infertility. Excess thyroid activity also increases the rate of bone breakdown in relation to the rate of building new bone. If hyperthyroidism goes undiagnosed for a long period of time, it may lead to low bone density and a higher risk of osteoporosis.

Hyperthyroidism in Pregnancy

It is much less common for a woman to develop hyperthyroidism and toxic thyroid excess *(thyrotoxicosis)* during pregnancy, but it does happen in about two out of every one thousand. Graves' disease is the most common cause of hyperthyroidism during pregnancy. It is an urgent medical condition because the thyroid-stimulating immunoglobulins in Graves' disease are able to cross the placenta and may cause thyrotoxicosis in the baby as well as the mother. Hyperthyroid states are sometimes missed in the early stages because some of the symptoms, such as nervousness, feeling overly warm, excess sweating, elevated blood pressure, and rapid heartbeat mimic the early changes of a normal pregnancy. Thyroid blood tests, along with checking for signs of excess thyroid (tremor, eyes protruding, hyperactive reflexes) help confirm hyperthyroidism. If you are pregnant and develop hyperthyroidism, I recommend that you have both an experienced endocrinologist and your OB physician monitor your progress.

Women with autoimmune thyroid disorders such as Graves' disease or Hashimoto's thyroiditis may notice that their thyroid symptoms are easier to control or may even diminish after they become pregnant. This is because the high progesterone levels of pregnancy suppress the mother's immune system so that the mother's body does not destroy the "foreign tissue" of the developing baby. This is one reason the autoimmune problems with Graves' disease flare up quickly after delivery and become hyperthyroid again when progesterone falls rapidly.

Postpartum Thyroid Disorders: Hypothyroidism, Hyperthyroidism, and Autoimmune Thyroiditis

Postpartum thyroid disorders occur in anywhere from 5 to 10 percent of women, a significant problem during our reproductive years. If the thyroid problems are associated with elevated thyroid antibodies, it is called *autoimmune postpartum thyroiditis,* and it may manifest as either hyper- (overactive) or hypo- (underactive) thyroid. This imbalance can lead to serious mood problems, including severe forms of postpartum depression and postpartum psychosis. Women with elevated thyroid antibodies prior to pregnancy are at much higher risk of developing severe postpartum thyroiditis after delivery that can lead to a serious postpartum psychosis. Autoimmune disorders of all types, but especially autoimmune thyroiditis, commonly return with a vengeance after delivery when progesterone levels fall and the immune-suppressing effects of this hormone are now gone.

Autoimmune postpartum thyroid problems often go undiagnosed because doctors today do not routinely test for thyroid antibodies, even though we have published reports in the medical literature about this problem going back many years. For example, a 1982 Japanese study found that over 5 percent of women had postpartum thyroid dysfunction, either hyper- or hypothyroid conditions. This translates to millions of women. A 1984 study of Swedish women found that the rate of hypothyroidism with positive thyroid antibodies was even higher, at almost 10 percent of reproductive-age women. They found that in women with hypothyroidism, microsomal antibodies were always present. The severity of the disease correlated closely to the level of antibodies measured during pregnancy and postpartum. Studies since that time have confirmed these findings, but doctors are still not seeing the importance of measuring thyroid antibodies.

There are many symptoms of postpartum hypothyroidism, but some of the more common ones are severe, unrelenting fatigue, markedly depressed mood, hair loss, dry skin, memory or concentration problems, difficulty losing weight, and constipation. These same symptoms may also occur from decreased production of the ovarian hormones in the postpartum phase as well as other causes, so you have to check all hormone levels. Be sure to ask your physician to also check thyroid antibodies.

It is possible to have both a thyroid problem and a postpartum depression or psychosis disorder. But since thyroid disorders can be indistinguishable from "psychiatric" disorders and also cause suicidal depressions and/or psychosis, it is crucial to check thyroid hormones thoroughly. You may only need thyroid medication, or you may need both thyroid hormones and antidepressants, or all thyroid tests may be normal and you may only need antidepressant medicine. We cannot assume that all "low energy, depressed mood" states are "just" due to postpartum depressions. Since antidepressants are more expensive and have more side effects than thyroid medications, it is important to rule out the thyroid first. In addition, if the cause of your symptoms is actually coming from the thyroid, or even from low estradiol, antidepressants won't "fix" this. The untreated thyroid malfunction will lead to additional health problems from the hormone imbalances, such as worsening depression or psychosis, high cholesterol, high blood pressure, hair loss, and weight gain.

Postpartum thyroid dysfunction is not limited to the immediate postpartum period. Effects may become permanent. Statistics show the magnitude of the problem. Dr. Premawardhana from the University of Wales in the United Kingdom recently found that permanent hypothyroidism developed in about 33 percent of the young women with postpartum thyroid problems. Another 20 percent developed hypothyroidism over the next three to five years, even though they had normal thyroid function in the first postpartum year. That means that over 50 percent of the women with postpartum thyroid problems had a lifelong thyroid problem within five years after delivery. This is a significant medical issue.

Juliana's story shows how crucial it is to correct thyroid problems early, and to monitor your complete thyroid function carefully and regularly.

After the birth of her third child, Juliana had a serious bout with postpartum hormone problems that almost cost her her life and that of her baby. She had had milder episodes of postpartum depression with her two earlier pregnancies, but neither she nor her family were prepared for what hit with the third. Within a few weeks, Juliana was having suicidal thoughts and hearing voices telling her to smother her new baby. She and her husband, Doug, were obviously frightened and he insisted she talk with her obstetrician. Her obstetrician referred her to a psychiatrist. She was immediately put on antipsychotic medication along with an antidepressant, but no hormone testing was done. She continued serious struggles with depression and intense thoughts of harming herself and her baby, despite three psychiatric hospitalizations and multiple medications—just since the birth of her last child.

Her husband and family were getting desperate. The psychiatrist was now recommending inpatient care again, this time for electroconvulsive (ECT) treatment. Aware of the risks, her husband was frightened about this approach. He was convinced that there were hormone connections in all this. "She only gets depressed after her pregnancies, so it just makes common sense to me that we should be checking her hormones, but no one will do that," he said. He didn't want Juliana to have ECT until this had been checked.

Although they lived about a day's drive from my office, a friend suggested Doug arrange a consult—Juliana clearly wasn't getting better, and it was now six months after her baby was born. To save time and make the initial visit more meaningful, there are certain lab tests I request ahead of time, particularly in a situation like this. Her lab results came back a week before her appointment, and just prior to the other doctor's decision to start ECT, although I was unaware of this development. As usual I gave directions for the lab to send a copy of the report to me and to the patient at the same time. Doug quickly saw how many of the hormone studies were significantly out of range. He talked to her obstetrician, who agreed the results were abnormal, but didn't recognize the *brain* effects of such profound imbalances. "This isn't a hormonal disorder," he told Doug, "it's psychiatric. She needs the psychiatric medicines and the ECT; hormones won't help." Her psychiatrist also realized the hormones were abnormal, but since the gynecologist did not want this treated, the psychiatrist felt Juliana needed to go ahead with ECT.

Doug called our office in a panic. "Is it really safe for her to have ECT with all these hormones out of whack?" I explained why it was not safe to have ECT until these hormone problems were addressed. Juliana had a severe postpartum thyroiditis with markedly elevated thyroid antibodies, and her TSH was so low it was barely detectable. She was seriously *hyperthyroid,* in addition to her significantly low estradiol and high prolactin, each of which alone can cause depression. By itself, hyperthyroidism is not a safe metabolic condition in which to do ECT. Excess thyroid *coupled with low estradiol* would further aggravate the potential for heart arrhythmias during ECT. With her psychosis getting worse and the family's concern for the safety of both Juliana and her baby, we immediately made arrangements for her to be seen and start treatment for the endocrine imbalances.

The complexity of her situation required a combined approach to address the thyroid disorder, her low estradiol and high prolactin, and the side effects of her psychotropic medications. She had what is called an *extra-pyramidal syndrome* (EPS) from the antipsychotic medicine Haldol. This caused her to have slowed movements, muscle stiffness, difficulty swallowing, a blank facial expression, and a restless crawly feeling, a horrible sensation similar to being buried in an anthill!

I was convinced that her psychosis was caused by the hyperthyroidism. I thought that, in all probability, she would not need the antipsychotic medicine if we could correct the thyroid excess. Since she lived so far away, I was concerned that we needed time to observe her responses and make certain she was not in danger of hurting herself or her baby as we made these changes. Her family kept her children while we worked to start new medications and taper off some of the psychiatric ones, especially the antipsychotic medicine that was causing so many side effects.

I knew that if I started her on a birth control pill right away, it would increase the thyroid binding proteins and keep some of the excess T4 and T3 from being such a problem. I also gave her medicine to treat the extra-pyramidal side effects of the Haldol. By the end of that first week, both her family and I could see a major difference. Her anxiety, depressed mood, and suicidal thoughts were lifting with the added estrogen in the birth control pill, and this also diminished the hyperthyroidism by shifting her excess thyroid hormone into a less active state. A lower dose of Haldol, plus the addition of Ativan, helped relieve the agitation, slowed movements, muscle stiffness, and the awful crawly sensation. She and her family could tell she had turned the corner.

It was a frightening time for everyone, and her treatment certainly required thought and a careful adjustment of medications to find the balance that saved her. I continued to work with her and her husband on the medication adjustments for another six months as her hormones changed. It was complicated and challenging, but a gratifying experience of everyone working together in a therapeutic partnership. She did not have another psychiatric hospitalization and did not need ECT. Within six months, she was able to go back to work. By the end of that year, she was off all psychotropic medicines. She remained stable on just the birth control pills.

As I write this, it has been six years since I first saw her and started her hormone therapy. She has had no further episodes of the severe depression or the psychosis, and no further need for antidepressant or antipsychotic medicines.

But there is an important update that illustrates another reason we must treat these postpartum hormone disorders aggressively. Women with postpartum thyroiditis are at higher risk for later development of thyroid cancer, so they need to be monitored regularly. Recently, we found a nodule on Juliana's thyroid, and sent her for a biopsy. Even though only in her mid-thirties, Juliana had thyroid cancer. She had surgery to remove her thyroid gland, and is now on full replacement thyroid hormones.

Even though antidepressants and antipsychotics may help depression and the abnormal thoughts of a psychosis, they don't treat endocrine problems that can have other effects and later health risks. Endocrine causes can be missed if hormone evaluation is not part of the workup for postpartum depression and/or postpartum psychosis. I find myself wondering whether such a comprehensive evaluation could have helped to prevent the tragedy with Andrea Yates and the deaths of her five children.

The chart on page 170 summarizes these important thyroid effects. If you think you may have a thyroid disorder, turn to Chapter 17 for a discussion of what to have tested, medications available, and how to work with your doctor to get started safely.

Oophoritis and Adrenalitis: Autoimmune Disorders Affecting the Ovaries and Adrenal Glands

Although you may not have heard of these terms, there is a wealth of published medical literature, particularly in the international journals, that addresses these overlooked autoimmune disorders that can lead to premature ovarian decline, infertility, chronic fatigue, fibromyalgia, and immune system disturbances. Most of the research I find that supports the existence of an autoimmune "attack" on the ovaries (oophoritis) comes from work done overseas in the past several decades. One of the difficulties is that we don't have a reliable method for anti-body testing for ovarian or adrenal antibodies as we have for thyroid antibodies. And without reliable measures of the antibodies, our understanding of these conditions is limited and it is difficult to prove their existence, particularly since it is hard enough to get many physicians to check levels of ovarian hormones using the reliable blood tests we *do* have. So you may have one of these disorders without a good way to test for them, other than checking levels of the hormones made by these glands, or checking levels of the pituitary hormones that oversee the function of the ovaries and adrenal glands.

The other key issue that makes diagnosis difficult is that symptoms are nonspecific. You can have the same symptoms from any of these autoimmune endocrine syndromes—adrenalitis, oophoritis, or thyroiditis. In addition, the symptoms are so varied and vague that doctors don't typically associate them as ovarian, adrenal, or thyroid in origin; they are more likely seen as part of a depressive syndrome. Some of the common ones I see are sleep difficulties (rest-less sleep, trouble falling asleep, waking early, multiple awakenings at night—all of which are also listed in the diagnostic criteria for depression!), impaired mem-ory and concentration, marked fatigue, bone loss, hair loss, muscle pain, joint aches, bladder problems, vasomotor instability, low blood pressure, loss of inter-est in sex, vaginal dryness, premature skin aging, increased allergies, and chemi-cal sensitivities. The symptoms appear everywhere in the body. No wonder our fragmented, specialty-based medical model makes it hard to find someone to put the pieces together and relate it to the ovaries!

When I evaluate a patient, it often comes down to looking at the entire pic-ture of symptoms and then using years of clinical experience and intuition to make a judgment that the *gestalt* suggests autoimmune oophoritis, thyroiditis, or adrenalitis. I may not, however, be able to *prove* it objectively given the limita-tions of existing lab tests. Sometimes two or three problems may be present. Keep in mind that women with an autoimmune disorder affecting one endocrine pathway may well have other glands affected.

Over the course of nearly twenty years' work in climacteric medicine and hor-mone evaluations, I have seen many young women I think have developed the clinical syndrome of autoimmune oophoritis, showing clear-cut, objective evi-dence of premature ovarian failure that appeared to be autoimmune but not a result of an autoimmune *thyroid* disorder. The ovarian hormone decline that occurs in the autoimmune oophoritis is similar to thyroid hormone decline that occurs in thyroiditis. Both of these autoimmune disorders produce symptoms that may be similar and overlap because of a combination of factors that include loss of optimal hormone production and the autoimmune response itself.

These women typically have a family history of autoimmune disorders. They probably had a triggering event that affected the immune system—such as exposure to environmental chemicals (pesticides and others), exposure to an infectious agent (viral, bacterial, or fungal illnesses), or exposure to a biological antigen (tick or spider bites). The women I have seen with this type of ovarian decline are typically much younger than the normal menopausal age, may still have FSH in the "normal" range, and will still have some degree of menstruation,

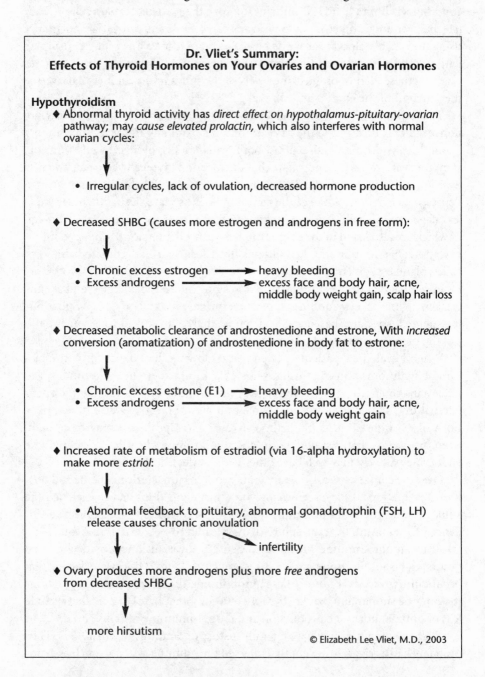

Dr. Vliet's Summary:
Effects of Thyroid Hormones on Your Ovaries and Ovarian Hormones

Hypothyroidism
- ◆ Abnormal thyroid activity has *direct effect on hypothalamus-pituitary-ovarian* pathway; may *cause elevated prolactin,* which also interferes with normal ovarian cycles:

  - • Irregular cycles, lack of ovulation, decreased hormone production

- ◆ Decreased SHBG (causes more estrogen and androgens in free form):

  - • Chronic excess estrogen ⟶ heavy bleeding
  - • Excess androgens ⟶ excess face and body hair, acne, middle body weight gain, scalp hair loss

- ◆ Decreased metabolic clearance of androstenedione and estrone, With *increased* conversion (aromatization) of androstenedione in body fat to estrone:

  - • Chronic excess estrone (E1) ⟶ heavy bleeding
  - • Excess androgens ⟶ excess face and body hair, acne, middle body weight gain

- ◆ Increased rate of metabolism of estradiol (via 16-alpha hydroxylation) to make more *estriol*:

  - • Abnormal feedback to pituitary, abnormal gonadotrophin (FSH, LH) release causes chronic anovulation ⟶ infertility

- ◆ Ovary produces more androgens plus more *free* androgens from decreased SHBG

    more hirsutism

© Elizabeth Lee Vliet, M.D., 2003

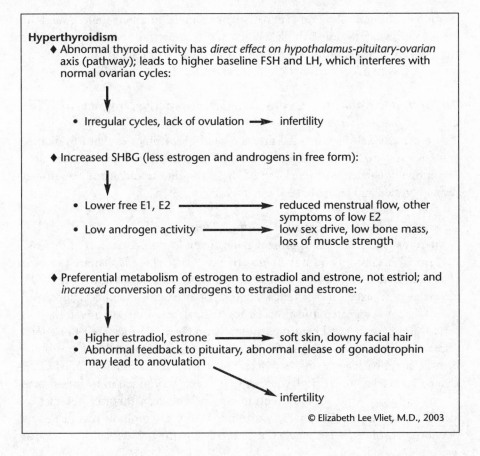

Hyperthyroidism
- ◆ Abnormal thyroid activity has *direct effect on hypothalamus-pituitary-ovarian* axis (pathway); leads to higher baseline FSH and LH, which interferes with normal ovarian cycles:

  - Irregular cycles, lack of ovulation ⟶ infertility

- ◆ Increased SHBG (less estrogen and androgens in free form):

  - Lower free E1, E2 ⟶ reduced menstrual flow, other symptoms of low E2
  - Low androgen activity ⟶ low sex drive, low bone mass, loss of muscle strength

- ◆ Preferential metabolism of estrogen to estradiol and estrone, not estriol; and *increased* conversion of androgens to estradiol and estrone:

  - Higher estradiol, estrone ⟶ soft skin, downy facial hair
  - Abnormal feedback to pituitary, abnormal release of gonadotrophin may lead to anovulation ⟶ infertility

© Elizabeth Lee Vliet, M.D., 2003

though it isn't regular cycles and healthy flow. Although there is still some menstrual function, ovarian hormone levels are lower than healthy levels.

An autoimmune attack on the ovaries can damage them and alter production and availability of ovarian hormones, causing complete premature ovarian *failure* (POF) or the milder form, premature ovarian *decline* (POD). True premature ovarian failure is defined by a high FSH (greater than 20) in a woman younger than age forty. She no longer has menstrual periods and has menopausal levels of the ovarian hormones. Premature ovarian decline (POD) occurs earlier in the process, with loss of ovarian hormone production sufficient to cause profound symptoms and even infertility, but without complete loss of menses or an FSH over 20. This is a part of the continuum that many doctors do not realize is there. Consequently, if the FSH is still less than 20, they tell women "you aren't menopausal." They overlook the point that most of the time it takes several years of declining hormone levels before the FSH will rise that high. You can have "low estrogen" symptoms that disrupt life, even if your FSH is only 10 or 12! Many fertility specialists consider an FSH over 10 to mean that you don't have enough remaining follicles for fertility treatment to succeed. My message continues: The medical community shouldn't get so caught up in the numbers that we miss the person and her suffering. I think the best way to determine whether you suffer from one of these syndromes is a complete evaluation of tests to look at the various aspects of endocrine function. I describe these in Chapters 16 and 17.

When the Adrenals Are Overactive or Underactive: Impact on Your Ovaries

Two other adrenal disorders fall into the category of illnesses that can disrupt your ovaries and lead to abnormal ovarian hormone levels. If you are feeling "hormonally challenged," be aware of these conditions and learn how to get properly tested and where to seek treatment.

Adrenal Corticosteroid Excess (Cushing's Syndrome)

Steroids produced by the adrenal glands include glucocorticoids ("cortisol," the "stress" hormone) and mineralocorticoids. Cortisol levels that are too high over time lead to high blood pressure, high cholesterol and triglycerides, high fasting glucose, excess insulin release and resistance to insulin effects, increased risk of diabetes, repeated infections (from cortisol's immune-suppression), thin skin, thinning hair, easy bruising, muscle weakness, and increased bone loss. Excess cortisol causes marked fat deposits around the middle of the body, breasts, upper back and arms, as well as a rounded puffy face that is called *moon facies*. Excess levels of cortisol, whether due to excess production by the adrenal glands or from corticosteroid medications, such as for asthma or allergies or arthritis, may lead to Cushing's syndrome. The most common reason people develop cortisol excess is actually due to taking corticosteroid medications, such as Cortef or prednisone.

One young woman I evaluated was given prednisone for optic neuritis, a painful inflammation of the optic nerve that can lead to blindness if not treated aggressively with corticosteroids. The optic neuritis resolved quite well with this treatment, but over the next few months she began developing more intense PMS, insomnia, hot flashes, irritability, fatigue, and menstrual headaches that she had not had before. A naturopathic doctor (N.D.) told her she had "adrenal exhaustion" and started her on a high dose of DHEA, 50 mg daily. She became more irritable, had greater difficulty sleeping, started craving sweets, developed severe acne, and began losing "handfuls" of hair in her brush each day. In a panic, she arranged a consultation with us to have all of her hormone levels checked to get to the bottom of her problems.

We did our complete laboratory workup, and her hormone levels showed she was in early ovarian decline, likely precipitated by the corticosteroid treatment. Both her estradiol and testosterone were too low, and her DHEA was excessively high from the supplements she was given. Thyroid and adrenal function tests were good. She did not have adrenal exhaustion; she had "ovarian exhaustion"! Her ovaries had been knocked down by the corticosteroids, and the effects were made worse by the DHEA supplements that caused the symptoms of androgen excess—hair loss, weight gain, insomnia, acne, and irritability.

I treated her successfully with an estradiol patch to boost ovarian function back to normal, which in turn led to her ovaries functioning better to make more testosterone. Since her ovaries were still making good levels of progesterone and she was having regular periods, she did not need supplemental progesterone. I tapered her off the excess DHEA. In nine months, her ovarian function normalized completely and she stopped using the estradiol patch. She is one example of many women we see with ovarian imbalance or decline from corticosteroid medication. I am not advocating that you avoid such treatment—there are clearly times it is critical. Just keep in mind that too much cortisol from your own adrenal glands, or from medicines, may interfere with your ovaries. Check hormone levels if you start having symptoms.

Cortisol levels can also be elevated due to less common causes, such as adrenal disease (Cushing's syndrome) or a pituitary disorder. High cortisol is actually more commonly caused by life stress, loss of optimal estradiol, illnesses, infections, chronic pain, surgeries, loss of optimal thyroid function, biological depression, high-progestin birth control pills, medications such as decongestants and steroids used to treat asthma and arthritis, to name some of the most common ones. These problems are best treated by addressing the underlying cause, such as changing medications or improving "stress relief" strategies. Your cortisol levels will most likely return to normal when these other problems are corrected.

I typically find that if the cortisol is elevated because of thyroid disorders or loss of estradiol, once we have restored estradiol and/or thyroid balance, the cortisol usually falls in line. If cortisol is high due to a suspected adrenal disease such as Cushing's syndrome, or to a pituitary disorder, your physician will likely suggest further testing. Once a specific adrenal or pituitary cause is identified, treatment can be individualized and directed to the cause. See Chapter 17 for more detailed information on testing and treatment options.

When Cortisol Is Too Low: Addison's Disease or Adrenal Insufficiency (AI)

Cortisol and other hormones produced by the adrenal gland are critical for survival. If the adrenal gland is making too little of these hormones it leads to serious illness and major disruptions in multiple body pathways, including the ovaries. If you have been under severe, unrelenting stress for long periods of time (many months to several years), your adrenal glands can lose their ability to respond properly with increased cortisol and you enter the phase called *adrenal insufficiency.* It is also called *adrenal exhaustion,* but this term is significantly overused. Fortunately, it is rather straightforward to test for adrenal insufficiency by first checking serum electrolytes and an eight A.M. serum cortisol.

The hallmark of true adrenal insufficiency (AI) is low cortisol (generally, an 8 A.M. cortisol less than 7 to 8), along with abnormally low sodium and abnor-

ADVERSE HEALTH CONSEQUENCES OF EXCESS CORTISOL

- Middle and upper body fat gain, enlarged breasts
- Hair loss
- Thinning skin with splotchy discolorations
- More fragile blood vessels, leading to easy bruising
- Elevated blood glucose, glucose intolerance, and insulin resistance, leading to increased risk of diabetes
- Increased total cholesterol, LDL, and triglyceride levels and lower HDL leading to increased risk of early heart attacks in younger women
- Disrupted formation of healthy collagen, the basis of healthy ligaments and tendons, leading to injuries and joint and back pain
- Fragmented sleep, leading to diminished growth hormone, decreased muscle repair at night, and daytime fatigue. If your estradiol is also low, it adds to these negative effects of high cortisol.
- Disrupted thyroid function, leading to less available T3, which is important for cellular metabolism throughout the body
- Suppressed immune function, leading to more infections and illnesses
- Increased need for antioxidants, vitamins, minerals as well as proper balance of macronutrients; yet if you are stressed and don't feel well, you may not pay attention to the nutritional balance most needed

© Elizabeth Lee Vliet, M.D., 2003

mally high potassium. AI may arise for unclear reasons not related to persistent, severe stresses, and is then called *Addison's disease*. True Addison's disease is uncommon, but it is a very serious medical disorder and needs proper treatment by an endocrinologist experienced with its complexity and life-threatening medical complications.

Addison's disease typically causes loss of menstrual periods or very light flow. This occurs due to ovarian suppression from the loss of optimal adrenal hormones, or as a result of the same illness that triggered the adrenal insufficiency. Women with very low adrenal hormones typically experience extreme fatigue, poor appetite, marked weight loss, brownish pigmentation of the skin (commonly elbows, knees, knuckles, and mucosa inside the mouth), muscle and joints aches, loss of pubic and underarm hair, thinning scalp hair, and low blood pressure. AI is almost always associated with severe *weight loss* rather than the weight gain seen with high cortisol. If you are overweight, it is very unlikely you have "adrenal exhaustion" and low cortisol, so be wary of people who tell you to take over-the-counter adrenal "boosters" for fatigue.

In Summary

There are many medical disorders and illnesses that affect the ovaries along with other systems. There is a great deal of overlap in the symptoms from imbalances of your thyroid, ovarian, adrenal, and glucose-insulin pathways. If you want a clear picture of *what* is out of balance and *how* to fix it, you must have a careful, complete, systematic hormone evaluation, rather than just relying on a list of symptoms to make a "diagnosis." I have shown you some examples in this chapter, although this is certainly not a complete list.

The health and function of your ovaries may be affected by many different factors, and you should get the ovarian pathways checked if you have problems similar to those described. Doctors often don't want to do this, saying it isn't necessary, it's too expensive, or the levels vary.

None of these reasons hold up when you look at the science today of how our body systems are affected if ovaries do not make optimal levels of their hormones. These excuses are not valid, either, when women are suffering and not getting answers to their problems.

It is *your* health at stake.

Push to get the answers and treatment options you need.

10

Ovaries at Risk: Unrecognized Problems from Surgery, Medications, and Herbs

Common Surgeries: Pitfalls for Your Ovaries

Over the last decade or so, I have evaluated hundreds of young women for symptoms they thought were related to hormone imbalance. The onset of these symptoms and menstrual cycle changes often followed a surgical procedure or illness.

One such procedure is a *bilateral tubal ligation,* often called just a "tubal" or BTL. Most of these women said they were not told that such problems were possible after such a "simple" procedure. When they sought explanations for symptoms, they were often told it couldn't possibly be related to having their tubes "tied." If you have experienced such changes after a tubal, you are not imagining it: There can be premature decline in ovarian hormone levels afterward.

Questions have been raised about post-tubal ligation syndrome since the 1950s. In fact, I found articles in the British medical literature published over forty years ago that described this problem (see Appendix II). In 1951, Dr. Williams and colleagues found that as many as 31 percent of women had abnormal uterine bleeding after a tubal ligation, and 16.5 percent ended up having a hysterectomy to control new bleeding problems. This was *triple* the rate of hysterectomy in the women who had not had a BTL. A number of studies in the 1970s found that hysterectomy rates were much higher (5 to 33 percent) in women who had a BTL than in women who had not. Specialists felt the disruption in ovarian function from the BTL led to the abnormal bleeding or other problems that eventually had to be controlled with hysterectomy.

Finally, a U.S. study, published in 2000, looked at menstrual cycle effects following BTL and supported exactly what I have seen in my patients all these years. The researchers compared 9,514 women who underwent tubal ligation between 1978 and 1987 with 573 women whose partners underwent vasectomy in that same time frame so that the women did not need to have a BTL for contraception. They found that women who had tubal ligations were more likely to report persistent cycle irregularities, painful menstrual periods (dysmenorrhea), and decreases in the number of bleeding days and in the amount of bleeding. These changes indicate a decrease in hormone levels, but this study unfortunately did not check ovarian hormone levels in these women. Without reliable hormone measures, they could not confirm the lower levels we see so commonly in our patients. In spite of the problems reported by the patients in this study, the authors concluded that BTL was "safe and effective," and the results provided "welcome reassurance" regarding tubal ligation since there were no changes in the menstrual cycle! In view of the problems listed above, I can't see how they reached that conclusion, but this illustrates why women today feel they are not informed about possible hormone problems after a BTL.

Why does this procedure cause hormone and bleeding problems? One theory is that the surgical process of cutting, cauterizing, or tying off the fallopian tubes also affects ovarian blood flow, leading to impaired function of the ovary and decreased hormone production. Many gynecologists tell me "it isn't possible" to interrupt the ovarian blood flow with a tubal ligation, and even if that did occur, it wouldn't affect hormone production by the ovary. Dr. John Cattanach, an Australian gynecologist, did an analysis of this hypothesis and published a plausible explanation of how a tubal ligation could lead to diminished estradiol production in the ovary afterward.

Tubal ligations are done at the isthmus, the narrow part of the fallopian tube. Dr. Cattanach explained that at the isthmus, the ovarian branch of the uterine artery is so close to the fallopian tube that the artery is "almost certainly occluded, or at least interrupted, by most of the usual forms of tubal ligation." That leaves only part of the other end of this artery to become the main blood supply for the entire ovary, which means both less blood flow and increased pressure in the artery. We know that whenever the arterial pressure is too high, as in hypertension, it can damage the small blood vessels, the arterioles. This damage means impaired oxygen delivery to the cells of the ovaries, which in turn can decrease hormone production. The chemical reactions in the ovaries that convert cholesterol to estradiol and progesterone require between 3.3 and 8 times more oxygen to make 1 mol (a unit of measure) of estradiol than to make 1 mol of progesterone. Decreased oxygen delivery shifts hormone production toward making *less* estradiol, while a normal amount of progesterone is still being produced.

When I measure hormone levels in the second half or luteal phase of the cycle in women who have had tubal ligations, I consistently find estradiol is *lower* than normal, while progesterone is in the upper end of the normal range, altering the usual ratio of these two hormones. This is exactly what Dr. Cattanach predicted, based on damage to ovarian blood flow. High progesterone when estradiol is lower than it should be is another cause of PMS and heavy menstrual bleeding, commonly described in many of the early studies of BTL and the recent U.S. study, as my patients also commonly describe.

As more time elapses after a BTL, the gradual decline in blood flow causes lower than optimal estradiol levels for most of the cycle. Lower estradiol begins to cause menopause-type symptoms, even in women who are "too young" for menopause. After a BTL, younger women may have irregular cycles, lighter menstrual flow, insomnia, mood changes, more PMS, or even hot flashes. I often hear these symptoms described by women who had a tubal ligation. I find that these young women typically have a high progesterone to estradiol ratio and also describe problems with painful, crampy menses. High progesterone levels stimulate more prostaglandin production by the uterus, and more prostaglandins mean more cramping, so I am not surprised to see more cramps and pain following a tubal.

I am not saying that you should avoid a BTL if you want reliable, permanent contraception. Certainly it is a safe, effective approach. But if you have the procedure, be aware that changes in your ovarian function and hormone production are possible afterward. Test hormone levels when you are feeling really good before you have a tubal ligation. If symptoms develop later, have your hormone levels rechecked and compare them with your earlier test results. Then you can choose to supplement your hormones rather than settle for a diagnosis of "stress" or depression. Statistics show that antidepressants are overprescribed for women. I think this is because physicians do not evaluate the endocrine issues. If you have good objective information to determine the *cause* of your problems, you can explore other options for feeling better, not just antidepressants.

Hysterectomy—Another Cause of Premature Hormone Loss

Another common surgery is the hysterectomy, or removal of the uterus. Many doctors recommend that for women under age forty-eight, the ovaries should not be removed, so that women will have their hormone production until natural menopause. At first glance that rationale makes intellectual sense, except when you consider that rarely do surgeons check hormone levels later to determine whether the ovaries still produce optimal hormone levels. Doctors just assume the ovaries continue to work fine after a hysterectomy. Even more patronizing, doctors tell women with one ovary removed, "Don't worry, the other ovary will take over and make enough hormones. You'll be fine."* Try telling *that* to a man who has lost one testicle.

Since the early 1970s, studies have shown that premature ovarian failure is far more common than we thought, even though the ovaries were left in place. Thirty to 60 percent of women have menopausal levels of estradiol and testosterone as early as two to three years following removal of the uterus. (I have included a number of these references in Appendix II should you have a hard time convincing your doctors of this real concern.) Most of these studies came from England, Germany, Italy, and other European countries. In the United States, this issue has not been taken as seriously. It is not clear to me why doctors here don't think follow-up checks of ovarian hormone levels are necessary.

Dr. John Studd, an internationally known menopause researcher from London, is a strong advocate for follow-up tests of women's hormone levels after a hysterectomy that leaves the ovaries. Dr. Studd says the majority of gynecologists and primary care physicians miss the diagnosis of premature hormonal decline after removal of only the uterus. He attributes this oversight in part to two fac-

---

*See *The Complete Guide to Women's Health* by Bruce Shephard, M.D. (New York: Penguin Group, 1990), page 301.

tors: the loss of menstruation as a marker of the phases of the ovarian hormone cycle, and to doctors' *assumptions* that "vague" symptoms such as insomnia, anxiety, low libido, and depressed mood occur because of psychological reactions to losing the uterus, to feelings of lost femininity, or fear of aging. This focus on assumed psychological issues completely overlooks the physical hormone effects on brain chemistry. There is confirmation of this endocrine connection to such symptoms: FSH is elevated in 25 percent or more of women who have had their uterus removed but still have ovaries. I certainly find these same objective confirmations in my evaluations of hormone levels in my patients.

Hysterectomy is often accused of causing depression, inability to function sexually, and a host of other problems. But the newer, carefully designed prospective studies do not support that removal of the uterus causes major depression or other psychologically damaging consequences in the majority of women. In fact, just the opposite has been found in a number of recent studies: The incidence of depression (as a mood state, not an illness) is about *half* the incidence found prior to surgery, with women showing *improved* psychological and physical well-being, including sexual enjoyment, after hysterectomy.

Surgery is usually done today only when there are clear indications it is needed, such as severe endometriosis, excessive bleeding, painful periods, intractable PMS, severe fibroids that cause abdominal distension, and pain with intercourse. We certainly see many patients who have low hormone levels and don't feel "back to normal" following a hysterectomy, but even these women are grateful the surgery took care of the bleeding or pain. Why the discrepancy between the general perception of hysterectomy versus the positive outcomes from studies like these?

I think the explanation lies in several facts:

1. Even after surgical menopause induced by removal of the uterus and the ovaries, only 25 to 30 percent of women start hormone therapy. Only about half take it for longer than five years. This means a huge number of women with no ovaries are going without any replacement of the very hormones needed for a myriad of body and brain systems. I don't believe it is the loss of the uterus; I think it is the loss of their crucial metabolic hormones that leads to so many problems.

2. Women who still have ovaries are assumed to be making enough hormones, but this is rarely ever checked objectively. The data shows that most of them, in fact, do *not* make adequate levels of ovarian hormones even though the ovaries are still there. Studies from Germany and England have even shown other objective evidence of inadequate estrogen levels even if ovaries remained—there were adverse cholesterol changes and loss of bone, respectively.

3. Even if women *do* start hormone therapy after a hysterectomy, most still do not get "optimal" replacement of their ovarian hormones. The usual approach is to simply give estrogen, usually Premarin. Testosterone is rarely

replaced. No hormone levels are checked; there is typically no individualization of type, route, or dose of estrogen. It doesn't have to be this way. I work hard to help my patients achieve optimal hormone replacement, and most are amazed at the degree of well-being that returns. I consistently find it isn't the removal of the uterus that causes so many problems; it is the lack of adequate hormone therapy afterward.

4. Whether with ovarian removal, or early ovarian decline, women lose most of their testosterone production as well as their estradiol. Testosterone enhances energy level, libido, sense of well-being and mood, bone and muscle formation, and also (along with estradiol) improves the vaginal tissue to relieve dryness that causes pain during sex. Even though medical studies going back to the 1950s show the benefits, and safety, of testosterone replacement, the vast majority of women who have had a hysterectomy *still* are not offered testosterone therapy.

5. Depression following hysterectomy is assumed to be a psychological reaction to losing the uterus. Dr. Studd's view is that "the more plausible cause of depression is the varying degree of ovarian hormone deficiency, which is often overlooked and untreated following hysterectomy." I certainly agree; my clinical experience clearly shows that depressed moods, low energy, sleep loss, anxiety, and loss of libido are alleviated with good hormone management. A long-term prospective study published in 1992 found no depression at four months after hysterectomy, but it did develop after twenty-four months. This again supports the concept that depression is *not* likely to result from an emotional reaction to hysterectomy but can occur as the ovarian hormones decline over time. Such a gradual decrease in estradiol and testosterone just may not produce noticeable symptoms for two or more years after the surgery.

What does this mean for you? If you are only thirty years old and have a hysterectomy, and even if you keep both ovaries, you can still develop menopausal hormone levels in your thirties, on average, within three years of the surgery. You can't be guaranteed to have fully functioning ovaries until natural menopause, on average about age fifty-one. In fact, even if the ovaries work well for many years, studies show that you will become menopausal four to five years earlier than average. But since no one is checking your hormone levels, the hormone cause of symptoms is missed. Fatigue, headaches, depression, insomnia, loss of sex drive, and other symptoms are more likely labeled depression, chronic fatigue, anxiety, or stress.

How do women become prematurely menopausal after a hysterectomy? The reasons are very similar to those described for the BTL. This time, the decrease in blood flow is more severe because the uterine artery has to be "tied off" (clamped) when the uterus is removed. Otherwise you would have uncontrollable bleeding. When this artery is tied off, it means a loss of over 50 percent of the blood flow to the ovary from the ovarian artery. The ovary still gets some blood flow from another, smaller artery in the wall of the pelvis, but this does not make up for what is lost from the uterine artery. You can imagine how difficult it is for the ovary to work optimally if blood supply is reduced over 50 percent.

If you have spent years suffering, not feeling well, and going from doctor to doctor trying to find a way to relieve symptoms and to feel better, all it takes to answer your questions is for a doctor to check your hormone levels! It is not difficult or overly expensive to do. You deserve to have your hormone concerns taken seriously and properly tested.

Common Medications: Unexpected Pitfalls and Problems for Your Ovaries

The Twenty-First Century "Tonic": Serotonin Boosters and Other Mood Managers, or "Just Give Her a Happy Pill"

Prozac (and its new packaging as Sarafem), Zoloft, Paxil, Celexa, and Luvox are the most frequently prescribed group of medications for women under fifty in the United States. Over 30 million Americans have taken these "serotonin enhancers" (SSRIs) at one time or another. For women especially, these drugs are doled out rather like the turn-of-the-century Lydia Pinkham's Tonic, a popular "women's remedy" for a host of ailments from anxiety, depressed mood, irritability, and premenstrual problems to headaches, insomia, low energy, muscle pain, excessive "worrying," and a variety of others.

Our twenty-first-century mood-altering medicines have a reputation for being so safe and effective that they are commonly prescribed for both FDA-approved reasons like depression and obsessive-compulsive disorder, as well as many off-label uses, such as chronic pain, bulimia, attention deficit hyperactivity disorder, borderline personality disorder, hypochondria, fibromyalgia, migraine headaches, social shyness, and most recently PMS and PMDD.

Since most of these conditions are more prevalent in women, we can see why now 65 to 70 percent of all SSRI prescriptions are written for women. Less than 10 percent are written by psychiatrists. In the United States, primary care physicians, gynecologists, neurologists, and rheumatologists prescribe most of these medicines. As a result of their use for so many conditions other than depression, and their being prescribed by nonpsychiatrists, there are some emerging concerns: Doses are now often larger than originally studied and medicines are commonly combined with many other prescriptions. The typical woman I see, even if she is in her teens, is already on an average of five to eight different prescriptions. The greater the number of medicines you take at any one time, the greater your likelihood of serious side effects and drug interactions.

When these drugs are properly used, they have significantly fewer side effects than older antidepressants like the tricyclics (TCA, such as amitriptyline or Elavil, Pamelor, doxepin, and others). I do not think they are really needed as often as they are prescribed, and they are definitely overused for women. In addition, their effects can mask other health issues, including other causes of similar symptoms. What about use of these medications over a number of years, as many women often do? Do they have subtle side effects not easily recognized? Yes. These medicines may cause weight gain, headaches, memory disturbance, and have effects on ovarian function that you, and possibly your doctor, haven't realized.

First of all, many younger women have symptoms such as those above for a variety of other reasons, not "psychiatric" in origin. They may, therefore, need different treatments instead of simply using psychiatric medications. Two common endocrine problems—low estradiol and low thyroid—discussed in previous chapters, cause many of the same symptoms.

Erratic menstrual cycles caused by declining ovarian hormone levels or thyroid disorders may cause mood swings or ups and downs in moods similar even to bipolar illness. Women are then prescribed mood-stabilizers such as Depakote (valproic acid), Tegretol (carbamazepine), Neurontin (gabapentin), or lithium. These medicines can disrupt neuroendocrine pathways that regulate the ovaries and alter thyroid hormone production. Lithium, for example, commonly causes hypothyroidism by interfering with the manufacture of thyroid hormones, and it also triggers potential autoimmune reactions in the gland itself. So if your mood symptoms were actually caused by an undiagnosed thyroid problem, you can see how your problems could get worse if you are put on lithium, based just on your symptoms.

Both SSRIs and "mood stabilizer" anticonvulsants such as Depakote, Tegretol, and others can increase release of the pituitary hormone prolactin via their action on the brain chemical messenger called *dopamine*. Prolactin is the hormone that regulates nursing after delivery. Another effect of prolactin is to suppress the return of ovarian cycles and ovarian hormone production, helping prevent another pregnancy while a mother is still nursing a new infant. If you take a medicine that increases prolactin even though you are not nursing, it can cause a higher than normal prolactin level for a nonpregnant woman, which leads to menstrual irregularity, a decrease in ovarian hormones, weight gain, headaches, depression, and even infertility. Most of the antidepressants today act on pathways in the brain that either directly or indirectly affect prolactin. If you take these medicines for a long time, they can increase prolactin, which in turn suppresses your ovaries.

SSRIs, or serotonin-reuptake inhibitors, boost serotonin by inhibiting reuptake by the nerve cell, a process that inactivates serotonin. Brain cells get flooded with available, active serotonin that increases the transfer of messages between nerve cells. These medications also may work by stimulating the growth of new nerve cells and connections, called *neurogenesis*. Increased serotonin activity at receptor sites in the brain and body is usually a desirable therapeutic action of these medicines, though too much serotonin activity can cause unwanted side effects such as fatigue, headaches, anxiousness, and insomnia.

Another downside of increased serotonin action is a decrease in activity of the chemical messenger dopamine, which inhibits prolactin release. If dopamine is too low, prolactin is no longer inhibited correctly in a nonpregnant woman and levels rise. Higher prolactin then decreases the normal FSH-LH regulation of the menstrual cycle, inhibits normal ovarian cycling and hormone production. Estradiol, progesterone, and testosterone can all decline, even if you are in your teens or twenties and far from menopause. When the SSRIs are prescribed year after year, you are more likely to have side effects from too much serotonin effect relative to dopamine. In addition, these drugs are so widely prescribed for all kinds of other problems—from migraines and PMS to premenstrual dysphoric disorder (PMDD)—that more women take them for many years and are more likely to develop undesirable side effects.

High prolactin also leads to weight gain, breast enlargement, milky discharge from the breast, headaches, fatigue, and depressed mood. So if you are on a tricyclic antidepressant or a serotonin-booster medication for a while and have any of these symptoms, it is important for your doctor to do a blood test for prolactin. If the level is too high, you should talk with your doctor about medication changes. For example, bromocriptine is a medicine designed to increase dopamine and reduce prolactin. Dopamine is a critical chemical messenger in the brain's sexual circuits, so if you lose dopamine activity, sexual response is blocked. This is how serotonin boosters cause loss of sex drive and interfere with your ability to have an orgasm.

A number of other medications commonly prescribed for women also act on these same brain pathways and can lead to increased prolactin:

Anticonvulsants, such as the mood-stabilizers I mentioned above, that are also commonly prescribed for seizures, migraine headaches, muscle and nerve pain syndromes. The anticonvulsant Depakote has another potential risk to your ovaries. Some studies have found it causes an increase in ovarian cysts and an increased risk of developing polycystic ovarian disorder (PCOS). This may happen due to elevated prolactin, or it may be through a different, unknown mechanism.

Antipsychotics such as chlorpromazine (Thorazine), haloperidol (Haldol), droperidol (Inapsine), thioridazine (Mellaril), thiothixene (Navane), risperidone (Risperdal), pimozide (Orap), quetiapine (Seroquel), and others.

Antinausea medicines such as Compazine and Reglan.

Shake off your complacency about these medicines, and review the potential problems carefully before you turn to SSRIs as "magic bullets." Many medications have more, and different, side effects in women than in men. Most testing was done on men because they don't have all the "noise" of hormone fluctuations that can confound a study. Yet it is precisely these hormone changes that can alter how women's bodies metabolize medicines! Many medications have been on the market for years without being subject to safety analyses by gender. As an example, let's take a look at some heart side effects that are more likely to occur in women.

Heart Side Effects of Common Medicines—A Hidden Danger for Women

Long QT Syndrome (LQTS), a disturbance in the electrical conduction system of the heart, is a new concern for women taking tricyclic antidepressants, SSRIs, antipsychotics, antihistamines, decongestants, and a number of other drugs. LQTS is much more common in women than men, and usually occurs at times in the menstrual cycle when estradiol is falling or low. The electrical impulse system of the heart keeps your heart pumping at a steady rate, so any disruption can lead to a potentially serious disturbance in heart rhythm called *torsade de pointes*. This abnormal heartbeat decreases blood flow to the brain and body and may cause fainting spells (syncope). Or, the abnormal heartbeat can degenerate into ventricular fibrillation, a very serious rhythm disturbance that can cause sudden death from cardiac arrest.

Why talk about this in a book about ovaries? Because many young women take multiple medications for mood, headaches, allergies, and other problems, which creates potential problems for the heart, even though it doesn't appear directly related to the ovaries. Even if you are not taking medications that affect heart rate and rhythm, you are more likely to have heart arrhythmias due to fluctuating and falling levels of estradiol. Women naturally have a longer QT interval in their heartbeat cycle than do men, which means they are more susceptible to these medication side effects. Hormonal imbalance added to multiple medications is an explosive mix that makes LQTS and torsade de pointes much more likely. That's another reason I am so concerned about the overprescribing of medications for women without baseline blood tests of the ovarian hormones. Doctors have assumed, incorrectly, that hormone levels don't matter. I hope I have shown you they *do*.

There are over fifty different prescription medications that can cause LQTS (and that doesn't include herbs that may also have this effect), including TCA antidepressants Elavil (amitriptyline), Sinequan (doxepin), Tofranil (imipramine), Norpramin (desipramine); SSRIs such as Zoloft (sertraline), Prozac and Sarafem (fluoxetine), and Paxil (paroxetine); "atypical" antidepressants such as Effexor (venlafaxine); antiarrhythmics (such as quinidine, Norpace, Tambocor, Pronestyl, and several others); antipsychotics (see earlier list of these that cause high prolactin); antibiotics (Biaxin, Tequin, Levoquin, Zagam, Bactrium-Septra, erythromycin); antimigraine medicines (Amerge, Imitrex, Zomig); the GI stimulant Propulsid; and some of the newer antipsychotics such as Risperdal.

The presence of an eating disorder (anorexia nervosa or bulimia, which can cause electrolyte imbalances) and dehydration are other risk factors that can lead to LQTS and torsade de pointes. If you have episodes of irregular heartbeat, fainting, or significant tachycardia after starting a new medicine, talk with your doctor promptly. Change occurs rapidly in our understanding of these medication effects on the heart. You can locate more detailed and updated information by checking the website *www.QTdrugs.org*, or by contacting the Sudden Arrhythmia Death Syndromes Foundation at 800-786-7723. As more women demand better information, new studies now include women as well as men to clarify how to use all medicines more safely. In the meantime, you can reduce your risk by learning about serious drug interactions and talking with all your physicians about *everything* you are taking, including herbs and supplements.

Other Common Medication Pitfalls Affecting Women

Antibiotics. Antibiotics are certainly necessary, and clearly lifesaving. But antibiotics are also widely *over*used today, often for minor problems that will get better on their own in a week or so, or would respond to simple remedies. Women who overuse antibiotics are at risk for frequent or persistent yeast infections that create many problems. You are probably aware of this antibiotic complication. But maybe you do not know that prolonged use of antibiotics might also alter hormone metabolism in the liver by increasing the metabolic breakdown of estradiol, progesterone, and testosterone.

You may not notice antibiotic-induced effects on your ovarian hormones because you are accustomed to daily variation throughout the menstrual cycle. But if you are using an estradiol patch or tablet, you may need a brief increase in the dose during antibiotic therapy to prevent the return of hot flashes, mood changes, or insomnia that results when the antibiotic increases the liver metabolism of estradiol. Likewise, if you take oral contraceptives, adding an antibiotic may increase the rate of hormone breakdown in the liver, which could mean your birth control pill is less effective for contraception, and you may have more spotting or breakthrough bleeding.

Beta-blockers. Beta-blockers are often used for migraine headaches, mitral valve prolapse, some types of anxiety, and to control blood pressure. While these are safe medicines overall, they have some unique problems for women, especially if taken for a long time. Beta-blockers can inhibit the conversion of T4 to T3, leading to symptoms of hypothyroidism. This can lead to significant problems that in turn disrupt ovarian function. Beta-blockers also impair glucose-insulin pathways, leading to problems with insulin resistance, and even diabetes. Women already have these problems at a higher frequency than do men, so you have a double whammy when medications have these side effects. Weight gain, marked fatigue, difficulty concentrating, and decreased sex drive are common with beta-blockers, even if your hormones are in balance. These medicines will intensify such symptoms caused by hormone imbalances.

High-progestin birth control pills. The progestins in birth control pills, particularly those with high progestin–low estrogen formulas, are common causes of fatigue, depression, headaches, low libido, muscle and joint pain, vaginal dryness, or vulvar pain. I have treated many young women for vulvodynia caused solely by several years of using a high progestin–low estrogen pill like Loestrin, Mircette, or Alesse. Progestin-only contraceptives like Depo-Provera or Norplant are often worse, because they contain no estrogen and act to suppress your own estradiol production.

Suzette is a woman in her early thirties who was experiencing severe depressive symptoms, including mood swings, irritability, and sudden tearfulness for no apparent reason. She also reported feeling tired all the time, hot flashes, insomnia, joint and muscle aches. "I feel like I've had a long bout with the flu," she said. Suzette had difficulties having orgasms, and had lost her interest in sex, causing a serious strain on her new marriage. What triggered all this? She noticed the problems began within a few months after her gynecologist started her on Loestrin to keep her periods lighter and reduce menstrual cramps. "I did pretty well at first," she said, "and then I noticed that my depressed mood, irritability, and low energy got worse and worse the longer I was on these pills."

I changed her oral contraceptive to Ovcon-35, with much less progestin and slightly more estrogen, which improved her symptoms. I told her to use a low dose of estradiol alone for the days between Ovcon pill packs to keep her estrogen from falling abruptly, which triggered her migraines. The estradiol didn't prevent a normal period, because bleeding would occur with the drop in progestin when she stopped Ovcon.

At her first follow-up appointment two months later, she said: *"I feel like someone flipped a switch on me. I don't have that deadened feeling, I don't feel depressed, I am not crying, my angry outbursts are gone, I sleep better, I have my energy, I don't have all those headaches, and I am getting my interest in sex back. It was remarkable to feel so much better in such a short period of time. It also surprised me that my joint pain was gone after you cut the amount of progestin I was getting. I never knew that what's in a birth control pill could make such a difference!"*

Her laboratory results showed other interesting findings related to the higher progestin content of Loestrin: Her eight A.M. cortisol was higher than normal, indicating a "stress response" activated by the low estrogen–high progestin pill. This returned to normal after she was on Ovcon for six months. Her free T3 and T4 thyroid hormones were lower than optimal, another effect of birth control pills, especially the high-progestin ones. Although her TSH was still in a desirable range, her thyroid hormones weren't as effective as they should have been because a higher percentage was attached to the binding proteins in the bloodstream, making them less active. These changes are common contributing factors to symptoms of depression, tiredness, and waistline weight gain when women are on the wrong birth control pills. This is another reason to integrate the evaluation of thyroid and ovarian hormone pathways.

Soy, Supplements, Herbs, and OTC Hormones: Pitfalls for Your Ovaries

Women today are inundated with articles, ads, and multilevel sales schemes pitching a myriad of herbs, soy-containing products, "natural" progesterone–"wild yam" creams, over-the-counter forms of DHEA, and melatonin—all touted as "magic bullets" for menopause, PMS, and perimenopause. Women have the mistaken belief, reinforced by clever marketing, that everything "natural" is automatically "safe" and without side effects. This is not correct. Remember, plants can produce potent poisons that humans have used for killing animals (and other people) for thousands of years. Many types of herbs and supplements have the potential to cause *harmful* effects, particularly if you already have a decline in your ovarian hormones, a thyroid disorder, allergies to plants and pollen, or any problem with liver metabolism.

Plant Estrogens (Phytoestrogens)

The phytoestrogens, found in several hundred different plants, are biologically weaker than the native human estrogens. Phytoestrogen effects at the human estrogen receptors are not the same as our own estradiol. Your body cannot make the identical ovarian estradiol from the phytoestrogens in soy or yams. All of the phytoestrogen chemical building blocks require chemical conversion in the laboratory because our body does not have the enzymes to make these changes. Taking phytoestrogen supplements does not restore what your ovary made. Even worse, high concentrations of phytoestrogens, such as soy isoflavones, can overwhelm your declining estradiol at receptor sites and interfere with the action and production of the body's "natural" estradiol, even though phytoestrogens are less potent than estradiol. In addition to these receptor effects, studies also show that high soy intake in *pre*menopausal women suppresses ovary production of estradiol and progesterone by 20 to 50 percent. That's a significant loss, especially if you already have symptoms of hormone imbalance.

Research from several countries shows that phytoestrogens and isoflavones compete with our own estradiol and progesterone at the body's receptor sites. For example, genistein, a soy isoflavone, has different binding strengths depending on which estradiol receptor (ER) is considered—for example, it has a sixfold greater affinity for the ER-beta than for ER-alpha. Genistein can act either as an estrogen *blocker* at low concentrations or an estrogen *enhancer* at high concentrations. At higher concentrations, the estrogen-enhancing effects of genistein have *stimulated* the growth of breast cancer cells. Soy isn't as innocuous as the ads claim.

If you have problems with your ovary hormones, eating a lot of soy can make matters worse. If you are trying to get pregnant, or having problems with infertility, soy supplements can interfere with ovulation and your hormone levels. If you have already lost significant bone, soy-induced ovarian suppression can cause further bone loss. In China and Japan, where diets are high in phytoestrogens, women do not typically describe hot flashes, but they *do* continue to have bone loss after menopause, and osteoporosis is a serious problem in most Asian countries today. Research indicates that phytoestrogens alone do not provide enough estrogen effect to protect against bone loss and decline in cognitive function.

If you have frustrating problems with nightly insomnia, already triggered by declining estradiol, too much soy intake can make your sleep problems worse by reducing your ovary's estradiol production. Low estradiol contributes to sleeplessness, anxiety, and high blood pressure, which can in turn be made worse by some herbs. Ginseng, for example, is often recommended by herbalists as a "nat-ural" source of estrogen and given to women to "balance their hormones." Yet ginseng can cause high blood pressure, insomnia, anxiety, or agitation in the usual supplement doses. Furthermore, based on recent studies, ginseng has little or no measurable estrogenic effect. It doesn't even do what many of the ads claim it does.

I am aware of studies that show increased soy intake is associated with lower cholesterol, higher HDL ("good") cholesterol, and lower blood pressure. But there is a drawback that you don't hear about. Soy isoflavones block your thyroid gland from converting T4 to the more active T3. The high intake of soy-based foods in Japan is one factor contributing to the high rate of hypothyroidism and goiter in that country. Studies from as early as the 1970s show soy isoflavones have marked antithyroid effects and cause hypothyroid disorders in infants fed soy formulas, but this is not mentioned in the current hype for adding soy foods to your diet—including all those protein drinks, protein powders, protein snack bars, and isoflavone supplement pills. Some of these negative effects of soy can be reduced by eating only *fermented* soy products (such as tempeh, miso, and tamari), which are more commonly consumed in Asian cultures. Most American women don't know this, and flock to soy supplements based on all the clever marketing claims, not knowing that the products sold in the United States are those more likely to cause thyroid problems. Don't forget, having optimal thyroid function is critical to the health of your ovaries. If your thyroid hormones aren't working properly, you won't have normal ovarian hormone production either!

There are now excellent double-blind, randomized, prospective placebo-controlled studies (the "gold standard" type of medical research studies) show-ing that isoflavone supplements have *no effect* greater than placebo on *any* of the menopausal symptoms measured, including objective measures of estrogen effect. These studies were interesting because the hot-flash frequency decreased in *all* participants, but there was *no difference* in flash/flush frequency between placebo and isoflavone groups. Earlier studies that did not include placebo com-parisons tended to overestimate the value of phytoestrogen products such as soy on reducing hot flashes without realizing why. This is a big factor with symptoms like hot flashes, since there has consistently been an unusually high positive response to placebo in studies on how to control hot flashes. Funding for both of these studies was provided by the company that manufactured the particular isoflavone supplement (Promensil), and one of the study authors served as a consultant to the company. It is unlikely that there was a bias *against* Promensil.

You have probably also read recently about the Asian high-soy diet being associated with a lower risk of breast cancer. A sales pitch for soy supplement pills and protein powder drinks usually comes along with such articles or adver-tisements. What's not often mentioned is that in Japan and other Asian coun-tries, there are additional factors that also contribute to their lower risk of breast cancer. Asian women generally drink very little alcohol. Drinking even two or three alcoholic beverages (wine, beer, or liquor) several days a week can increase breast cancer risk to four times greater than in women who don't drink alcohol. Asian women have a far lower fat intake, particularly animal fats that are a risk factor for breast cancer. They are far more physically active throughout their lives than are American women, and studies clearly show that regular exercise lowers risk of breast cancer.

Even more ominous for young women, red clover (or soy) isoflavones can *cause infertility,* as seen in a variety of animals. Be careful about using these products in your childbearing years. I think important information like this is left out because companies want to make money selling you supplements, regardless of whether you need them, whether they work, or whether they do harm. Millions of women are using these products every day, so that's why I reiterate the potential negative effects.

Lessons from Women's Experiences

Rose is a thirty-three-year-old woman who came for a consult describing "severe vaginal burning, painful intercourse, lack of lubrication, and diminished orgasm." At her first appointment she said, "I have been through the mill—I have been to about a dozen different doctors including two different gynecologists and a urologist, who put a scope up my bladder. One GYN checked an estrogen level and told me it was normal, but it was just done once on the day I went to the office and no one asked what cycle day I was on. After I read your book, I realized the cycle day was important to understand the test result. I went to a vulvodynia specialist and all they did was give me a prescription for citrate and glucosamine and said I could have surgery to remove the damaged tissue. I certainly didn't want surgery, so I tried the glucosamine and it has helped a little but I still had the burning. I felt like they were just treating the symptom, not getting at the cause. Another doctor told me it was happening because I was in a stressful relationship. I didn't know what to think by then."

I explained to Rose what her lab studies showed about potential causes of her vulvar pain. I also told her about the many endocrine and metabolic factors causing vaginal and bladder pain problems in women. I think it is damaging to just write them off to "relationship problems." As we discussed her problems further, an interesting fact came to light. After reading that soy was really good for you, Rose began eating a lot of soy foods, taking soy isoflavone supplements, buying tofu and eating it instead of meat, and she even stopped drinking regular milk and switched to soymilk. This was about two years before she started having vulvodynia. "I heard soy was so good," she said, "I changed everything to soy and I cut fat out of my diet and was eating only about 10 percent fat, if that much. I was so good at watching the fat, I was doing better than what they recommend at Pritikin!" So what affected her ovarian hormones and, in turn, contributed to the vulvar pain?

I explained earlier that a high intake of soy phytoestrogens actually decreases your estradiol and progesterone production, anywhere from 20 to 50 percent. Since Rose was getting in her thirties, her ovaries were slowly decreasing their hormone production anyway, and the soy-induced inhibition just added to this loss. In addition, women need 20 to 30 percent fat intake for the body to have the necessary "building blocks" to make steroid hormones (estradiol, progesterone, testosterone, DHEA, cortisol). Your liver manufactures cholesterol from the fats in the food you eat, and from triglycerides. This occurs even if you don't eat foods that are themselves high in cholesterol. Rose was eating such an extremely low-fat diet that her body simply didn't have enough fat to make the normal amount of ovarian hormones. Then, all that soy in her diet "competed" at the estradiol receptors with what little estradiol her body was making.

Rose's serum estradiol levels were abnormally low throughout her menstrual cycle, both before and after ovulation, but her DHEA and progesterone levels were still quite good and well into the normal range. Her thyroid and adrenal function were excellent. The loss of adequate estradiol was the primary cause for her vulvar pain. She later sent a letter saying how much better she felt, and commented that she was shocked that no one had checked her hormone levels before this. She ended her letter with, "My health was regained by me listening to my own inner guidance and intuition of what was right for me, because I thought this was somehow a hormone problem."

Sue Ellen is now thirty-eight. Five years ago, she began having night sweats, hot flashes, severe fatigue, insomnia, irritability, and mysterious crying spells a week before her period. When I saw her, she said, "I am tired of being tired. I'd like to feel energetic again. I am tired of feeling so cold all the time, and feeling so irritable. I'd really like to have my sex drive back, both for me and for my husband. Sometimes I feel sick, totally weak, and lose my mental functions. I'm tired of having to restrict my foods so much because they say I have all these food allergies. I'd like to know if I really have them, because sometimes just having to watch what I eat all the time is another major stress in my life. I'd like to age gracefully and not look so dried out and wrinkled at my age!

"Since all this began, I've seen several doctors and several alternative practitioners. The M.D.'s all just told me the typical 'it's normal to be tired and not sleep well when you have three children,' and I thought the alternative practitioners were going to be helpful, but I quit seeing them after spending too much money and seeing no improvements. The last person I saw was a naturopath who put me on Progon B (progesterone) sublingual capsules. When I tried to talk with her about my total lack of libido and my skin problems, she just said it was caused by stress. I was so upset, I stopped seeing her after that."

On the Progon B, Sue Ellen had serious skin breakouts, acne flare-ups, eczema of her ankles and elbows, boils on her buttocks, several episodes of pink eye, and frequent sinus infections. She had other upsetting skin changes: a "brownish" pigmentation around her mouth, and an "orangish" cast to her skin. Her face wrinkled more than usual; her scalp was dry, flaky, and itchy; and she said she felt "dry all over." She couldn't have an orgasm easily, and was especially bothered that her libido had "completely disappeared."

Sue Ellen's evaluation showed a number of causes of her multiple symptoms: Her estradiol level was extremely low at 36 pg/ml; her testosterone was too low at 23 ng/dl; her DHEA and progesterone were still in the healthy normal ranges, which meant an excess of both of these hormones relative to her low estradiol and testosterone. Progon B gave her an excess of progesterone, and when this was *added* to her own body's progesterone and DHEA, it caused the acne, other skin eruptions, and her worsening allergies. Remember, progesterone suppresses your immune system. To complicate matters, she was taking the progesterone under the tongue (sublingually), which makes the excess even greater than if this same amount had been taken orally and swallowed. Excess progesterone effects caused her low libido, irritability, and blood sugar fluctuations.

She also took so many vitamin and herbal supplements that she had side effects from these, too. For example, high doses of vitamin A and beta-carotene commonly cause an orange discoloration of the skin. She was taking excessive doses of the B vitamins, vitamin E, and omega-3 and -6 essential fatty acids. Her other supplements included chaste berry (Vitex), nettle, dandelion, Siberian ginseng, licorice, horsetail, rosemary leaf, gingerroot, and yellowstock root. All these phytoestrogens helped lower her estradiol even further, leading to dry skin, sinus infections, vaginal dryness, low libido, insomnia, night sweats, fatigue, and irritability. I frequently see women who are seriously overdoing it with excess vitamin doses and multiple, potentially conflicting, herbs and supplements. Be careful about interactions and watch the *combined*, total daily doses in multiple products.

Additional Herb and Supplement Cautions

There are several additional cautions for women who have ovarian hormone imbalances:

- *Saint-John's-wort* should **not** be taken with prescription hormones, as it decreases the effectiveness of the hormones by 50 percent. This is due to the way the herb increases liver metabolism of the hormones. If you take Saint-John's-wort with a birth control pill, you risk losing the contraceptive effectiveness because of the drug-herb interaction. Unless you want a "Saint-John's" baby, you best forget taking this herb.
- *DHEA.* I do not recommend taking over-the-counter DHEA. Most over-the-counter products contain doses higher than women need and can lead to excess androgen side effects such as weight gain, sweet cravings, acne, facial hair, loss of scalp hair, irritability, restless sleep/insomnia, agitation, anxiety, and muscle spasms. In addition, many women with ovarian or thyroid hormone imbalances need to be sure that their bodies are not already making *too much* DHEA, such as in PCOS, before adding this hormone. You need

reliable blood tests, not saliva tests, of *all* your hormones before deciding whether DHEA is needed.

- *Melatonin.* Studies show that this popular sleep aid has some adverse effects for women. Daily use of melatonin by women causes cortisol levels to rise, but not in men. High cortisol causes more fat around your waist and upper body, interferes with immune function, and may also impair fertility. Taking melatonin every night for sleep also commonly leads to headaches, tiredness, and depression during the day. If you are having trouble sleeping, don't just pop melatonin pills. You need a thorough medical evaluation of the cause.

In Summary

Adverse medication effects, as well as drug-drug interactions and herb-drug interactions are far more common than most people, physicians included, realize. Be aware that all of these seemingly innocuous medicines and herbs may affect your ovarian and thyroid hormone balance. In addition, if you have had surgery involving the uterus or ovaries, insist on having your hormones properly checked when you start having symptoms. Good studies show that these common surgeries *do* cause earlier loss of optimal ovarian hormones in a significant percentage of women.

Remember, herbs may be wildly popular today, but many are metabolized by the same liver pathways that metabolize prescription medicines. Taking them together can significantly change the rate of breakdown of one or the other. In Section IV, there is a list of commonly available herbs and their potential adverse effects. Several reputable sources for additional information are listed in Appendix II. *The Comprehensive Database of Natural Medicines* is an excellent authoritative guide based on solid worldwide research. It is published by a team of pharmacists who also publish *The Prescriber's Letter* for health professionals. Let your doctor know about any herbal supplements you take, just as you would any other medications, so that if you develop problems, he or she will have all the information needed to properly evaluate your symptoms.

In addition, keep in mind that physicians see many patients each day. They may not always remember, or think to ask you, what supplements or herbs you take. Doctors need gentle reminders now and then. *At every appointment, always tell your physicians all the supplements, herbs, or over-the-counter products you take. Bring to your appointment a list of what is in each one. This is for your safety.*

SECTION III

*Your Ovaries
and
Your Body*

11

Ovaries out of Balance:
Patterns in Women's Lives

Introduction

The patterns in women's lives and cycles have intrigued and fascinated me since my days in a college endocrinology course. The endocrine-reproductive system was my favorite in medical school. In my clinical years, I was struck by patterns in the way patients described what was happening to them. This became more striking when working with PMS in 1983, a time when menstrually related problems were not taken very seriously in most medical settings. I was a full-time medical school faculty member seeing patients and developing a curriculum in what we now call *mind-body medicine*. Once other physicians learned of my interest, they referred many young women for evaluation.

Most were in their teens and twenties. I was struck by the similarity in the descriptions of their symptoms whether they had ever heard of PMS or not. I couldn't help but see common patterns in what they described. One sixteen-year-old described having "horrible" mood swings the week before her period. "I feel like I am losing control, I crave chocolate, and I drink [alcohol] more. I am depressed, bloated, and sleepy, and I feel so tired. I also get constipated, my breasts swell, and hurt, and I ache a lot. I don't usually have headaches, but I get them along with all this other stuff. It goes away when my period starts, but I feel like I am going to explode until then."

It was similar with a twenty-nine-year old: "About a week before my period, I start getting really cranky and edgy, I snap at people and don't mean to, and then I feel bad about myself," she said. "I don't sleep well, I feel like my appetite is out of control, and I can't seem to get enough to eat. It seems like all I want to eat is junk food and ice cream or at least something sweet. I get these times of feeling dizzy and lightheaded in the afternoons or late morning, and then I feel anxious and hyper. I feel so bloated and sluggish and don't feel like doing anything much at all. Once my period comes, I feel fine again."

And even a fourteen-year-old had similar problems: "My mother wanted me to see you about this because she thinks my hormones are out of whack," she said shyly. "It feels crazy talking about this, but I get scared because the week before my period is such a nightmare. I am so mean nobody wants to be around me. My friends say I'm a real bitch. I fly off the handle at everybody, I'm out of control, I cry for no reason, I'm screaming at everybody, and I feel like I have to scratch myself until this tension goes away. Sometimes I feel like I want to pull my hair out, it's so awful. I don't like telling anybody how I feel because they'll think I'm crazy. I'm fat and puffy and achy and I feel totally miserable. I sneak all this chocolate because I can't seem to leave it alone, and then my face breaks out and I don't want to be around anybody. I can't sleep at night and I can't stay awake at school. I feel like my body is some alien thing and I hate it. But it's weird, because when my period comes, it all goes away like it wasn't ever there. Makes me feel like I was in a bad dream for a couple weeks. Then I wonder if I imagined it all. But it keeps coming back the same time every month."

A thirty-five-year-old described her experience as an "overall achy feeling, like I have the flu. I feel depressed, irritable, and mad at the world. I am much more anxious, and I often cry for no reason and then feel silly. I get these aches and cramps in the lower part of my abdomen and have this backache that really gets me down. I have a lot of water retention, and I get constipated and that makes me feel even more bloated and miserable. But I am so hungry I eat too much, and it drives me nuts because I crave chocolate so much. I have this dull headache a lot of the time, and I don't sleep well. When my period comes, it all clears up and I feel normal again."

Today, after thousands of PMS consults, the patterns are similar from woman to woman, no matter what her age. Symptoms start at ovulation or a few days later, and magically vanish with bleeding or a few days after menses begin. I have also observed *cyclic* patterns in other uniquely "female" syndromes such as irritable bowel symptoms, bladder pain or recurrent infections, vulvodynia, interstitial cystitis, and endometriosis, to name a few; and in disorders more common in women than men, such as asthma or fibromyalgia, chronic fatigue, migraines, depression, or anxiety problems. I have found a common thread in women with these disorders: low estradiol production often accompanied by low testosterone, whether or not they still make healthy levels of progesterone. Let's look more closely at the patterns.

Premenstrual Syndrome (PMS)

Most women who have menstrual periods (or remaining ovarian cycles if they have had a hysterectomy) have some physical or emotional cues that tell them their periods are about to begin. When these cues and physical changes become bothersome, we call them *symptoms*. Mild to moderate PMS symptoms may strike as many as 95 percent of women at some point in their lives. Five to 10 percent of women have symptoms severe enough to significantly disrupt their daily lives and relationships. This is not a trivial health issue.

Close to two hundred symptoms have been associated with PMS. Because the ovarian hormones help to regulate the function of almost every system in the body, PMS symptoms can appear just about anywhere, from your hair to your eyes to your sinuses to your heart, lungs, intestinal tract, muscles, joints, skin, immune function, and sexual response as well as the more obvious and expected effects on the reproductive system. Nothing is immune to the cyclic changes in the hormones from our ovaries!

In my medical practice, there are many women who have PMS symptoms severe enough to interfere with optimal function at home, at work, and in relationships. The symptom patterns fall into several main categories, listed with sample symptoms:

1. *Brain-mood symptoms: depression, irritability, angry outbursts, anxiety, agitation, crying spells, feeling out of control, problems with memory or word retrieval, concentration problems, fuzzy or "foggy" thinking, insomnia.*
2. *Appetite changes, food cravings: most common—sweets or chocolate, also salty foods; food binges are common; increased desire for alcohol (for reasons similar to the hormonal-metabolic changes that trigger the sweet cravings).*
3. *Physical changes: constipation, headaches, dizziness, backaches, abdominal pain, pelvic pain, cramps; others include racing heartbeat, sweating, palpitations, nausea, tremors, shortness of breath, asthma attacks, blurred vision, more frequent migraines.*
4. *Fluid retention: bloating, breast fullness, swelling of hands or feet, feelings of fullness in the sinuses, ears, or head.*
5. *Hair-skin problems: acne, oily skin, oily hair; other common complaints include more allergies, outbreaks, hives, urticaria, or herpes outbreaks.*
6. *Changes in vitality: low energy, fatigue, lack of motivation, desire to be alone, loss of interest in usually enjoyable activities, social withdrawal.*

Women also experience changes that signal the decline in ovarian hormones, even if it occurs long before the "normal" age of perimenopause. When women have a hysterectomy but keep their ovaries, they often describe the body-brain markers of a residual ovary cycle. They still have breast tenderness, bloating, food cravings, and constipation, among others. Or they describe a few days of restless, fragmented sleep, abrupt emotional shifts, crying easily, loss of energy, feeling mentally foggy, or having anxiety attacks and palpitations like they did during the first few days of bleeding, when estradiol is at its lowest. Yet these women are often told they "couldn't possibly" have PMS after a hysterectomy. Many physicians seem to forget the ovaries are still there and have a cycle with hormone shifts. Another cause of PMS is that the ovaries' hormone production declines sooner after hysterectomy due to the interruption in ovarian blood flow when arteries are tied off.

Now, do we call it PMS, or the newer term *premenstrual dysphoric disorder* (PMDD, a more severe form of PMS), *pre*menopause or *peri*menopause? One reason this is confusing is that these terms are used in different ways among physicians, the media, and scientific articles. Generally, but not always, **premenopause** refers to a woman *still menstruating* regularly. **Perimenopause** refers to a woman beginning to have *erratic, inconsistent periods* with changing flow-patterns (i.e., long and heavy one month, lighter and shorter the next), changing cycle lengths, a rising FSH, fewer ovulatory cycles, and skipped periods. PMS refers to the physical and emotional symptom cluster occurring between ovulation and menses, which then ceases for a symptom-free interval each month. It is important to keep in mind that **PMS (and PMDD) may occur in both pre- and peri-menopause, since women still have their ovary cycles.**

Menopause technically means "cessation of menses" and loss of the ovary cycles. Yet, it is difficult to pinpoint the last period until a woman has gone an extended time without them, usually at least a year. If we use the commonly accepted definition of PMS, it doesn't occur after menopause because there are no more natural cycles. However, menopausal women taking cyclic progesterone or progestin hormone therapy can have PMS-like symptoms when they start and stop the progestogen. *Postmenopause* refers to the years after the complete cessation of menses. Health books and articles typically write as if chronological age is the *primary* indicator of when to expect menopause changes. We must know the *endocrinological* age to determine if you are menopausal or not. The problem is that *chronological* age doesn't necessarily correlate well with the endocrinological age. I have twenty-three-year-old patients who are hormonally menopausal and women at age fifty-eight who are not. We *must* measure objective hormone levels rather than *age* as the basis for a decision.

What Are Some of the Causes of PMS?

I think of PMS as a neuroendocrine disorder that begins with physiological hormonal shifts, particularly declining estradiol, which affects multiple brain centers and chemical messengers regulating functions throughout all body systems. The changes in chemical messengers that occur with hormone shifts can also be aggravated by when and what we eat, what we drink or smoke, what medicines and supplements we take (or what vitamins and minerals we may be missing!), chemical exposure, sleep, and stress.

Hormonal Fluctuations: A Key Factor

A major link between hormones and mood symptoms is the *degree of fluctuation, or rate of change,* in hormone levels. Most medical studies do not address this crucial factor. The more rapid the rate of fall, or rise, in any of the ovarian hormones, the greater the impact on multiple chemical messengers in the brain. Falling estradiol decreases several mood-elevating messengers—endorphins, serotonin, and dopamine—and also leads to an increase in monoamine oxidase (MAO) enzymes that break down (inactivate) the mood-lifting chemical messengers. These combined effects contribute to the depressed, irritable, anxious mood so typically described by millions of women during this time of the cycle. Falling estradiol may also set off a burst of norepinephrine in the brain's alarm center, activating the fight-or-flight response and adding to the feelings of anxiety and irritability as the estradiol falls. The fall in progesterone prior to bleeding intensifies the drop in endorphins that can make you depressed and irritable. Since progesterone acts like Valium by activating GABA pathways in the brain, when it falls naturally or you stop using it, there is rebound anxiety and irritability, just as you would experience if you abruptly stopped taking Valium.

What we hear from women corresponds to what we know from studies of brain function. Many women describe their worst days in the cycle as the day prior to bleeding and the first day. This is exactly when estradiol falls sharply and is at the lowest point of the cycle. Progesterone has also fallen. Both of these hormone changes can trigger mood effects. No wonder you feel tearful and have fragmented sleep, anxiety attacks, palpitations, and irritability. These are the brain's response to the physical hormone change. It doesn't mean you are crazy or have a psychiatric disorder; it means that some women are simply more sensitive to these hormone changes than others.

PMS does not appear to be a deficiency of progesterone before menstruation, as proposed by Dr. Katharina Dalton, the British physician who popularized the use of natural progesterone (as opposed to synthetic progestins) as a PMS treatment several decades ago. Her hypothesis was that PMS was due to "estrogen dominance." Dr. Dalton, and subsequent physicians who have written books based on her work, have sold a lot of progesterone products with this idea. But this is a *theory,* not based on actual measures of hormone measures, by cycle phase, to confirm a true deficit of progesterone and an excess of estradiol.

Nothing in our scientific understanding of reproductive hormones or wisdom gained from listening to women supports the idea that PMS is caused by a deficiency of progesterone. Rather, everything in both the science of hormone actions and the pattern of symptoms points to a cyclic rise and fall in progesterone as a major *cause* of PMS. Dr. John Studd in London has confirmed this in several well-done studies.

Think about it. PMS doesn't occur before puberty or after menopause or in cycles in which you don't ovulate (which is what causes the rise in progesterone), or if the ovaries are removed. But as soon ovarian progesterone rises, or you take a progestin for ten to fourteen days a month, classic PMS symptoms return. In fact, it is the very PMS symptoms in a *cyclic* HRT regimen after menopause that is one of the reasons women don't like taking hormones and stop. Many women say to me, "I felt great on the estrogen, but I had to give up that good feeling because I felt so horrible when the progesterone was added!" Mood swings, depression, irritability, bloating, breast tenderness, increased appetite, food cravings, feeling "fat," and no libido all began when progesterone was added, and were not present during the estrogen-only phase.

In over fifteen years of testing hormone levels, by menstrual cycle phase, of women with PMS, I have never found this hypothesized condition of "estrogen dominance." In women with low levels of progesterone in the luteal (PMS) phase of the cycle, I also found *low estradiol levels.* By the time women reach the stage

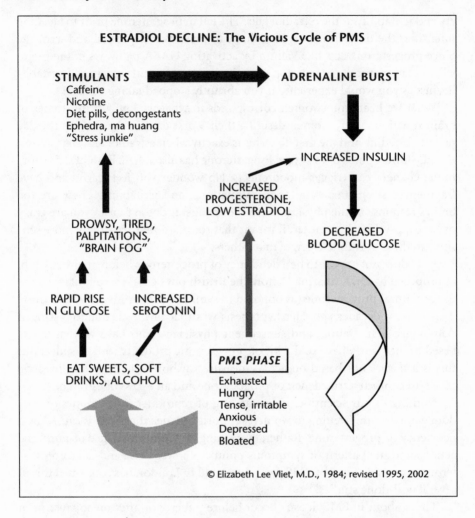

ESTRADIOL DECLINE: The Vicious Cycle of PMS

STIMULANTS ➡ ADRENALINE BURST
Caffeine
Nicotine
Diet pills, decongestants
Ephedra, ma huang
"Stress junkie"

INCREASED INSULIN

INCREASED
PROGESTERONE,
LOW ESTRADIOL

DROWSY, TIRED,
PALPITATIONS,
"BRAIN FOG"

DECREASED
BLOOD GLUCOSE

RAPID RISE   INCREASED
IN GLUCOSE   SEROTONIN

EAT SWEETS, SOFT
DRINKS, ALCOHOL

PMS PHASE

Exhausted
Hungry
Tense, irritable
Anxious
Depressed
Bloated

© Elizabeth Lee Vliet, M.D., 1984; revised 1995, 2002

of anovulatory cycles and low progesterone, the ovaries have already declined in production of estradiol, and testosterone has usually decreased as well.

Dr. Dalton used high doses of progesterone suppositories, or troches, to treat PMS. She reported that many women in her program found relief from their premenstrual symptoms. This is likely because such high doses of progesterone have the same effects on the brain as a big dose of Valium or Xanax. Much of the neuroendocrine science that deals with ovarian hormones and the brain emerged years after Dr. Dalton first proposed her theory. Pharmacological studies show that large doses of progesterone have a Valium-like action on the brain by binding at the GABA receptors, so it stands to reason that some women would feel relief from premenstrual anxiety and tension, although many become depressed and lethargic.

The majority of PMS researchers and clinicians, however, have not found

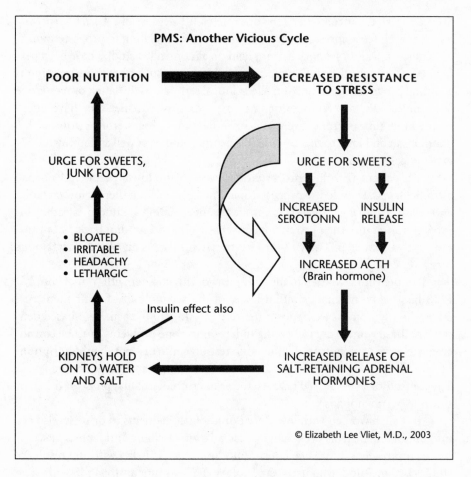

PMS: Another Vicious Cycle

© Elizabeth Lee Vliet, M.D., 2003

progesterone successful, and many women with PMS become markedly *worse* taking only progesterone. In double-blind, placebo-controlled studies published in recent years, progesterone treatment is not any better than placebo in relieving PMS symptoms. This confirms what I found in my clinical practice when experimenting with Dr. Dalton's progesterone recommendations. I stopped because too many women became profoundly depressed and gained weight when given those high doses of progesterone.

More recent controlled studies, such as those described by Dr. John Studd's group in London, clearly show that it is actually *estradiol* supplementation in the luteal phase of the menstrual cycle that gives the most impressive symptom relief for PMS. I found this out many years ago from hormone-testing my patients. The laboratory results showed why: My patients didn't have a deficit of progesterone. They had unexpectedly low estradiol and quite normal progesterone levels. Current research further shows that progesterone *decreases* serotonin, while estradiol *boosts* serotonin, which confirms my clinical findings and those Dr.

Studd reported. Since higher serotonin helps lift depression, it isn't surprising women often feel depressed when estradiol is low in relation to progesterone.

Thus, Dr. Dalton's theory has not held up as controlled studies have been performed. The controlled studies report very different results from those practitioners using progesterone in uncontrolled clinical settings. In the latter, progesterone is recommended to everyone for PMS, regardless of whether they have documented low progesterone levels or not. So take the "progesterone gurus" with a grain of salt and look to the more solid scientific studies as well as your own body experiences for sound information.

For a patient with low progesterone levels in the luteal phase and normal estradiol levels, I would use progesterone. And conversely, if there is low estradiol and relatively normal luteal phase progesterone, creating a reduced estradiol-to-progesterone ratio, then it only makes sense to boost estradiol back to optimal ranges as a first step. The key for effective treatment is an objective hormone measure.

All of the young women in the beginning of this chapter with "out of control" PMS had below normal estradiol levels in the second half of their menstrual cycle when symptoms were most intense. According to the usual age-based definitions, these women are too young to have hormone problems or to be considered pre- or perimenopausal. Hormone testing confirms that their descriptions of symptoms matched the science, based on estradiol and progesterone levels. Their estradiol levels indeed reached the endocrinological first phase of the transition to perimenopause.

I treat such women with low-dose estradiol supplements to bring levels back into optimal menstrual cycle ranges, instead of prescribing antidepressants, as is more commonly done. They consistently improve. This fits with the results of studies by Dr. Studd, who used estradiol patches or implants for PMS with great success. The women describe improved mood, diminished irritability, better sleep, improved libido, a higher energy level, diminished food cravings (especially for sweets and chocolate), and reduced mood swings. Only a few require antidepressants once hormone levels return to healthy ranges.

Cyclic Acne

We've all heard that chocolate, caffeine, and fatty foods "cause" acne, but there really isn't such a simplistic connection. What about hormones? Seems reasonable, especially since most women from puberty to menopause notice acne outbreaks most often the seven to ten days before their period. How do hormone changes affect your skin in ways that lead to acne?

Let's first look at what acne is. Glands just under the skin secrete a waxy, oily substance called *sebum* that helps keep skin supple and moist, preventing dry, wrinkled skin. If sebum builds up around the hair follicles of the skin, it causes the follicle to get plugged with debris—sebum particles, bacteria, dead skin cells, dirt from the air, excess makeup, etc. This leads to clogged pores that become whiteheads, blackheads, and pimples. If our white blood cells start attacking this pile of debris in the hair follicle, it can then lead to the accumulation of swollen, red pockets of pus and debris we call *pustules,* or *cystic acne.* If these pustules or cysts continue to increase in size and become more inflamed, they are painful.

Increased sebum production sets off unwanted acne. Other causes include ethnic background, family genetics, what you eat and drink, what you put on your face, and how you take it off and wash away the accumulated debris of dust and dirt from daily activities. You are familiar with these causes, so let's explore some of the hormonal imbalances that increase sebum production.

Stress is one, because it increases cortisol, which in turn revs up your oil-producing glands, and also tends to increase the adrenal glands' output of androgens. The rise in progesterone after ovulation is another trigger of increased sebum production and outbreaks of acne. Excess male hormone production (testosterone, DHEA, androstenedione), as in PCOS and during perimenopausal estradiol decline, is another. Why? During years of optimal ovarian estrogen production, the estradiol decreases the sebum production, which keeps acne in check. During both adolescence and perimenopause, the androgen balance is usually higher in relation to the amount of estradiol, and there is often a greater percentage of the androgens in the free, active fraction. This is why perimenopausal women often feel they are returning to adolescent acne! Excess insulin production in obesity, Syndrome X, and PCOS contributes to further excess production of androgens, making acne even worse.

Women can get an excess of androgens and not realize it. *Charlotte* is a soft-spoken young woman in her early thirties who came for an evaluation of possible hormonal factors in a disfiguring outbreak of painful cystic acne. She was distraught and had a great deal of difficulty getting physicians to take her seriously. The photos of her face show one of the worst cases of cystic acne I have ever encountered. The acne was on her upper chest and back as well. She was becoming a recluse because she was embarrassed about her face, describing it as "like someone had put my face through a meat grinder."

Prior to this outbreak, she consulted a family physician for insomnia and night sweats. She was told she was in early menopause. The doctor gave her a combination hormone injection without measuring her hormone levels. She said, "Within a few weeks my face became covered with huge, painful pimples that had erupted into these enormous pus-filled cystlike things all over my face. They were much worse than anything I had ever had in my life." No connection was made between her hormones and acne.

After several months of different specialists, "countless remedies," and feeling dismissed and discounted, she still had no relief from the painful acne. Investigating further, she asked her family physician for a copy of her medical records and checked these against her insurance bills. Although there was no record in the doctor's notes of the injection, the insurance bill listed an injection that contained estrogen, vitamin B12, and, to this young woman's surprise, testosterone. Reading about the effects of testosterone, she found levels too high can cause cystic acne in women. She said, "Now I had confirmation of the cause of my problems but I still had the affliction. The horror in the mirror caused me unbearable pain." I cannot adequately portray the enormous degree of despair, humiliation, discouragement, and depression in this young woman from the ordeal.

When I saw her, her testosterone, DHEA, DHEA-S, and androstenedione were all very high, and her estradiol much too low for a woman her age. I started her on an aggressive, integrated treatment to restore her hormone balance and resolve the acne. A year later, her hormone balance is normal, her PMS is gone, her acne has cleared, with no further outbreaks, though there is some scarring.

Her story illustrates three important points: First, even common, "ordinary" acne can indicate a serious underlying endocrine imbalance that physicians must take seriously and evaluate properly. Second, women with PMS and the other hormone-triggered problems need systematic baseline hormone levels *before* being given something as potent as an injection of hormones, especially testosterone. Third, patients must know what medications are prescribed. Ask questions and write it down. Charlotte might have been spared humiliating and unproductive encounters with other physicians had she known she had been given a high dose of testosterone shortly before her severe acne outbreak.

Endometriosis: New Insights and Emerging Concerns About an Old Problem

Endometriosis is an enigmatic, painful disorder that is far more common than statistics convey because it manifests itself in many ways and is notoriously hard to diagnose with certainty, short of having laparoscopic surgery. It likely affects more than 5 million women in the United States alone, yet only a small percentage are accurately diagnosed. The vast majority experience its debilitating effects without explanation. For women who are properly diagnosed, it is often a long, arduous process involving multiple physicians over many years before anyone considers endometriosis. "Endo," as it is often called, is a complex health problem. It can lead to infertility; causes severe, persistent, debilitating pain for many; and is a disruption in quality of life and relationships. It is also costly—to the women, their employers, and their insurance carriers.

Endometriosis is on the rise today. But why? This is not simply due to better diagnostic techniques. It is related to connections I have been describing in this book: exposure to endocrine-disrupting environmental chemicals and their damaging effects to the reproductive system, the thyroid, and immune system. There are significant emerging connections between endometriosis and exposure to environmental chemicals, as well as links to thyroid disorders (particularly autoimmune forms like Hashimoto's), premature ovarian decline, mitral valve prolapse, chronic fatigue, and susceptibility to chronic infections. Let's look at some crucial issues between environmental chemicals and this mysterious, debilitating disorder. This is an overview of critical issues. Read more in materials from the Endometriosis Association, which is conducting landmark research on links between endometriosis and organic pollutants like dioxin (see Appendix II).

What Is Endometriosis and Why Is It a Problem?

Endometriosis is *not* a simple disease. Endometriosis is tissue (endometrium) that should be lining the *inside* of the uterus but is growing *outside* the uterus in the pelvis or abdomen. These little blobs of endometrial tissue, medically called *endometrial implants,* or *endometriomas* if they are bigger and cystic, can cause severe pain because the endometrium outside the uterus bleeds with the menstrual cycle hormone changes as if it were inside the uterus. When the lining of the uterus is where it is supposed to be, the menstrual blood is easily released through the cervical opening, into the vagina, and out of the body. Normal menstrual bleeding does not cause pain. But when the endometrial tissue lies outside the uterus, in the pelvis or abdomen, the blood has no way to be released from the body and accumulates. Blood in the pelvis is a major irritant to the other organs, causing inflammation and pain. Endometrial implants outside the uterus also release inflammatory chemicals, such as cytokines, that stimulate more pain and inflammation. Over time, there is chronic irritation of pelvic tissues, more inflammation, causing sticky adhesions and scarring that further intensifies pain.

Some of the newest research, discussed at the World Endometriosis Conference in February 2002, describes another wicked way endometrial implants outside the uterus increase pain and inflammation: They produce their own estrogen (estrone and estradiol) from adrenal androgens via an enzyme system called the *aromatase pathway.* This means that even if your blood levels of estradiol are low, or you take drugs to reduce ovarian estrogen, these little devils can still make estrogen anyway to feed their own growth! Normal endometrial tissue inside the uterus does not have this "estrogen factory" pathway.

Endometrial implants may seed almost anywhere, even beyond the pelvis. The most common sites are in the lower pelvic area called the cul de sac, on the major ligaments supporting the uterus, on the bladder, on the outside of the uterus itself, on the ovaries, on the outside of the bowel wall, or scattered along the side walls of the pelvis. Small bits of endometrial lining have been found as far outside the pelvis as the lungs and spinal cord. In cases of periodic collapsed lung during menstruation, the women were found to have endometrial implants causing this mysterious link with the menstrual cycle. In fact, in the studies of monkeys who developed endometriosis after dioxin exposure, the endometrial implants were scattered throughout both lungs, which contributed to the animals' death.

Small endometrial implants may also migrate to the cauda equina, or "tail" of nerves at the end of the spinal cord, causing excruciating low-back pain that is notoriously difficult to diagnose and treat. Endometrial implants can also burrow deep into the muscle wall of the uterus, which is known as *adenomyosis.* Such implants bleed into the uterine muscle during menstruation and cause menstrual "cramps" so painful, intense, and sharp that the pain may cause you to faint or vomit. Endometrial-type adenomyosis implants can even wedge in the connective tissue (septum) between the rectum and vagina, causing intense pain with bowel movements during menstrual periods.

The relationship between the amount of endometriosis and the degree of pain is puzzling. Some women with severe pain have minimal endometrial implants in the pelvis. Other women have extensive endometriosis throughout the pelvis with little or no pain. Most are somewhere between these extremes, and commonly experience pain with intercourse, bowel movements, or menstruation. Some of the degrees of pain may occur because of implant location rather than amount. Discrepancies may also result from what triggers the endometriosis. For example, the monkeys exposed to dioxin had an extremely aggressive form of endometriosis and appeared to be in severe pain. Organic pollutants causing endometriosis may also damage pain-regulating pathways.

Endometriosis causes many different problems, depending on where it hides in the body and how it responds to hormone changes and other factors. The puzzling array of symptoms is one reason it is so hard to diagnose. Sometimes symptoms aren't even the same from one menstrual cycle to the next. A diagnosis is first made clinically, based on a high index of suspicion about the classic symptoms. Ultimately, however, the diagnosis must be definitively made during exploratory surgery of the pelvis. Such surgery can be done with an instrument called a *laparoscope* (laparoscopic surgery), or the surgeon may decide to open the abdomen (laparotomy).

How Do I Know Whether I Might Have Endometriosis?

Infertility is one serious consequence of endometriosis, affecting 30 to 40 percent of women with the disease, according to the Endometriosis Association. Even before fertility problems are recognized, however, a woman has probably experienced pelvic and abdominal pain. There are three "red flags" that should alert you and your doctor to possible endometriosis, and the need for laparoscopic evaluation by an experienced surgeon:

- *Severe, crampy pain with your menstrual flow each month* (dysmenorrhea)
- *Pain with intercourse* (dyspareunia)
- *Pain with bowel movements (occurs primarily during your menstrual periods, but can occur at other times due to adhesions from endometrial implants and scarring on the outside of the bowel)*

The Endometriosis Association Research Registry shows over 96 percent of women with endometriosis have dysmenorrhea or pain throughout the menstrual cycle; 80 percent report pain with bowel movements or alterations in bowel movements during menses; while almost 60 percent of women have severe pain with intercourse. Over 82 percent of the women in their registry also describe fatigue and exhaustion. I strongly suspect from my work with endometriosis patients that the low levels of estradiol and testosterone are significant causes of the low energy.

What Causes It?

Endometriosis is one of the better-studied clinical problems for women, yet it remains one of the most mysterious. Why do some women have extensive disease yet few symptoms, while others have relatively little disease and severe or incapacitating symptoms? One of the oldest theories, proposed by Dr. John Sampson in the 1920s, is that endometriosis resulted from menstruation flowing backward (called *retrograde menstruation*) through the fallopian tube into the pelvic cavity, instead of into the cervical opening, the vagina, and then out of the body. Although this theory has not been proven, it has remained one of the most widely reported "causes" of endometriosis. One problem with Dr. Sampson's theory is that it doesn't really explain how endometriosis can be found in such far-flung spots as the lung or along spinal nerves. In addition, *all* women have at least some degree of backward menstrual flow, and yet all women clearly do not develop endometriosis. The retrograde menstruation theory simply does not explain it fully.

Over the years, researchers have looked at genetic, immune, and lifestyle factors. Dr. David B. Redwine, a gynecologist in Oregon who made endometriosis a serious focus of his clinical work and research, feels that our traditional theories of cause and our traditional medical treatments with drugs have addressed only a small piece of the endometriosis picture. Dr. Redwine and others have a broader view than the traditional "backward menstruation" theory, and propose that girls are born with endometriosis rather than developing it after menstruation begins. This view theorizes that endometriosis develops when embryonic tissue destined to migrate to the area of the uterus fails to complete the journey, landing in areas of the pelvis outside the uterine cavity. The tissue lies dormant until the hormone cycles of puberty begin, and then the outside endometrium is activated to follow the menstrual cycle pattern as is the endometrial tissue inside the uterus. Dr. Redwine and others feel that endometriosis is *constant* in amount, rather than the standard medical teaching that it progressively increases with years of menstruation. If this theory is correct, it means endometriosis is actually a congenital disorder that occurs during fetal development, and could have a number of causes. This helps explain how chemicals like dioxin can cause the disease—by disrupting normal fetal development of the reproductive system and interfering with endometrial tissue development.

Current research demonstrates that endometriosis can have a variety of appearances, not just the "chocolate" or dark reddish-black color described as the "classic" color of endometrial implants. Pale, whitish endometrial implants, as well as other colors, can be present from birth. Researchers think their color changes over time following puberty. The darker, blackish or chocolate-colored endometrial implants are found more in women in their thirties, the implants surgeons see and remove more frequently because they are readily identified. The white or yellowish endometrial implants can be widespread but more difficult to see with the usual laparoscopic techniques. Dr. Redwine developed specific surgical techniques that markedly improve the detection rate, and allow a more thorough removal of the implants. Many more endometriosis specialists around the country now use these techniques.

The theory that endometriosis is a congenital disorder actually fits well with newer research showing that dioxin, and probably many similar organic pollutants, cause endometriosis. These same compounds damage the developing thyroid gland, immune system, and other hormonal target tissues. Here is a way that all of these "mysterious" conditions may share a common trigger. The dioxin link was published in the fall of 1993, from the Endometriosis Association's pioneering research on monkeys mentioned earlier. This same connection was made earlier in a 1985 Canadian study by Dr. James Campbell, but it had been overlooked until the Endometriosis Association raised awareness of the dioxin link. Dr. Campbell's group demonstrated that another group of environmental pollutants called *PCBs* also caused endometriosis in monkeys.

The first clue that environmental chemicals caused endometriosis came from a colony of Rhesus monkeys that were part of a study to assess possible damage from the dioxin compound called *Agent Orange,* a chemical defoliant used in the Vietnam War. The endometriosis was an unexpected finding since it is extremely rare in monkeys and apes. Researchers were stunned to find endometriosis implants in about 80 percent of the animals that received concentrations of dioxin compounds over the years. The higher the concentration of dioxin, the more severe the endometriosis. Animals exposed to the higher doses developed such an aggressive form of endometriosis that they died from it, also an unusual finding.

Here are two of the most frightening aspects of this research: (1) Endometriosis did not develop until *years* after the initial exposure. In the case of dioxin it was over ten years later, so the causative link is difficult to pin down. (2) Even the highest concentrations in the studies were miniscule: 25 parts per *trillion* of dioxin in the monkeys' water supply, about the same as the average American is exposed to in common foods contaminated with the chemical. To put this in perspective, it is similar to you spitting once into an Olympic-size swimming pool and trying to measure the effects of your saliva on the depth of the pool. It is pretty staggering that such a miniscule amount causes such profound damage, and even death, from the disease it triggers. This is one of the silent health crises facing women today, because we do not realize the degree to which we are exposed to these chemicals.

Our increased exposure to these hormonally active environmental chemicals plays a bigger role in our health than medical professionals recognize. Newer research also links dioxin exposure to insulin resistance, in both women and men, and a number of scientists have suggested that endometriosis, like PCOS, may be caused by insulin resistance. Excess insulin has been identified as a risk factor for later breast cancer. We simply must pay attention to these damaging chemicals, and work together toward a ban on the most dangerous.

Even with all of this research, we can't say with certainty what causes endometriosis, or whether there is one primary cause, as once thought, or many. The most likely explanation is that it has several causes, one of the most potent being exposure to the POP chemicals, especially during fetal development, childhood, and even adulthood. The more collective risk factors in your history, the more likely you will develop endometriosis.

RISK FACTORS FOR ENDOMETRIOSIS

- Family history of endometriosis
- History of maternal exposure to DES and/or other xenoestrogens
- History of exposure to dioxin, PCBs, organochlorines in utero, in breast milk, and/or in early childhood
- Obesity, with excess estrone
- History of heavy and/or longer than average menstrual flow
- History of elevated thyroid antibodies
- History of recurrent, chronic yeast infections
- Possibly, the presence of mitral valve prolapse

© Elizabeth Lee Vliet, M.D., 2003

The Ovary and Your Bladder

Bladder problems are one of the least discussed of women's health issues, especially among younger women. We see the "adult diaper" commercials featuring older women and we can't conceive of having similar problems. If you have premature ovarian decline and lower than optimal estradiol levels, you may experience urinary leakage, frequent urges to urinate, painful intercourse, and urinary, vaginal, or vulvar burning even in your twenties.

The linings of the urinary bladder, urethra, and vagina all have estrogen receptors, just like other organs and tissues in the body. The cells of the urinary bladder and lining of the urethra are sensitive to the rise and fall in estradiol levels during the monthly cycle, in pregnancy and perimenopause, as well as to the loss of estradiol at menopause. Many changes result from the decrease in estradiol: more sensitivity to the usual stimuli for the urge to urinate, loss of smooth muscle strength so you can't hold it when you have to go, decreased pain tolerance, and changes in the pressure of the bladder and urethra (urodynamics) so that the urethra can't close properly. Together these changes cause more "leakage" problems. When your estradiol is too low, the cells lining the bladder, urethra, and vagina also become fewer, thinner *(atrophic)*, and are easily torn or damaged with friction *(friable)*. This means urination, friction from sex, or pressure from tight clothes can hurt and sometimes cause bleeding.

Nerve endings contain estrogen receptors. The pain threshold is higher with normal estradiol levels. When estradiol decreases, the pain threshold is lowered, and the nerve endings become more sensitive. Increasing pain causes more urges to urinate, more burning during urination, and more vaginal burning. There are also estrogen receptors in cells that make collagen, the major protein in the connective tissue that helps support our entire urinary and genital system. Loss of estradiol at any age leads to decreased collagen and skin wrinkling, as well as a loss of the collagen support that holds the bladder in place and allows the urethra to close.

Due to these hormone-triggered changes, women are much more susceptible to the problems summarized in the box on page 211. Bladder and vaginal problems are common for women of all ages, and it is appalling that we lack more controlled studies concerning the hormonal effects on these problems. I have heard many medical presentations on issues like interstitial cystitis, vulvodynia, and other problems, but no one mentions checking hormone levels or even using hormone treatments to improve the symptoms. Hormone connections are more likely discussed if a woman is menopausal, but are almost never taken into account for younger women who may also be suffering similar consequences of low estradiol.

Early Estrogen Decline and Vulvodynia: A Young Woman's Painful Saga

Grace was only twenty-three and newly married when I saw her. Her mother encouraged the consult to see if hormone factors played a role in her severe vaginal pain. She described having vaginal burning during intercourse that was so painful her husband was afraid to attempt sex. She had no vaginal lubrication with arousal and was rarely able to orgasm. She was suffering from the pain, and it threatened her new marriage. Her gynecologist told her she had a "hang-up" about sex and should see a sex therapist because there wasn't anything wrong physically. After such a humiliating encounter, she was embarrassed and hesitant to talk, even to a woman physician with her mother there for support.

Her vaginal pain had been getting worse since age eighteen. She started taking birth control pills at sixteen to prevent heavy menses and painful cramps. She was taking Loestrin 1/20, a high-progestin pill with one of the lowest amounts of estrogen. Another specialist recommended Premarin vaginal cream, but this caused so much burning she had to stop using it. Several significant factors in her history provided clues to the cause of her problem. She was concerned about weight gain on the pill and drastically cut down her dietary fat when she became a vegetarian. Vegetarian diets are typically high in soy and low in protein, iron, and vitamin B_{12}. Her ferritin (iron stores) was low at 8 (desirable level is

---

BLADDER AND VAGINAL EFFECTS OF ESTRADIOL DECLINE

- Vaginal and vulvar dryness, itching, burning, stinging pain (several disorders: vaginitis, vulvodynia, vestibulitis)
- Pain with intercourse (dyspareunia)
- Recurrent bladder infections/inflammation (cystitis)
- Urethral infections (urethritis)
- Recurrent vaginal infections (vaginitis)
- Incontinence (loss of urine—several types, see description)
- Painful urination (dysuria)
- Urinary frequency
- Urinary urgency

© Elizabeth Lee Vliet, M.D., 2003

60–100), and her B_{12} level was low, as expected in women with predominately plant sources of protein. The higher fiber of a vegetarian diet decreases absorption and increases elimination. She did not use alcohol or tobacco, and exercised regularly and reasonably.

Remember, the important connections in the development of her vaginal pain: high-progestin birth control pills, high intake of soy phytoestrogens that compete at the estrogen receptors preventing binding of estradiol, a low-fat diet that prevents the body from making enough estradiol from cholesterol, low B_{12} levels, and low ferritin. All of these contribute to a burning type pain (neuropathic) because all of these factors are needed for normal nerve function and pain regulation.

The loss of adequate estradiol, coupled with the negative effects of the progestin, caused the vaginal dryness, pain, and difficulty having an orgasm. Her vulvodynia pain got worse each month when she stopped the active birth control pills and took the placebo pills to have a period. Since her own ovarian estradiol was suppressed by the Loestrin, her low-fat diet, and the high-soy intake, she was especially vulnerable to the drop in estrogen when she stopped the active pills each month. Practically speaking, she had almost no estradiol during her bleeding days. No wonder she was in such pain.

I prescribed a 0.01 percent (0.1 mg/gm) hypoallergenic estradiol cream *without* preservatives, and told her to apply the cream on her external vulvar and clitoral area nightly to restore the tissue estradiol. I also suggested she use low-dose Vagifem estradiol tablets in the vagina to improve pH and lubrication, also reducing the dryness and burning. Most important, I changed her birth control pill to Orthocyclen, which is higher in estrogen and lower in progestin.

At a follow-up appointment several months later, she said, "Everything feels much better, the pain is much less. I am amazed that changing my birth control pill and finding a vaginal estradiol tablet I could use would make such a dramatic difference!"

The Premarin cream did not help her, even though it contained estrogen. All FDA-approved commercial estrogen creams, including Premarin, contain a chemical preservative that causes burning and increases pain when sensitive tissues are damaged by loss of estrogen. Many patients who cannot use commercial products are able to use an estradiol tablet or cream made for them by compounding pharmacists who can eliminate any preservatives or dyes (see Appendix II for pharmacy resources).

There are a few nonhormonal causes of the pain as well. If your estradiol is low and the nerve endings feel "on fire," the substances below will likely make the pain much worse.

Food triggers. Many foods contain chemicals such as citric acid, salicylic acid, and oxalates that intensify bladder and vulvodynia pain. Some experts recommend that women avoid a long list of foods: caffeine, alcohol, tobacco (nicotine), chocolate, spices and spicy foods, apples, bananas, acidic foods (citrus fruits, tomatoes), Nutrasweet, saccharine, sharp cheeses, coffee, tea, carbonated beverages, chemical preservatives (found in many foods and beverages), lima beans, lentils, and yogurt. These foods produce metabolic by-products that can irritate bladder or vaginal tissue, cause pain and spasm, as well as increase the urge to urinate, in turn aggravating incontinence. Alcohol and tobacco are potent bladder irritants, and they also significantly interfere with the metabolism and effectiveness of prescription hormone therapies.

Diets too low in fat reduce absorption of prescription hormones, while diets high in fat increase absorption if taken at mealtime. Thus, the availability of any given oral hormone therapy is affected by when it is taken in relation to a meal, the type of meal, and the food additives present. Think about the typical diet of many women "on the run" and you realize just how many "triggers" people consume. I am surprised at how many of my patients worry about chemicals in meat, yet think nothing of polluting their bodies with cola beverages that have a wide variety of chemical irritants, not to mention calories from sugar.

Keep a dietary diary and note any patterns with the foods that cause a flare-up of bladder or vulvodynia pain. Make necessary modifications and clean up your diet.

Dyes. Tartrazine-based dyes (a common one is FD&C yellow #5, but there are many others) in medications, foods, and beverages have a molecular makeup similar to salicylate, the chemical name for aspirin. Many people allergic to aspirin are also allergic to tartrazine but don't know it. You may not know it is in a product or food either. FD&C yellow #5 and green and red dyes based on tartrazine are ubiquitous in thousands of common products, including foods, beverages, and vitamins. They are added to herbal products, many prescription medicines, and even medications to treat asthma and allergies.

These dyes have metabolic breakdown products excreted in the urine that are a potent trigger for "irritable bladder" that aggravates incontinence, or causes burning bladder pain like interstitial cystitis. Such dyes may also aggravate vulvodynia. I have seen reactions from rashes and wheezing to severe bladder spasms, all traceable to dyes in medications. Over the course of my medical career, I have found this a more common problem than I was taught to expect. If you have bladder sensitivities and an "irritable" bladder (or bowel, or even allergies in general), try to eliminate these chemicals in your food, beverages, and medicines. Many doctors don't check these issues, so *you* need to know such connections exist. If something seems to bother you and aggravate symptoms, ask your doctor to change your dose or brand of medicine to one without dyes. See what happens. You may be pleased with the results.

Preservatives. Propylene (or polyethylene) glycol (PEG) is a preservative used in many commercial hormone and steroid creams—both prescription and over-the-counter—to prolong shelf life. It is also in some antibacterial and antifungal creams used to treat vaginal infections. PEG and similar preservatives can cause itching and burning. It is also found in estrogen vaginal creams used to treat vaginal itching and burning. PEG can be very irritating, especially if the tissues are already inflamed and sensitive from low estradiol. If you have persistent problems with vaginal or bladder burning after starting one of the creams, talk with your physician or pharmacist and check your medication for these dyes, chemical binders, and PEG. The PDR (*Physicians' Desk Reference,* edited and published by Medical Economics) is now required to list dyes and other inactive ingredients in a particular medicine. Most libraries have a PDR, or it is available for purchase at any bookstore. Many food manufacturers will furnish a complete ingredient list if you write their consumer information office.

Chronic Bladder "Infections": Is It Really an Infection or My Hormones?

Lots of young women have problems with bladder or urinary tract infections (UTIs). Burning, frequency, and urgency can have many causes. Not all are due to yeast or bacterial infections. I am concerned about the trend of women calling doctors' offices for help with "bladder infections" and getting repeated courses of antibiotics that merely create resistant bacteria and set you up for chronic yeast infections without correcting the underlying cause. Make sure you see your primary care practitioner for a vaginal exam, culture, and urinalysis before you start on antibiotics. Many women with "chronic yeast" infections don't actually have yeast; the symptoms may come from a variety of causes.

It is important to check your hormone levels if you have problems with burning, frequency, urgency, or leaking of urine. Estradiol levels play a role in chronic bladder problems in younger women, as well as during and after menopause. Estradiol blood levels below about 60 pg/ml are a significant contributing factor in persistent vaginal and urinary problems, and can be a factor in chronic bladder problems in younger women, as well as before and during menopause.

Glucose intolerance and early diabetes are two other common endocrine causes of urinary problems in women, especially if you are overweight. In the early stages of diabetes, before your fasting glucose remains too high, you may have frequent yeast infections, burning during urination, leaking of urine or increased frequency. If you have a family history of diabetes, marked weight gain, or an increase in craving for sweets, talk with your doctor about checking for diabetes. In my patients, two endocrine changes—low estradiol and early stages of diabetes—are the most frequent *unrecognized* causes of persistent urinary problems. Assess the possible hormone causes and address this problem directly, perhaps first with a vaginal estradiol cream or by using hormone therapy, rather than continuing the vicious cycle of "infection-antibiotics."

Interstitial cystitis (IC) can be excruciatingly painful. The statistics are staggering. About 1 in every 250 women suffers from some form of this disorder, yet *fewer than 1 out of 5 have been properly diagnosed.* Over 75 percent of women with IC cannot have sex due to pain, which obviously takes a toll on relationships. About 50 percent of women with IC are so affected they cannot hold down a full-time job. And about 33 percent have been abandoned by a husband or lover as a result of this disorder. The characteristic symptoms of IC are, unfortunately, nonspecific and may occur in other kinds of bladder disorders: increased urination, sudden strong urges to void (urgency), intense pain becoming worse as the bladder fills up and often decreased by voiding (one woman called it "like passing fire"), pain with intercourse, urinating multiple times at night *(nocturia)*. There are many causes proposed, but no definitive answer. Some theories include overuse of antibiotics, a dysfunctional bladder lining (epithelium), manifestation of an autoimmune disorder, toxic substances in the urine, or a chronic persistent infectious agent—all of which damage the bladder lining and lead to the characteristic tiny hemorrhages in the bladder wall.

The obvious connection to women's hormones is ignored. Look at some of the medical data and the startling connections that support loss of estradiol as an overlooked factor in the development of IC:

- In a 1993 study of 374 IC patients, researchers at Scripps Institute found that the mean age of onset for IC is forty-two years, and 44 percent of the patients had hysterectomies prior to onset of IC. Women in their forties are often beginning the first phase of estradiol decline leading to menopause. Following hysterectomies, even with the ovaries left in place, about 60 percent of women have an earlier ovarian decline of estradiol due to the effects on blood flow to the ovaries.
- Surveys of women at any age who suffer from IC have found that flare-ups tend to occur after ovulation, just before menses, and postpartum. All are times when estradiol levels fall.

- Young women who develop IC have several common characteristics: prolonged use of high progestin–low estrogen birth control pills, ovarian suppression with low hormone levels, and decreased menses (whether from diet, smoking, drug or alcohol use, excessive exercise, or any other causes).
- IC also often begins following pregnancy, particularly with prolonged nursing, which keeps prolactin higher and suppresses return to optimal menstrual cycle levels of estradiol.

If you are suffering from persistent bladder pain and other approaches offer no relief, have your physician test blood levels of estradiol and other ovarian hormones. If your ovarian hormone levels are low, see Chapter 16 for treatment options. A decline in estrogen may not be the whole story, but it is a crucial piece. To ignore this connection is a glaring ommission. There are also a number of nonhormonal treatments for IC (see Appendix II for information on the IC Foundation, and other resources).

"Leaky Bladders"—Young Women Can Be Affected, Too

Continence is the ability to hold urine in the bladder and control urine flow. After toilet training, most of us control urination urges unconsciously as we go about our daily activities. Accidental loss of urine, or difficulty controlling the start and stop of urine flow, is called *incontinence*. A widespread misconception is that urinary incontinence is inevitable as we get older. Not true. Nor is it true that it "can't" happen to younger women. Grace, the twenty-three-year-old newlywed who also developed vulvodynia, was having urinary "leaks" when she laughed, jogged, and had sex, likely the result of the low estrogen–high progestin birth control pills. Younger women can also develop incontinence from damage to the pelvic-floor muscles and nerves following difficult vaginal deliveries of large babies or pelvic surgery such as a hysterectomy. For perimenopausal and menopausal women, the loss of estradiol causes loss of muscle tone and elasticity of connective tissue that leads to incontinence. For women late in life, incontinence carries an additional significance: Loss of bladder control is one of the most frequent causes for nursing home admission.

There are several types of incontinence, with different characteristics and causes.

Stress incontinence is one you often hear about, and patients are frequently confused about it. Stress incontinence does *not* refer to emotional factors causing loss of urine. It means loss of bladder control due to the *physical* stress of increased pressure in the abdomen from activities such as laughing, coughing, sneezing, orgasm, jogging, or straining to have a bowel movement. This type of incontinence is not caused by bladder spasms; it results from weakness or loss of tone in the bladder muscles from many causes: damage to the bladder muscles in childbirth, ligaments and muscles weakened by age, or loss of hormone or nutritional components necessary for healthy tissue, to name a few major ones.

Thirty-five to 40 percent of women experience postpartum stress incontinence for as long as six to twelve weeks after childbirth. This is due to trauma to the bladder muscles and the sudden drop in hormone levels after delivery. Stress incontinence is not usually associated with urinary frequency and urgency.

Urge (urgency) incontinence is the sudden urge to urinate and the inability to hold your urine long enough to reach the bathroom. It is usually caused by bladder spasms. It can also be caused by medical conditions such as herniated intervertebral disks, bladder infections, fibroids exerting pressure on the bladder, or loss of normal estradiol effect on urinary and reproductive tissues. Urge incontinence is also aggravated by increased urine formation from excessive fluid intake, alcohol, diuretics ("water pills"), caffeine, and/or tobacco. See a physician for a thorough evaluation since bladder cancer may also cause urge incontinence and should be considered before treatment starts. Many cases of urge incontinence do not have a clear-cut physical cause, but still respond to treatment.

Overflow incontinence is the accidental loss of urine from a chronically full bladder. A common cause is a *cystocoele,* a vaginal hernia or bulge due to weakened vaginal muscles. It occurs after childbirth, hysterectomy, or menopause. The bulge from the cystocoele creates a mechanical obstruction and prevents complete emptying of the bladder. A woman then loses small quantities of urine when she stands, sits, or bends. Other causes include: loss of adequate estradiol and diabetes-induced damage to the muscles and nerves that control the bladder, as well as herniated lumbar discs. Overflow incontinence problems happened to me at twenty-eight, before I was correctly diagnosed with a herniated disc. I can certainly relate to the embarrassment of incontinence episodes and the frustration of getting help. In my situation, removal of the herniated disc, which took

COMMON CAUSES OF URGE INCONTINENCE

- Urinary tract infections
- Bladder inflammation
- Loss of adequate estradiol (many causes, not just menopause or hysterectomy)
- Spinal nerve-root disorders (e.g., disc disease)
- Pelvic irritation
- Chemotherapy
- Spinal cord injury
- Pressure from uterine fibroids
- Emotional stress that suppresses ovarian function
- Excessive use of alcohol, tobacco, caffeine, stimulants

© Elizabeth Lee Vliet, M.D., 2003

the pressure off the spinal nerves, restored normal nerve function and the incontinence resolved.

Overflow incontinence is treated by identifying and resolving the underlying cause. A pessary, a device inserted into the vagina as a supportive structure, is sometimes used to lift the bladder away from the obstructed outlet, or bladder surgery can repair a cystocoele. An estradiol-releasing vaginal ring (Estring) provides both mechanical and hormonal support that can also help reduce the leakage.

You need to distinguish which type of incontinence you have because effective treatments are different. For example, stress incontinence is often relieved by bladder surgery, but urge incontinence is not. Loss of urine at night can result from a combination of continence dysfunctions. Some are responsive to hormone therapy with estradiol creams, rings, or vaginal tablets that restore the estrogen effects on bladder lining, smooth muscle of the bladder and urethral, and the connective tissues supporting the bladder. All are factors to explore with your doctor. Prompt and accurate diagnosis is crucial.

In Summary

PMS, endometriosis, cyclic acne, vulvodynia, bladder pain—all have the potential to significantly disrupt your life. All have important, overlooked hormone triggers that need to be checked. All are treatable, and generally respond well to the kinds of approaches I mentioned here and in Chapters 16 and 18.

There is also good news about incontinence. Regardless of your age, it is a problem that can be treated with a variety of medications or surgery, as well as alternative approaches that include everything from biofeedback to magnets. Never think incontinence is something you have to "put up with." With current knowledge about causes and a variety of diagnostic and treatment options—not always drugs and surgery—more than 50 percent of incontinence patients are cured, another 35 percent markedly improve, and the remaining 15 percent are more comfortable. See a knowledgeable, caring, and competent physician, or contact one of the resources in Appendix II to locate an appropriate professional near you.

Don't sit home and suffer in silence.

12

Ovarian Hormones and the Brain:
It's Not Just Stress or Your Imagination!

Introduction

You hit age thirty, your health is good, you exercise three or four times a week, and wham! Out of the blue, you are anxious, have an upset stomach and clammy skin. Or you suddenly have palpitations and pounding sensations as if your heart was going to literally jump out of your chest. "What's going on? Am I having a panic attack? A heart attack? I'm too young." The family doctor examines you and diagnoses panic disorder (PD). Or he says you have generalized anxiety disorder (GAD) and need to relax and reduce stress. You leave the doctor's office wondering just how to "relax and reduce stress." You go about your daily routine and then, a few weeks later, just as your period begins, it happens again. *What is this?*

PPD. PMDD. MDD. MDI. BPD. OCD. GAD. PD. ADD. ADHD. There is a veritable alphabet soup of psychiatric disorders common in women of reproductive age, especially in their thirties and forties. Over the last three decades, there have been enormous advances in scientific findings about the biological basis of these disorders, as well as the role of serotonin, norepinephrine, dopamine, and the brain's other chemical messengers and receptor actions. But science has not paid enough attention to the essence of women's biology—ovarian hormones, and how they trigger mood and anxiety problems. Current brain science understandings have not yet filtered down to general medical settings and treatment approaches used for women. Most of these clinical syndromes are still viewed as "only" psychiatric disorders, and treatment is almost inevitably a prescription of antidepressants.

From ancient Greece onward, we find a long history of inadequate study and incorrect conclusions about women's emotional life and the causes of "abnormal" emotions. First of all, the definition of *abnormal* was based on what was considered "normal" for males, not considering that "normal" for women's emotional expression may be quite different. And physicians still have not recognized the hormone connection in mood syndromes in women, even after a few thousand years of observation.

The ancient Greeks thought women's moods resulted from a "wandering uterus" (the Greek word was *hyster*). This is the origin of the word *hysteria* (and its negative connotations) applied to emotional, excitable, anxious women. During the Middle Ages, women healers who dealt with psychological problems and relieved illness and suffering with herbs were considered to be witches, and burned at the stake. Some five hundred years later Freud erroneously concluded that women's psychological disturbances were due to "penis envy." American psychiatry in the 1940s and 1950s labeled all psychoses "schizophrenia," failing to recognize that mania or depression *or endocrine disorders* could also produce the same abnormal thought patterns, hallucinations, or delusions. In the 1980s and 1990s, American psychiatry focused on the "serotonin connection" and developed "serotonin boosting" medicines that are now prescribed like candy for women of all ages, in numbers far greater than for men. The obvious hormone link has been overlooked or dismissed.

British psychiatrists and gynecologists presented different explanations for such mood problems in women *decades* before these concepts made it across the ocean to the United States. Manic-depressive illness (MDI) and major depressive disorder (MDD) were recognized as distinct from schizophrenia even though both these mood disorders, in their severe forms, can cause delusions and hallucinations. Several leading gynecologists and menopause researchers in Great Britain, such as Drs. Campbell, Whitehead, and Studd, described postpartum depression (PPD), PMS, PMDD, and perimenopausal depression related to the decline in estradiol. They did not simply focus on serotonin imbalance as a primary cause. Dr. Studd's group successfully treated women with estradiol implants or patches for years, yet few psychiatrists or gynecologists in the United States use that option. Women here are given more expensive serotonin drugs that also have more side effects.

Ovarian Hormones and the Brain

Estradiol, progesterone, and testosterone receptor sites exist throughout key areas of our brain, spinal cord, and peripheral nerves. In the brain, these hormone receptors are concentrated in the cortex and the limbic system areas. There are multiple connections between the limbic system and all the other parts of the brain and spinal cord. The rise and fall of estradiol, progesterone, and testosterone increases or decreases chemical messengers such as serotonin, norepinephrine, endorphins, and others that give directions to the limbic system areas regulating changes in mood, sleep, memory, pain, and appetite.

Hormones have many actions and sites in the nerve cells to modify the ways nerves function. Hormone levels affect the *number* of neurotransmitters produced as well as the *sensitivity* of neurotransmitter receptors. The brain clearly responds to withdrawal, or absence, of our ovarian hormones with a variety of physical and "psychological" effects. Reflect on the changing hormone levels at puberty, during our cycle, in pregnancy, after delivery, and at menopause, and you can see how many body systems are affected!

First, let's clarify some terms you often encounter in the press. Mood *symptom* usually refers to a brief period of mood change not severe enough or long-lasting enough to qualify for a formal diagnosis of mood *disorder*. Mood disorder generally refers to a group of physical and emotional changes severe enough and sustained enough to indicate an illness, based on criteria agreed upon by researchers, that needs evaluation and treatment. For example, about 90 percent of women in many different cultures experience mood changes or symptoms with their menstrual periods, postpartum, and during perimenopause. Only 5 to 10 percent, on average, experience symptoms severe enough to be considered a disorder, requiring more comprehensive treatment.

The same is true with anxiety, a widely used term with many meanings. Some people use it to refer to a mood: "I'm feeling anxious." Others use it to describe a characteristic or trait: "She's always anxious and uptight." It can mean a brief symptom: "I had an anxiety attack over my bounced check." It can also mean a sustained pattern of physical and emotional changes called *Generalized Anxiety Disorder,* or *Panic Disorder.* In these chapters, I am generally referring to fairly short-lived, episodic anxiety *symptoms* that occur in relation to changes in physiological variables such as levels of glucose, thyroid hormones, estradiol, testosterone, and progesterone.

Estrogen Effects

There has been an explosion of research interest, and exciting new findings, about how hormones affect the brain. Estradiol, produced by the ovary, has wide-ranging effects on brain function through many different pathways and mechanisms that we are just beginning to understand. One of the most significant effects of estradiol is its role in serotonin production, which influences such diverse problems as mood changes, insomnia, anxiety, appetite, pain, and headaches. In women of any age, declining estradiol is a cause of reduced serotonin production, reduced serotonin receptor density, and changes in serotonin activity at receptor sites. A *rise* in progesterone also decreases serotonin. Loss of usual serotonin activity in the brain helps explain why depressed, irritable, anxious moods occur in many women before their periods or during perimenopause. Low estradiol effects to reduce serotonin activity are made worse if women smoke or don't eat well. The hormone connection in younger women's problems—PMS, postpartum depression, insomnia, headaches, and anxiety symptoms—make even more sense when you consider all the dietary, environmental, and lifestyle factors I described earlier that can cause premature decrease in estradiol and also decrease serotonin.

Numerous worldwide studies over the past two decades show reduced serotonin levels as a primary cause of depressed mood, increased irritability, increased anxiety, increased pain sensitivity, eating disorders, obsessive-compulsive disorders, and disruption of normal sleep cycles. Low brain levels of 5-hydroxyindoleacetic acid (5-HIAA), a serotonin breakdown product, are found in women and men who attempt or commit suicide. In fact, decreases in other measures of serotonin activity in perimenopausal women correlate with a peak of suicide in this age range—a peak of suicide *not* seen in men. Serotonin also decreases as we get older, with prolonged stress, cigarette smoking, overuse of alcohol or cocaine or other stimulants, exposure to pesticides and other chemicals, and dietary deficits of the vitamins, cofactors, and amino acids used to make serotonin. Many factors affect serotonin balance, but the loss or decline in estradiol appears to be a critical gender difference that contributes to greater rates of depression, anxiety syndromes, and suicide in women.

Serotonin is not the only chemical messenger in the brain affected by estradiol. It also affects endorphins, our body's natural painkillers, and mood elevators. Endorphin production is highest when estradiol peaks at midcycle or during the last stage of pregnancy. Endorphins fall sharply when the placenta is delivered after the birth of a baby, causing both estradiol and progesterone levels to plummet. Endorphin withdrawal produces effects similar to heroin or morphine withdrawal: irritability, tearfulness, anxiety, stomach upset, diarrhea, and sweating. The drop in endorphins that occurs with falling estradiol and progesterone at menses and postpartum, as well as declining estradiol with perimenopause and menopause, plays a *contributing* if not a causative, role in anxiety, insomnia, depressed mood, headaches, and pain symptoms that many women describe.

Putting together all the serotonin and endorphin connections, estradiol has multiple effects on the brain that together act as a natural antidepressant and nerve growth promoter. It also has all the effects summarized in the chart on page 222. With all this activity in the brain, you can see how estradiol plays a major mood-lifting role, maintains our sense of well-being, and helps boost our energy level. Perhaps if we paid more attention to our "natural antidepressant," women wouldn't need so many prescription drugs or have to experiment with so many herbal preparations!

Testosterone Effects

Testosterone is also a "woman's hormone," made by the ovary before menopause, and to a much lesser extent by the adrenal gland (see Chapter 2). Testosterone receptors are found in several areas of the brain. As we all know, this hormone is crucial for sex drive because it activates the brain's "sexual circuits" in both women and men. EEG brain wave studies show that testosterone has a general activating or stimulating effect on brain pathways much like the antidepressant imipramine or the stimulant amphetamine. These effects are one way testosterone improves a woman's sense of well-being and energy level. Lose your optimal testosterone, and you lose more than your sex drive—you feel sluggish, tired, "blah." Too much testosterone, however, can cause nervousness, agitation, anxiety attacks, insomnia, and restlessness in the same way amphetamines do, even before you see it cause excess facial hair or acne. That's one reason it is crucial to restore estradiol first, to help balance the testosterone effects on the brain and body.

A certain level of estradiol must be present in the brain for testosterone to function properly because the brain testosterone receptor appears to be created by the presence of estradiol. Without enough estradiol to "prime the pump,"

SUMMARY: ESTRADIOL AND YOUR BRAIN

- Increases production and/or prolongs action of serotonin
- Enhances CNS availability of norepinephrine and dopamine
- Inhibits the monoamine oxidase (MAO) enzymes, which prolongs the mood-lifting actions of serotonin, dopamine, and norepinephrine
- Increases production of the enzyme needed to make acetylcholine, a crucial memory-enhancing neurotransmitter
- Increases blood flow to the brain
- Regulates contractility of blood vessels (vasomotor tone)
- Regulates sleep centers
- Regulates body temperature
- Raises pain threshold, which improves pain tolerance
- Increases dendrite connections between nerve cells in memory centers, which improves memory function
- Enhances attention and concentration mechanisms, increases sensory perception for fine touch, olfactory, and visual stimuli
- Involved in growth hormone release at night
- Prolongs neuron responses to excitatory amino acids in the cerebral cortex, cerebellum, hippocampus, hypothalamus, midbrain, and pons
- May alter seizure threshold (direction of change is dependent upon type of seizure)

© Elizabeth Lee Vliet, M.D., 2003

testosterone cannot attach or function properly in brain centers to stimulate sexual arousal. In women who have had breast cancer, and are not taking estradiol, studies show that providing supplemental testosterone may only partially improve their sexual desire and ability to have an orgasm.

No matter what your age, if testosterone is lower than normal, its impact is enormous. Understanding this basic biology has helped many women and their significant others overcome relationship difficulties when a partner felt unwanted or no longer attractive. It is rewarding to hear patients describe how they feel with natural testosterone supplementation: "Gosh, I feel like my old self again. I have my energy back. I'm interested in sex again" (see Chapter 16 for more information on natural testosterone).

Progesterone Effects

Progesterone has interesting effects on the brain, acting as an estrogen "blocker" to reduce estradiol binding at receptors. This action is similar to tamoxifen, the antiestrogen breast cancer drug. Progesterone decreases testosterone effects by several mechanisms, including a decrease of estradiol and testosterone receptor activity in the brain, called *down-regulation*. Progesterone competes with testosterone passing from the blood into the brain, competes for binding at testosterone receptors, and also decreases the conversion of testosterone into its most active form. In fact, progesterone is one of the most potent naturally occurring "androgen blockers" of all the ones identified. With all these effects that block testosterone, it isn't surprising that your sex drive plummets the premenstrual week of your cycle, when progesterone is naturally high, or when you are taking high-progestin birth control pills or large doses of progesterone for PMS. Women taking menopausal hormone therapy also describe loss of libido during the progestin or progesterone phase of their therapy. *Low* estradiol further intensifies the libido-blocking and depressant effects of progesterone. Both estradiol and testosterone have mood-*elevating* effects, so it's easy to see why you feel grumpy, irritable, or tearful whenever progesterone decreases the binding of estradiol and testosterone at brain receptors.

Progesterone can cause mood changes in other ways. There are several important progesterone breakdown compounds that attach to the brain's GABA receptors just like antianxiety medicines (Xanax, Valium, Ativan, Klonopin, and other benzodiazepines). Our brain makes its own natural anxiety-relieving chemical, called *endozapine,* which normally attaches to the GABA receptors to help alleviate anxiety. If you don't make enough endozapine, prescription medicines like Valium or Xanax can help replace it, and thereby relieve anxiety symptoms. Taking benzodiazepine medicine to replace endozapine is similar in concept to replacing lost thyroid hormone with thyroid medicine. Several progesterone metabolites act like endozapine at GABA receptors to produce a calming, sleepy sensation. But for some women, this GABA effect causes a depressed mood, just as we see with the depressant effects of benzodiazepines, leading to low energy, blunted sex drive, and decreased memory and concentration. Because the effects of progesterone are more inhibitory than excitatory, researchers have described its combined effects on the brain as depressant. Experiments show that it isn't just women who experience these sedative and depressant effects of progesterone, men given progesterone experience them, too.

Postpartum Anxiety, Depression, and Memory and Sleep Problems

Physicians since the time of Hippocrates have described postpartum depression as being triggered by the abrupt fall in hormones that occurs with delivery of the placenta after the baby is born. Our "modern" medical model has been slow to accept endocrine causes, focusing instead on serotonin and other neurotransmitter imbalances as primary causes. Since the clinical syndrome of postpartum depression has *symptoms* similar to other types of depression, doctors often overlook hormone changes as possible factors that may need treatment to relieve the depression. This problem is especially true since many researchers in postpartum mood disorders receive funding from the manufacturers of antidepressants, and *only* study these drugs, not hormones. To me, it isn't surprising that symptoms can be the same in depressions that have different causes, since many different triggers affect the same brain pathways.

Studies over many years show that women with one postpartum depressive episode are at high risk for a similar depressive syndrome with subsequent pregnancies. Women experience drops in estradiol with every menstrual cycle, but the drop when the placenta is delivered is over two thousand times greater. For example, estradiol levels in the last trimester are in the neighborhood of 20,000 pg/ml, but a few days after delivery, it plummets to about 100 pg/ml. And that's only one of many hormone changes after delivery. Talk about falling off a hormone cliff!

Although many physicians are not interested in these hormone changes, women who experience postpartum depression are quick to connect the rapidly falling hormones to their profound depressed-anxious mood and fragmented sleep. Hormone treatment of postpartum depression has been widely studied and used in England for many years, but the problem that faces women in the United States is finding a doctor who considers these hormone connections important, and who will use hormonal treatment approaches. Treating the patient with antidepressants is more convenient, and easier, but doesn't really address the underlying cause. Sometimes, as you see in the women's stories I share, the consequences of overlooking the hormone issues can be serious.

Following the birth of her daughter, *Leslie* developed severe anxiety, insomnia, scattered thinking, and trouble focusing on her work. She was told she had a "generalized anxiety disorder" and was treated with Klonopin. No one did an endocrine workup to test for hormonal changes that could also cause such symptoms. She struggled through each day, feeling sleepy and tired on the Klonopin, but at least it kept her anxiety symptoms under control so she could return to work. A few years later the marriage crumbled. Her husband filed for divorce, seeking custody of their daughter, claiming that Leslie was on the "addictive" medicine Klonopin and unable to care for the child. She wanted to get off the Klonopin to thwart her husband's tactic of using a psychiatric disorder as grounds for custody. She saw a naturopath who unfortunately prescribed progesterone cream and DHEA supplements that further aggravated her underlying low estradiol and excess free testosterone, making her anxiety, fatigue, and headaches much worse. Taking daily progesterone also prevented return of her normal ovarian estradiol production and further contributed to her depressed mood and lack of energy. The naturopath also recommended multiple soy isoflavone supplements that also interfered with estradiol and progesterone production. She was in a horrible downward spiral.

She came to us for a comprehensive hormone evaluation. Her anxiety symptoms began in the postpartum phase when her estradiol plummeted after delivery. When I saw her, the anxiety symptoms were clearly cyclic, and worse when her estradiol dropped abruptly with ovulation. Because of the incorrect hormones and supplements she had been given, along with all the stress and a very thin body, her own estradiol was further suppressed and far below optimal. The blood tests confirmed that her estradiol was less than *one third* of a normal healthy level for a woman her age. My evaluation found two other overlooked hormonal imbalances that can cause marked anxiety and insomnia: excess thyroid activity (*hyper*thyroid) and excess free, active testosterone relative to her low estradiol. When there is too much thyroid or testosterone, it overstimulates brain pathways that mimic the physical and emotional experiences we call anxiety. She also had a very high level of NTx, which indicates excess bone breakdown—additional evidence that estradiol was far too low and her thyroid was overactive. Leslie also had a B_{12} and iron deficiency that further added to the anxiety, insomnia, and fatigue. These are a lot of metabolic-hormonal issues that were not getting addressed with the prescriptions and supplements she had been given.

Her prematurely low estradiol was easily remedied with an estradiol patch, along with twelve days of natural progesterone every other month and vitamin B and iron supplements. It is unfortunate that Leslie was misdiagnosed as having a primary anxiety disorder when the proper medical/endocrine evaluation was not done. Without this complete evaluation, important hormonal problems were not getting proper treatment. I listed the several *primary medical* conditions that triggered her *secondary psychological* (anxiety) symptoms. Her anxiety and insomnia symptoms were relieved by hormone therapy. She was finally able to taper off Klonopin and eliminate the medicine that caused daytime tiredness and difficulty concentrating.

Leslie won full custody of her daughter when she showed medical documentation of her abnormal hormone levels, the revised diagnosis based on objective laboratory studies, and her new hormone treatment that relieved her symptoms. Getting proper treatment with estradiol, instead of the Band-Aid approach to symptoms with Klonopin, also stopped her excess bone breakdown, helping to reduce later risk of osteoporosis.

Where Are We Now?

I have worked with postpartum hormone connections for many years and have successfully used a variety of hormone approaches for women suffering significant postpartum depression, anxiety, and sleep disruption. As with Leslie, many women do not need psychotropic medicines if hormone balance is restored. But some do still need antidepressants or anxiety-relieving medicines, so we combine these with hormone approaches tailored to each woman. I have consistently found that with the foundation of proper hormone management, however, women frequently do not need standard doses of antidepressants, often only half the usual dose or even less. Patients often say that my clinical observations and their obvious improvements are discounted by other doctors, citing no "proof" that the hormones play a role in mood symptoms or recovery. But these women say, "The proof lies in how well I feel and that I have tapered off other medicines that cause side effects." Recent objective studies, however, provide "hard data" on this hormone connection that may convince skeptical physicians. The next section describes some of the key studies on the hormone-mood connection.

Hormone Crashes and Withdrawal: More Profound Than You Realize

When there is a tremendous drop in estradiol, from predelivery to postpartum levels, it is like your brain falling off a cliff to the rocks below. Such a precipitous fall in estradiol creates an "estradiol withdrawal syndrome" that appears to be a critical factor in setting off brain changes that lead to postpartum psychosis and/or major depression. An estradiol patch is like having a parachute that lets you glide gently and safely to the ground. If we can prevent the drastic fall in estradiol after delivery, we help blunt the dramatic decrease in mood-lifting serotonin and endorphins and the surges of anxiety-provoking norepinephrine.

Drs. Bloch and Schmidt did an interesting study to support, or "prove," that the "estrogen withdrawal state" can trigger mood or psychotic changes. They mimicked the high hormone levels of pregnancy in a group of women, and then put them into "hormone withdrawal," creating the same response in the brain and body as with the delivery of a baby. They found over 60 percent of the women with a history of postpartum depression developed significant increases in depressive symptoms when hormones were withdrawn, but *none* of the control group did. Here, the "controls" were women who did not have a past history of postpartum depression. Their conclusion states quite clearly: *"The data provide direct evidence in support of the involvement of the reproductive hormones estrogen and progesterone in the development of postpartum depression in a subgroup of women."*

In 1996, Dr. John Studd led a pivotal double-blind, placebo-controlled study in England investigating the effectiveness of transdermal estradiol for women with severe postpartum depression. Sixty-one women with a major depression that began within three months of childbirth were randomly assigned either placebo treatment or an active treatment with transdermal 17-beta estradiol, using 200 mcg daily for three months followed by three months of estradiol with added cyclical progestin at a dose of 10 mg daily for twelve days each month. The women were assessed monthly by self-ratings of depressive symptoms and by a clinical psychiatric interview. Based on the objective rating scale scores, the women in both groups were severely depressed at the pretreatment evaluations. During the first month of therapy the women receiving estradiol improved faster, and to a significantly greater degree, than those receiving placebo patches. The control group improved over time, but, on average, their improvement was much slower, and their scores did not fall below the major depression threshold level for at least four months. Most of the women with the estradiol patches did not need antidepressant medication. Dr. Studd and his team concluded that transdermal estradiol is an effective treatment for postpartum depression, recommending further research studies on dosage and duration of treatment.

A March 2000 medical publication described the results of Finnish researchers, led by Dr. Antti Ahokas, using an open trial of 17-beta estradiol to treat women who met diagnostic criteria for postpartum *psychosis,* the most severe form of postpartum psychiatric disorders. Serum estradiol levels were measured at baseline and weekly for six weeks. The baseline estradiol levels for these patients were lower than the threshold we use to indicate ovarian failure. All of the patients exhibited high scores on the psychiatric symptom scale. The researchers used doses of estradiol designed to restore healthy menstrual cycle levels. During the *first week* on the 17-beta estradiol treatment, psychiatric symptoms diminished significantly, with mean scores dropping from 78.3 to 18.8, a remarkable change! By the end of the second week serum estradiol concentrations rose to approximately the values normally found during the follicular phase of the menstrual cycle, and at these higher levels of estradiol, the patients became virtually free of psychiatric symptoms. Dr. Ahokas's group concluded that boosting the low estradiol levels led to complete reversal of the psychiatric symptoms in all patients. The one woman who then discontinued her estradiol suffered a recurrence of psychotic symptoms. The results matched the positive results I see in my own practice when using estradiol patches in this manner.

In 2001, Dr. Ahokas's group evaluated the effect of *sublingual* 17-beta estradiol for the treatment of women with postpartum depression. They again found that the severe depressive symptoms were quickly alleviated by estradiol therapy in women with postpartum depression who have low estradiol levels at the outset. Dr. Ahokas said, *"In spite of multiple contacts with health providers, women with postpartum depression often remain unrecognized and untreated."* In the United States, internists, family medicine doctors, and OB/GYNs are the highest prescribers of antidepressants in the country—and none of these physicians routinely do hormone tests, nor do most psychiatrists. This helps you understand why it is so difficult for American women to get hormonal treatments for postpartum depression. Dr. Ahokas's study found that women's depressive symptoms diminished significantly within the first week of the eight-week treatment period, which is a far more rapid response than with the standard antidepressant therapies. By the end of the second week, the researchers found that the scores on standard depression ratings were compatible with complete recovery in nineteen of the twenty-three patients. These are remarkable statistics, better than antidepressant recovery rates.

Dr. Ahokas's group found what I repeatedly see in my own practice: Correcting the hormonal balance with bioidentical forms of 17-beta estradiol creates a rapid, positive effect on mood and sleep for these mothers, many of whom did not respond to traditional antidepressant treatments. If a new mother's mood and sleep patterns are improved quickly, it obviously helps Mom, Dad, and baby! Another study from the University of Zimbabwe was published in 1999, and pharmacists reported, "Estradiol patches are now being used in the prevention and treatment of postpartum depression." If estradiol patches can be used to treat postpartum depression in Zimbabwe, you'd think we could do a better job in the United States!

The Finnish researchers described one drawback to sublingual estradiol: This form of delivery causes extremely rapid absorption, and the effects only last a short time because of rapid metabolism. Sublingual estradiol must be given several times a day to maintain stable blood levels, something I also commonly see in my patients. A transdermal patch gives more gradual delivery, keeping estradiol steadier over a few days. This is a significant improvement over the roller-coaster effect of sublingual estradiol.

A study, conducted by the Clinical Psychopharmacology Unit of Massachusetts General Hospital, and published in 1995, described high-dose oral estrogen treatment of seven women with histories of postpartum psychosis and four with histories of postpartum major depression. None had histories of depression or psychosis during *nonpostpartum* times, and all were free of mood symptoms throughout their current pregnancy. These women were at high risk for a recurrent episode of depression or psychosis postpartum due to their past history. Estrogen treatment was begun immediately after delivery. With the estrogen, only *one* woman developed a relapse of her postpartum mood disorder. All others remained well and required no antidepressants or other psychotropic medications during the one-year follow-up.

With all of the scientific evidence now available, it is not sufficient to tell a woman who is significantly depressed or anxious following her delivery that she's "just stressed" as a new mother, or that she feels conflicts about being a mother, or that she just needs a serotonin-booster medicine. Physicians in all specialties treating women with postpartum depression must do complete laboratory tests of the ovarian, thyroid, adrenal, and pituitary hormones, and then incorporate treatment approaches that correct imbalances.

Other Brain Effects: Hormone Triggers of Anxiety, Racing Heart, Flutters, and Palpitations

Many women are puzzled about hormone shifts that cause *brain* symptoms such as anxiety, or *heart* symptoms such as palpitations, rapid heartbeat, and flutters. Actually, there is a simple, straightforward connection: Hormone levels rising *or* falling too fast trigger a burst of norepinephrine that sets off the central alarm center in the brain's limbic system. Falling estradiol, for example, is like someone pulling the cord on a hotel fire alarm; the signal is relayed to the central alarm center that sends the warning to all the rooms of the hotel. The brain's alarm center, called the *locus ceruleus,* does the same thing. The flood of norepinephrine makes you feel "anxious," and sends a signal to the heart to pump faster and get the body ready for an emergency. This causes the heart pounding, skipping, or fluttering sensation. Signals are sent to other parts of the body to either shut down (bowel) or speed up (metabolism) and get you ready to "fight or flee." If you are sleeping, this surge of norepinephrine bolts you awake; it is also the trigger for the "hot flash" and sweats that can hit at the same time as the anxiousness and racing heartbeat. This cascade of events spreads over the body from the simple hormone-triggered release of brain chemicals.

Have you noticed *where* in the menstrual cycle these palpitations or panicky episodes occur? If your physical symptoms (heart flutters, heart racing or pounding; feeling queasy or nauseous; sweating; feeling anxious for no apparent reason) come at times of the menstrual cycle when estradiol is low or falling (around ovulation, a day or so before your period starts, or the first two or three days of bleeding), they are likely the hormone-triggered brain-body reactions. If you are someone who is very sensitive to the *rate* of hormonal changes, this same "alarm" response can occur with a rapidly *rising* level of estradiol or progesterone, as in pregnancy, or when starting hormone therapy or birth control pills.

Hot flashes used to be considered *psychological,* a figment of your imagination. We now know this is a *physiological* reaction when low or falling estradiol triggers reactions in the brain and blood vessels that fire off norepinephrine (NE) in the limbic system, disrupting normal function of the heat-regulating center in the hypothalamus, signaling the arteries to dissipate excess heat. The dilation is accompanied by sweating. The body temperature begins to drop, and a chilly sensation sweeps over you. If it happens at night you wake up, often soaked in sweat. If estradiol falls abruptly, this same series of events occurs in younger women, just as happens with menopause.

Serotonin helps maintain sleep and decrease anxiety, so a drop in this chemical messenger also adds to nighttime awakenings and aggravates adrenaline-induced feelings of irritability, tension, palpitations, and chest discomfort. It is wise to have palpitations and chest pain evaluated to rule out underlying cardiac disease, especially if you have several risk factors, but if the cardiologist tells you "nothing is wrong," that simply means you don't have cardiovascular disease. It *doesn't* mean you are imagining these sensations. Don't jump to the conclusion that, if it isn't cardiovascular disease, it must be "just stress," as many doctors tell women. Physicians must consider that for women fluctuating hormone levels cause these same heart-related symptoms. As you get older and estradiol production declines, a fall in this key hormone before menses triggers an even more pronounced physical response. It's a new, more intense feeling that makes you sit up and take notice. Women say they know "it's a physical, chemical kind of thing," but are told "it's just stress, it's all in your head," as if they are imagining it. While it is true that the chemical changes originate "in your head," it is *not* your imagination. It is very real. These sensations are physical reactions of hormone changes hitting brain centers.

Understanding Hormonally Triggered Migraines

Women are all too often told that hormones don't cause headaches! Yet from puberty to menopause, 60 to 70 percent of women with migraine headaches have episodes triggered by the drop in estradiol before the menstrual period or around ovulation. For women susceptible to migraine or other vascular headaches, the monthly fall in estradiol can set off spasms in the blood vessels and changes in serotonin that trigger the headache. Estradiol falls sharply around ovulation and again rather dramatically about Day 22 to 24 of your cycle, reaching its lowest point on Days 1 to 3 of bleeding. The estradiol level remains low for the first four to five days of bleeding, a reason for the increase in migraines during the early days of menstrual flow. Female migraine sufferers are more likely to be affected by hormone triggers the week they stop birth control pills to have a period, or postpartum, when estradiol, serotonin, and endorphin levels drop sharply. For menopausal women on hormone therapy, headaches can be set off by stopping estrogen for Days 25 to 30, or by starting the progestin phase of HRT.

It's true that there is a genetic predisposition for migraines. Most doctors, and most migraine sufferers, also recognize the usual classic migraine triggers such as red wines, aged cheeses, foods with MSG and nitrites or sulfites, histamine, alcohol, caffeine, chocolate, barometric pressure weather changes, stress, "rebound" from pain medication, and sometimes dairy products. *But the falling estrogen trigger, recognized for over thirty years, continues to be overlooked in almost 99 percent of women with migraines,* even though this hormone trigger can be alleviated in fairly simple ways (see Chapter 16).

Hormone Effects on Migraine Mechanisms

Migraine headaches often include a number of phenomena, such as aura, visual changes, sensitivity to light and sound, nausea or vomiting, numbness or tingling of face and arms, along with the throbbing head pain. Doctors used to think all these phenomena were due to circulation changes: blood vessels becoming first constricted (vasoconstriction) and then dilated (vasodilatation). Newer research shows migraine is a state of central nervous system "hyperexcitability," making you more susceptible to episodes of spontaneous firing (depolarization) of neurons, followed by dampening down of neuron function, which then causes changes in blood flow. Whole textbooks are devoted to the subject of migraine headaches, so my focus here is only on the important hormone connections that can set off the migraine cascade.

Estrogen and Progesterone Effects on Headache

The high frequency of migraines occurring at the onset of menses has been observed for several thousand years. It wasn't known which hormone was the primary cause until the mid-1970s, when Dr. B. W. Somerville did a series of studies that clearly demonstrated that estrogen and progesterone have very different effects on migraines. The migraine attack was triggered by the premenstrual drop in *estradiol,* not progesterone. The table on page 231 summarizes some of the ways falling estradiol can set off migraines, particularly if added to dietary, stress, weather, and medication triggers.

MECHANISMS OF ESTROGEN EFFECTS ON HEADACHES

- Falling estrogen decreases the amount of available serotonin (5-HT), as well as the number of certain 5-HT receptors, important in decreasing migraine pain. The drop in serotonin levels causes cranial blood vessels to spasm painfully. Adding estrogen to serotonin-boosting medications has a synergistic effect to boost serotonin.
- Falling estrogen causes a decrease in the pain-relieving beta-endorphins in the brain, spinal cord, and body tissues.
- Estrogen withdrawal (either naturally in the cycle or by stopping hormone-containing medication) causes a rebound in dopamine (DA) that can intensify pain.
- Estrogen decline causes vasoconstriction by contracting the muscles in the artery walls, aggravating pain of vascular headaches.
- Falling estrogen causes a burst of norepinephrine (NE) release in the brain's locus ceruleus, which increases vasoconstriction and diminishes blood flow to the area of the brain involved in vision, thus producing the aura.
- Increased NE release further intensifies pain.
- At the same time, a decrease in estradiol lowers the pain threshold, making nerve endings more sensitive to painful stimuli.

© Elizabeth Lee Vliet, M.D., 2003

The role of progesterone and progestins. Studies show that synthetic progestins in birth control pills or hormone therapy regimens can increase the frequency and severity of migraine, vascular, and muscle-tension headaches for some women. In my clinical experience, progestin-only types of contraceptives like Norplant and Depo-Provera are among the worst offenders. These products without any estrogen have a high rate of causing daily tension headaches as well as vascular headaches like migraines, even in women who did not have headaches prior to using these contraceptives. In combination birth control pills with both estrogen and progestin, it is the pills higher in progestin and lower in estrogen that are more likely to cause headaches as a side effect. If I prescribe an oral contraceptive to a woman with migraines, I use a pill such as Ovcon-35, Orthocyclen, or Yasmin, which have better estrogen and a lower dose of progestin that is still high enough to decrease heavy bleeding and provide contraception.

Progesterone, even though it is a natural hormone made by the ovary, has mixed effects in headache syndromes. It may be both positive and negative, so its role is more difficult to define. A normal effect of progesterone is to retain fluid and constrict blood vessels. In headache-prone women, these effects can combine to trigger a migraine when progesterone is rising. This is especially true if estradiol is lower than the optimal balance of these two hormones. In other women, progesterone's calming effects relax muscles in the head and neck that tense with stress, so some women may have fewer headaches in the progesterone phase of the cycle. Progesterone also acts as an anesthetic when levels are high (as in the last trimester of pregnancy). Like the benzodiazepines, high doses of progesterone have anticonvulsant and sedative effects at brain centers that can decrease headaches for some women.

There are several possible explanations why progesterone may make headaches worse in some women. Progesterone decreases estradiol binding at serotonin receptors, creating a "low-estradiol" headache trigger. Progesterone stimulates the production of prostaglandins that cause spasm of the smooth muscle lining the artery walls, another migraine trigger. If stopped abruptly, progesterone produces withdrawal symptoms similar to those of benzodiazepines, barbiturates, and alcohol. Progesterone withdrawal can cause throbbing headaches that can be mistaken for migraines. You need to decrease progesterone gradually if you are taking it for PMS or for hormone therapy at menopause, especially if taking more than 200 mg a day (based on oral dose).

I use progesterone in migraine sufferers as I do other therapies: I pay attention to what *you* say about your headache pattern in relation to hormone cycles. I integrate your observations with hormone pharmacology, and we work together to identify the best hormone and other medication options. Since progesterone effects can differ so much from one woman to the next, it's a good idea to track your personal cycle pattern to see when headaches occur and whether hormone changes appear to aggravate your headaches. Then you can work with your physician to find the most appropriate hormone options for you.

Overall, I have found that progesterone in high doses does *not* help prevent migraines. In women who still have headaches when taking natural progesterone, I use the lowest dose that will protect the uterine lining (see Chapter 16), and divide the total daily amount into smaller portions given several times a day. I also find that for some women the non-oral forms of progesterone, such as Crinone vaginal cream, or injectable progesterone in oil, also reduce headache frequency better than oral progesterone.

Pregnancy effects on migraine. The dramatic hormone shifts and high levels in pregnancy can affect migraine headaches in several ways. Some women develop migraines for the first time during pregnancy. Seventy percent of women who have migraines *without* aura report *relief* of migraines when they are pregnant. Women who have migraines *with* aura often find their migraines *intensify* with pregnancy. Still other women experience headaches different in quality and intensity from those prior to pregnancy. The pattern is variable and depends, to some extent, upon the phase of pregnancy. Women whose migraines get worse typically report that this occurs during the first trimester, when both estrogen and progesterone are rising rapidly and the placenta produces hormones independently of the ovaries. Women who experience relief show improvement most often *after* the first trimester, when progesterone levels have dropped and estradiol levels are higher and more stable. Since migraines tend to be worse with fluctuating estradiol levels, you can see how migraines may improve during pregnancy with the absence of a cyclic hormonal up-and-down pattern and the increased levels of estradiol and endorphins. These same effects explain women's reports of enhanced mood and feelings of well-being in pregnancy, which appear to be related to the mood-elevating effects of the high estradiol levels augmenting serotonin and endorphins.

How Do Oral Contraceptives Affect Migraine?

Until recently, it was thought that women with migraine headaches who used birth control pills had a slight increase in risk of stroke. However, early studies from around the world were done with women who took the older, high-dose oral contraceptives rather than today's lower-dose pills. In 1993, the International Collaborative Group for the Study of Stroke in Young Women reanalyzed the earlier data and did not confirm the initial reports that migraine headaches might increase the risk of stroke in young women using oral contraceptives. The new data review determined that cigarette smoking was the primary risk for stroke in women with migraines; this risk increased in *smokers* taking birth control pills.

Physicians have also been taught that oral contraceptives aggravate migraines, but this is another incorrect generalization. Whether headaches are aggravated or relieved with oral contraceptives depends on the estrogen-to-progestin ratios in the pill. Current studies, and my clinical experience, have shown many women actually achieve relief with the right hormone ratio in an oral contraceptive and if they do not stop the pill to have a period each month, thus allowing continuous, stable hormone levels.

Earlier studies concluding oral contraceptives increased migraines did not look carefully at when in the pill cycle the headaches occurred. For example, researchers often did not ask whether the headache occurred while on the active hormone-containing pills (which would likely mean the pill did make the headaches worse), or whether the headaches occurred in the placebo cycle (which would indicate *hormone withdrawal* as the cause). Forty to 60 percent of women with migraines who take oral contraceptives experience headaches in the last seven days of the pill pack (i.e., placebo pills) supporting rapidly *falling* estradiol levels as the trigger. In four double-blind, placebo-controlled studies there were no differences in headache frequency between women on birth control pills and those taking a placebo. Dr. Stephen Silberstein, a well-known migraine specialist, emphasized in an article that appeared in *Neurology*, in March 1992: "Estrogens and OCs are not contraindicated in migraine patients. In fact, they may actually be indicated for certain women." Some physicians still think women with migraines should not use oral contraceptives, but this belief has not been supported by recent international data analyses.

The variation in birth control pill effects summarized in the box on page 234

POTENTIAL BIRTH CONTROL PILL EFFECTS ON MIGRAINES

- Headaches can increase. This is typically seen with pills having varying hormone content, such as Tri-Levlen, Ortho Tri-Cyclen, Triphasil. Increased headaches are also seen with high-progestin pills such as Loestrin, Alesse, and Mircette, and with progestin-only contraceptives such as Norplant, Depo-Provera, or the pills Micronor, Nor-QD, and Ovrette—*if they are not prescribed with estradiol to balance the progestin.*
- Headaches can be *eliminated or* significantly decreased. This is more common with *monophasic* (constant dose) pills with lower progestin content, such as Ovcon 35, Modicon, Orthocyclen, Yasmin, and Diane 35, particularly if taken continuously with no break for menses. Studies show as much as 60 to 80 percent improvement in migraines when women use steady-dose combined estrogen-progestin contraceptives taken continuously.
- Birth control pills can contribute to the first appearance of a migraine, usually in women with a significant family history. This response suggests that the progestin is too high, and a pill with a better hormone balance should be found. If the headaches continue, then I would not use BCPs and would look for other options.
- New or different symptoms, such as aura or visual changes, can occur. This change is potentially serious and should be discussed immediately with your physician. It usually means you should stop BCPs right away.

© Elizabeth Lee Vliet, M.D., 2003

is another indication of the crucial need for *individualized* therapy. There is no one right answer for all women. You must work closely with knowledgeable specialists to make the best use of available products to find the right balance of estrogen and progestin for you (see Chapter 16 for more information).

Hormones and Seizures

Over the years I have encountered women with seizures that were clearly affected by their menstrual cycle. This letter, from a young woman's brother in Illinois, illustrates many important points.

Dear Dr. Vliet,

I am writing to you in response to a [newspaper] wire article about you and your practice. The problem is with my sister. Back in January of this year [1996], while she was on her job as a nanny, she had what appeared to be a black-out. She became disoriented about the date, time, and place. She left the child on the floor, and left the house. They found her later that day but she did not remember anything that happened. She scheduled an appointment with a doctor [I assume an internist] who ran a battery of tests and found nothing. She was released with a perfect bill of health. The very next month she had another episode while visiting Tucson. She became disoriented and was putting salt and pepper on her cereal. Again, she remembered nothing. This time she went to see a neurologist who also performed a battery of tests and found nothing. She was released again. Shortly after this, the association was made with the fact that the episodes were occurring at the beginning of her period. She made an appointment with an OB/GYN who gave her a checkup and released her with a clean bill of health. We were worried but did not know what to do.

Well, on Memorial Day, it happened again and this time she was not as lucky. She was driving my father-in-law, who incidentally happens to be a D.O. [doctor of osteopathy] physician in Arizona. According to my father-in-law, she began to have a seizure while approaching a red light. She was frozen solid with her foot on the gas. He tried to remove the key but could not. She sustained minor injuries from the impact but the car was totaled and my father-in-law is in the hospital in Illinois awaiting neck surgery for two ruptured disks and replacement of most muscles and ligaments of the area. My sister had wandered away from the accident but was taken to the emergency room after she was found. She did not feel any pain and had no memory of the accident. Another battery of tests was done and the doctor was told of the relationship to her period. She was released with minor injuries related to the accident. This time she was in and out of a prolonged spell that lasted two days. My parents took her to the University of Chicago Hospital where yet another battery of tests were performed. They said nothing was wrong and she had to be released. She is currently awaiting an appointment with another neurologist at the University of Chicago. This is why I am appealing to you. We have come close to exhausting all avenues and the doctors say she is fine. The fact is, if she were fine, my father-in-law would not be in intensive care. They were extremely lucky that the accident was not fatal. If nothing can be done, she would have to remain in the constant care of my parents indefinitely. The doctors seem to be ignoring the fact that it must be related to her periods. Can you offer any help?

My office staff described our approach to evaluating the hormone triggers of such episodes. Her family decided to send her for our evaluation. We discussed the abrupt fall in her estradiol and progesterone at the onset of her periods as one trigger of her seizures. Her EEG did not show seizure activity, which wasn't surprising since the test was not done during her menses, and this was the *only* time she had seizures. Her neurologist started her on the anticonvulsant Tegretol, but even with this medicine, her family reported, she was still having seizures with onset of her periods. I prescribed a trial on a steady-dose birth control pill to suppress ovarian cycles, stop the rise and fall in ovarian hormones, and give a steady estrogen-progestin amount each day. She took the pills steadily for four to six packs, which reduced the number of times her hormones fell if she stopped the pills to have a period. I also prescribed a Climara patch to keep the blood level of estradiol steady during her period, which eliminated the estrogen drop that appeared to precipitate her seizures. She has done well on this regimen for five years, without *any* further menstrual seizures, and is cleared to drive again. Sometimes finding the right treatment just takes a little common sense, some thinking "outside the box," tracking patterns with the menstrual cycle and listening to observations from patients and their families.

Hormones and Memory: "Now What Was It I Was Going to Do?"

"Where did I put my keys?"; "What did I come in here to do?"; "I feel like I'm losing my mind." I hear these comments every day from women, young and old. It isn't just at menopause that you can't think of words or you forget where you *put* your to-do list, much less what was on it! You feel scattered in your thinking and can't focus like you used to. You worry about Alzheimer's. Familiar? Don't worry, you aren't alone, nor are you imagining it. You probably don't have attention deficit; more likely you are experiencing a subtle decline in the important ovarian, and possibly thyroid, hormones that oversee the brain's memory centers. Estradiol plays a significant role in preserving normal nerve cell growth, repair, and function, and science shows the ways this hormone oversees normal memory function.

Dementia means generalized loss of the brain's ability to retain, perceive, integrate, retrieve, and act appropriately on information. Collectively, we call these tasks *cognitive function*. Dementia is not one disease; it is a group of brain diseases with a hundred or more different causes. Dementia is not a normal part of aging. It is an *illness* that affects about 10 percent of the population. Some types of dementia are treatable, and reversible if the cause is caught early. For example, untreated hypothyroidism or B_{12} deficit can lead to marked impairment of cognitive function or even full-blown dementia.

Alzheimer's disease is a different type of irreversible dementia with no known cure that leads to inexorable loss of all brain function, then death. Some medications, including estradiol, may delay the progression of brain damage. In women who already have Alzheimer's disease, recent studies show that estradiol may slow the progression by as much as two years. In women who do not have the disease, studies from several countries show that estradiol can reduce later risk of developing Alzheimer's disease by 40 to 50 percent. Milder forms of memory changes that women describe during postpartum, pre- and perimenopause, and after menopause are generally not the more serious illness of dementia. But if hormonal decline is one contributing factor that helps explain memory loss in women, physicians must consider this issue and address it before permanent damage occurs.

Some Basics About How Memory Works

The complex components of our memory system were only recently delineated. Memory functions are primarily in the limbic system, which includes the *hippocampus, mammillary bodies, septal region,* and part of the *thalamus.* There is still much to clarify about how memory processes work, but so far it appears to be a system of "storage centers" located in both hemispheres of the brain. Having storage centers in different areas of the brain is like backup for your computer. Memory is not completely lost if one hemisphere of the brain is damaged or injured, which shows that memory function is different from other brain functions—most have specific locations in one hemisphere or the other, not both.

Most people think of verbal memory, but the brain has mechanisms for remembering specific types of sensory memories as well: sound (auditory), sight (visual), touch (kinesthetic), smell (olfactory), and other sensory perceptions. These sensory memory centers are also widely distributed throughout the brain. Since memory is so crucial to survival, it makes sense that the brain has evolved multiple areas for memory storage of all kinds of information needed to keep the organism alive and functioning.

To simplify, memory is either short-term or long-term. We use short-term memory in day-to-day situations. For example, you hear a telephone number or a name and remember it just long enough to use it. When the name or number or piece of information is something you want to remember longer, you convert it to long-term memory. The hippocampus and mammillary bodies are the primary centers involved in converting short-term to long-term memory. This conversion involves an actual physical change in the brain with the creation of new connections between nerve cells. Estradiol stimulates growth of these sprouts, called *dendrites,* to make more new connections between neurons, and this helps memory. This physical change can also involve the creation of actual "memory molecules" that contain specific codes for information. Short-term memory is affected first by memory robbers such as estradiol decline, nutritional deficits, or dementia-type illnesses. Later, with more and more damage, long-term memories are lost. The key role of the sex hormones in memory function is one of the mechanisms that help the species survive.

Advances in Neuroscience: Estrogen Effects on Memory

Estrogen deficiency plays an important role in causing memory loss and even some dementias. Dr. Barbara Sherwin, at McGill University in Canada, has spent almost three decades researching estrogen effects on the brain. Her studies show improvements specifically in verbal memory in healthy postmenopausal women on estrogen compared to those who are not. Dr. Sherwin and her colleagues also evaluated surgically menopausal women and found those treated with estrogen did significantly better on several measures of cognitive function than those given a placebo. Other studies of surgically menopausal women show that taking estradiol specifically enhances short-term verbal memory. None of these women had any type of dementia; they were all healthy but considered impaired in their memory abilities. Yet the improved performance in women on estrogen therapy was statistically significant and fits with what patients say when their hormone levels are restored to optimal levels.

In an ongoing study of 8,879 female residents of a retirement community in California, researchers found that estrogen users had a 40 percent lower risk of dementia (or only about 60 percent of the risk of Alzheimer's) than that seen in women who did not take estrogen. These preliminary results were published in 1998. The USC investigators further found that the higher the dose of the estrogen, the lower the risk of Alzheimer's. The risk of dementia also *decreased more* the longer women took estrogen: Women who took estrogen seven years or more had a 50 percent lower risk of dementia than those not taking ERT.

In 1994, Japanese researchers showed ERT gave measurable improvement on measures of recent memory, distant memory, attention, orientation, personality, mood, sleeping, and eating behaviors in women with documented Alzheimer's. Serum estradiol levels with ERT matched those of healthy, younger women right before ovulation. These results suggest that the estradiol and serum levels achieved with therapy must reach a certain threshold or minimum level to reap the benefits on memory and other cognitive functions. The positive changes disappeared after estrogen therapy stopped, strongly suggesting estrogen's major influence on cognitive functions. At the end of the study, the families of these patients saw the improvement and requested that estrogen therapy continue long-term.

In 1999, Yale researchers found that even a three-week course of ERT changed brain activity in postmenopausal women performing memory tasks in a randomized double-blind, placebo-controlled clinical trial. Brain activity changes in the ERT group, documented on MRI, mimicked brain activation patterns typically seen in younger women. Dr. Karl Mortel found that among women with cardiovascular disease (CVD), those taking estrogen showed improved blood flow to the brain and improved cognitive function. His work fits with other research showing estradiol's *relaxing effect* on arteries, leading to increased dilation and better blood flow to all organs in the body.

Worldwide research and my own clinical experience shows clearly that the brain is a target organ for estradiol action in women. Regardless of age, we must consider the effects of estradiol decline on memory and thinking when we are evaluating women. Psychological symptoms, like memory changes, are not *only* caused by stress; they also have physical, endocrine causes as well. We don't yet know the entire spectrum of estrogen's effects on memory and cognitive pathways, but there are a number of intriguing hypotheses about how it works, summarized in the box on page 239. On a humorous note, when someone in my office forgets something, another staff member will often ask (on the basis of experience), "Did you forget your patch this morning?"

ESTROGEN EFFECTS ON MEMORY AND COGNITIVE PATHWAYS

- 17-beta estradiol, the primary estrogen produced by the ovary before menopause, has specific receptor binding sites in many different areas of the brain. These receptor sites appear to be quite specific for the native human form of the molecule. (All of my clinical work with patients strongly supports these basic scientific findings in animal models and studies of human brain cells in tissue cultures.)
- Estradiol promotes growth of new dendrites between nerve cells, making more synaptic connections. More synapse connections mean nerve cells can handle more incoming signals. Progesterone breaks down these nerve cell connections.
- When estradiol declines, synapse density in the hippocampus (memory and learning center) decreases as well. Denser synapses allow better cell-to-cell information flow.
- Estradiol enhances the ability of nerve cells to absorb *nerve growth factor (NGF)*. In animals without ovaries, those who did not receive estrogen had a marked (56 percent) decline in the number of nerve cells; the animals given estrogen had only a slight decrease in nerve cells.
- Estrogens regulate memory-regulating (cholinergic) nerve cells in the basal forebrain of rodents. The basal forebrain is one of the regions of the brain involved in cognitive function and one of the areas that degenerates in humans with Alzheimer's disease.
- Estrogens increase the production of choline acetyltransferase, an enzyme needed to make acetylcholine (ACh). Estrogen thereby prevents the marked loss of ACh found in patients with Alzheimer's. ACh is the brain's most important chemical messenger for storing new memories in the brain, regulating memory retrieval, and cognition. Loss of the cholinergic nerves and chemical messengers is the most marked brain change in Alzheimer's disease.

© Elizabeth Lee Vliet, M.D., 2003

Multiple Sclerosis: New Insights on Hormone Connections

Multiple sclerosis (MS) hits young women hard, much harder than men. Approximately 75 percent of MS sufferers are women, most between the ages of fifteen and fifty, with an average age of onset at twenty-eight to thirty years. With these patterns, it has long been suspected that there are important hormonal factors contributing directly or indirectly to MS. MS is the most common nontraumatic neurological disease of young adults. It is an immune-mediated disorder that targets the central nervous system, causing inflammation, loss of the myelin protective coatings around nerve cells (demyelination), death of axons, and formation of scar tissue. The cause of MS is unknown, but it appears to involve a variety of genetic, hormonal, immune system, and environmental factors, such as excitotoxins, chemical pollutants, and/or infectious agents.

MS causes puzzling symptoms that come and go. At first, you wonder if you are imagining the visual changes, muscle weakness, loss of bladder control, and numbness or tingling of hands, feet, legs, or arms that can be fleeting in the initial stages of the illness. These same symptoms can have a hundred or more different causes, including hypothyroidism, menopausal loss of estradiol, diabetes, and a variety of vitamin deficiencies, to name a few. If symptoms disappear and don't return for months or years, people do not realize there *could* be the potentially serious problem of MS. The brain abnormalities of MS are more widespread than once thought, causing problems like memory loss and difficulty with concentration, focus, and attention—all of which may also be mistaken for other disorders.

MS involves important gender-related issues. Pregnancy has a short-term, favorable effect on MS, followed typically by a serious relapse in the immediate postpartum period for 65 to 70 percent of women, as hormone levels fall sharply after delivery. This observation suggests that ovarian hormone loss plays a role in the relapse. There is a much higher incidence of cognitive impairment in menopausal women with MS compared to men of the same age with the disease, an observation that points to estradiol and possibly testosterone having a stabilizing effect. Since estradiol is well documented to improve memory and other brain functions, current research suggests that hormone therapy for menopausal women with MS can help reduce cognitive loss.

There are important links between the endocrine, nervous, and immune systems that are played out in both the onset and progression of MS. MS patterns during pregnancy have led to important clues for some causes as well as possible therapeutic approaches. Some studies show that higher estrogen levels protect against some of the progression of central nervous system damage. Other data suggests that times of low estradiol and progesterone during bleeding days of the menstrual cycle, and during menopause, are times women are more likely to have MS flares, with 25 to 30 percent of women experiencing more intense MS symptoms at these times. Breast-feeding, which also suppresses estradiol production, also seems to affect the progression and severity of symptoms of MS.

Osteoporosis is another medical issue for women with MS. There are several reasons for risk of bone loss to increase: from corticosteroids used to treat MS; from decreased physical exercise resulting from fatigue and loss of muscle strength; reduced heat tolerance keeps many MS sufferers from getting sun, which in turn means a possible vitamin D deficiency. Women with MS are not screened with DEXA tests for bone density, nor are they offered treatments with bone-building medications. One survey conducted at Mt. Sinai in New York found that 80 to 85 percent of women with MS were not tested for bone density, whether they were menopausal or not. In the same survey, only 1 percent of the women with MS took medications like Fosamax or Actonel to preserve bone. I find it tragic that there is such widespread failure to diagnose and treat bone loss.

In all areas of MS management, there are issues unique to women. Women often have a harder time getting a correct early diagnosis, in part related to many studies that doctors have a stereotypical view of women as hypochondriacs and think women have more stress-related problems or are "just" depressed. This deeply ensconced physician attitude leads to a greater possibility of the diagnosis of MS in women being missed in its early stages. Once MS is diagnosed, medications for management of symptoms and to modify the course of the disease have potentially more adverse effects for women than men. Hormone therapy, when used, can have different effects and benefits depending on what forms are used. The approaches for women with MS need to take into account types and routes of hormones most likely to avoid side effects that could aggravate symptoms of the disease. There are many challenges for MS sufferers, and our health care system needs to make significant improvement in the approaches tailored for women's unique needs.

Hormonal Decline: An Unrecognized Cause of Fatigue

Chronic Fatigue Syndrome (CFS), a more severe degree of fatigue, has many causes and contributing factors. Ovarian hormone levels play an important, overlooked role, even if this is not the only factor involved. Milder forms of fatigue and loss of vitality, or "zest," are even more dramatically affected by decreases in ovarian hormones. Fatigue that makes it hard to get through the day is described by 70 to 80 percent of women experiencing such hormone changes, whether they are adolescents with Polycystic Ovary Syndrome, postpartum women with low ovarian hormones from suppression by nursing, women infertile from premature loss of ovarian hormones, or perimenopausal and menopausal women with naturally declining ovary hormone levels. Thyroid hormone dysfunction is another common hormonal cause of fatigue and loss of vitality. All of these issues need careful evaluation.

Estradiol and testosterone have significant activating or stimulating effects on energy levels. Losing optimal levels of these key metabolic hormones makes you tired, lethargic, and sluggish even if you don't have full-blown CFS. Sleep disruption comes with low estradiol and is another connection between ovarian hormones and persistent fatigue. These sleep changes can begin eight to ten years *before* you stop menstruating. Sleep deprivation robs you of normal daytime energy, contributing to persistent fatigue, and also causes suppression of the immune system, which makes you more susceptible to infections and allergies that make you tired. In addition, a wide variety of endocrine disruptor compounds can further interfere with the normal function of your ovarian and thyroid hormones, leading to fatigue and low energy (see Chapter 5).

Most physicians check the adrenal and basic thyroid hormones in people with CFS, but they do not check women's ovarian hormone levels. Yet 60 to 70 percent of patients with CFS are women. That statistic alone should make every-one think it crucial to investigate changes in the ovarian hormones as a factor in this enormous female preponderance in the incidence of this disorder. In all of the medical articles I have read on CFS, *I have not seen one that adequately addresses this issue.*

In one study that shows 60 percent of CFS patients being female, the average age of onset is 41.9 years. This is the same time frame that ovarian decline com-monly begins. Another study found that 90 percent of patients with fibromyalgia were female, with an average age of 44.0 years, again the perimenopausal stage. Nothing was mentioned about hormones in either study. The amazing thing is that there were two female physician investigators in one of these studies. Yet not one comment about checking women's hormones in future research was made. Doctors treating women seem to ignore the basic scientific advances in under-standing the many metabolic effects of the ovarian hormones on every organ system in the body. Everywhere in medicine, clinicians have blinders on when it comes to incorporating an awareness of the key hormones that make a woman's body different from a man's.

Many physicians are skeptical that CFS is a "real" disorder, and the condition is controversial. Researchers have been unable to identify a cause, predict a course, or find effective treatments. CFS appears to be one of a cluster of neuroendocrine disorders that includes Fibromyalgia (FMS) and Multiple Chemical Sensitivities (MCS). Although there are many theories about causal factors in these condi-tions, there is no *one* cause clearly demonstrated in the research to date.

One theory has been that viral infections like Epstein Barr, cytomeglovirus, herpes, and others can lead to a viral infiltration of the thyroid gland (thyroiditis), ovary (oophoritis), or adrenal gland (adrenalitis) creating a subsequent decline in the optimal functioning of these hormone-producing organs. Viral-induced loss of endocrine gland function can lead to subtle forms of hypothyroidism or adrenal decline causing fatigue, and subtle forms of ovarian decline that cause infertility and fatigue syndromes. These types of viral syndromes (thyroiditis, oophoritis, adrenalitis) are commonly overlooked in most medical settings, especially for women. Viral illnesses are known to trigger later development of autoimmune disorders affecting many endocrine organs, another potential link between a viral illness and subsequent appearance of CFS, FMS, or MCS. The viral theory offers one possible connection that could explain the marked female preponderance of cases.

Other stressors to the body's immune system are implicated in CFS. Persis-tent low-grade infections such as mycoplasma (a cause of "walking pneumonia") can lead to CFS symptoms but are hard to detect unless a clinician specifically tests for mycoplasma. Environmental pollutants (such as "sick building syn-drome"), toxic chemicals ("Gulf War" syndrome, insecticide toxicity, DES expo-sure in utero), and even low-grade toxic effects from chronic use of common household chemicals can lead to immune suppression causing symptoms of

CFS. Some of these chemicals also damage endocrine tissues like the thyroid gland, ovaries in women, and testicles in men, causing disruption in hormone production. Prolonged stressful situations also suppress the ovaries, and can lead to the neuroendocrine changes associated with CFS, FMS, and MCS. Illnesses like depression and generalized anxiety stress the immune system and play a role in CFS. We also know that declines in both thyroid and ovarian hormones can affect the onset of these mood symptoms. Proper testing can identify many of these potential overlooked causes for fatigue and immune changes.

Louise was thirty-seven when she developed a severe, persistent fatigue in the postpartum phase. "I've had a horrible struggle with total exhaustion and hormonal problems since the birth of my daughter eight years ago," she said. "I had preeclampsia [toxemia of pregnancy] and then a severe hemorrhage after the placenta came out. I was healthy before all that. Now I am totally exhausted all the time. My doctors told me I had chronic fatigue, but they said there wasn't anything to do about it. I live in a constant brain fog, my memory is terrible. I don't sleep well, and I don't have the energy to exercise. I am still having periods, so my doctor said it couldn't be hormonal. I can feel the ovulation twinge most of the time, but my periods have changed in that they aren't as long and the cycles changed from short to long. I just know it is connected to my hormones somehow."

Her blood pressure was very good at 110/68, so I did not think hypotension is a cause of her fatigue. She was not overweight, her cholesterol profile was very good, and her thyroid tests, including antibodies, were all negative for evidence of thyroid disease. Her eight A.M. cortisol was slightly higher than desirable at 25 as a "stress" response, so she certainly didn't have "adrenal insufficiency." Her serum ferritin, a measure of iron stores, was lower than optimal, but not so low that it was a major factor in her fatigue.

While her adrenal and thyroid hormones were checked numerous times, none of her physicians ever checked her ovarian hormone levels. A pharmacist checked saliva levels of her hormones and told her she was "estrogen-dominant and deficient in progesterone." She was given a progesterone skin cream to use twice a day, but had to stop this because it made her fatigue markedly worse. This wasn't surprising, in light of the progesterone effects on the brain that I described earlier. When I checked the more reliable serum hormone levels, the primary cause of her fatigue became clear. Her estradiol on Day 1 was significantly low at 27 pg/ml, and her Day 20 estradiol was low at 61 pg/ml (it should be 200–250 pg/ml or so). Like many younger women with this pattern of low estradiol, she still had a healthy luteal phase ovulatory rise in progesterone (15.2). Her N-telopeptide level was too high at 65, indicating rapid bone breakdown, even though she was only thirty-seven. This further confirmed that her estradiol level was lower than optimal. No wonder she was so tired. She didn't have enough estradiol to provide the metabolic fuel for her muscles, brain, and body. After eight years of struggling, she finally had some test results that made sense in understanding her symptoms.

Her ovarian hormone production had not "bounced back" following pregnancy and the postpartum hemorrhage. She was not clinically depressed. The continued loss of these vital hormones had caused her fatigue and other neuroendocrine symptoms. I took a fairly simple approach and suggested a steady dose of estrogen-dominant birth control pills using Orthocyclen. At each of her three-month follow-up appointments, she described feeling more and more like her old self. At her one-year appointment, her fatigue symptoms had completely resolved, along with the brain fog. Once we had reliable hormone levels to clarify the cause of her problems, it became a straightforward approach to helping her get better.

Margie was twenty years old when I first saw her, and she was struggling with severe fatigue, confused and fuzzy thinking, mood swings, night sweats, and PMS since age seventeen. She was a professional ballet dancer and having difficulty with her training schedule because of her profound fatigue. "I am too young to feel so old!" She didn't eat well, restricting calories to keep her weight down, causing loss of her regular menstrual periods. Her ovarian hormone levels showed disturbing results: an estradiol less than 10 pg/ml on Day 2 and only 60 pg/ml on Day 20, a testosterone level of 10 ng/dl—all far too low for optimal energy, normal muscle growth and repair, and bone preservation. It was clear why her dancing suffered. Her low bone density was consistent with the hormone findings. By putting her on the Ovcon birth control pill and improving the quality of her nutrition, she had better hormone and food fuel. Her energy returned, her PMS was controlled, her mood stabilized, and her bone density is building appropriately again for a young woman her age. She no longer needs the antidepressants that a previous physician prescribed, which actually made her fatigue worse.

At forty-six, *Annette* had been having restless sleep, low sex drive, marked fatigue, premenstrual sweet cravings, and depressed mood for the last five years. The fatigue and insomnia had gotten so bad she had difficulty working full-time. Her doctor had started her on Mircette, a low estrogen–high progestin contraceptive pill, to help regulate her periods. Her fatigue, mood, and sleep problems got worse the longer she was on it, although it did help reduce her cramps and heavy periods. Then she saw her family physician who started her on Zoloft for the depressed mood, but this made her even more tired during the day, so she stopped this and the Mircette. She consulted an alternative practitioner who told her she had "adrenal exhaustion" and recommended adrenal hormones, even though her eight A.M. serum cortisol was high, not low.

Annette's comprehensive hormone evaluation revealed several reasons for her problems: extremely low estradiol, low testosterone, and elevated thyroid antibodies that suggested the beginning of Hashimoto's thyroiditis. Her low bone density and high NTx indicated she likely had had low estradiol for a while. I suggested Yasmin, a pill with a better ratio of estrogen and progestin that would help keep the cramps and heavy bleeding under control but not cause the unwanted side effects she had with Mircette. I also suggested she start a low dose of thyroid hormone to slow down the progression of her thyroiditis. Six months later, Annette was jubilant: "I have my energy back, that awful fatigue is gone, and I am able to work full-time."

The full syndrome of CFS requires severe, persistent fatigue plus four of the following eight symptoms: myalgia (muscle pain), arthralgia, sore throat, headache, sleep disruption, malaise following exercise, tender neck, and cognitive difficulty (memory, concentration, focus difficulties). However we define the disorder of CFS, many of these same symptoms are a result of declining ovary or thyroid hormones. Decline in women's ovarian hormones may not explain all cases of CFS, or why CFS occurs in males, but if some 70 percent of the patients with CFS are women, it makes sense to check ovarian hormones. I think we should also check the major hormone levels in men with CFS, although I have not seen a formal study of that connection. The male patients I have evaluated for CFS had low testosterone and/or DHEA, so I think women, and men, must look into these possible hormonal factors in CFS.

In Summary

Hormones and brain. Brain and body. They are inextricably linked. If you have "brain" symptoms, you need a careful evaluation of the endocrine, nutritional, and metabolic factors that can cause such symptoms before you allow health professionals to write off your problems as "stress" or a "psychiatric" disorder. Antidepressants are fine if biological depression is truly what you have. But if hormone loss, such as estradiol, is causing your mood changes, fatigue, memory loss, and insomnia, then antidepressants won't be the answer. So take into account the connections described here. Have your hormones checked before you simply pop a Prozac or Paxil pill.

The Perils of PCOS, Obesity, Syndrome X, and Diabetes

Introduction

In spite of an obvious epidemic of obesity evident all around, most doctors still do not take an aggressive approach to diagnosis and treatment of PCOS, Syndrome X, or diabetes, particularly in young women. This chapter explores the many ways these serious metabolic syndromes lead to obesity and rob you of your health. Reduce your risks while you are young, *before* diabetes develops. Not just because PCOS, Syndrome X, and diabetes affect your fertility. Not just because they cause short-term concerns like acne, excess facial hair, and excess weight. PCOS, Syndrome X, and diabetes are deadly diseases. All three cause heart attacks and premature death in women in their thirties and forties. They increase risk of serious depression. They increase risk of uterine cancer. They increase risk of early breast cancer. They increase risk of early stroke.

You may say to yourself, "I'll skip this. . . . I'm too young to worry about diabetes!" Well don't. What was once called *adult-onset diabetes* has become a serious health crisis in *children* in the United States. I see more and more obese adolescent girls who are already diabetic. Women in their twenties, eager to start a family, find out the hard way that obesity can cause infertility, just as extreme thinness does. In some of these girls, PCOS is also damaging their ovaries and hormones much earlier than anyone realizes. PCOS is clearly on the rise in this country, in large part for the very endocrine-disrupting reasons discussed throughout this book. I am shocked at the number of calls from mothers of girls as young as nine and ten, asking for hormone evaluations because of ominous body changes, even before their menses start. I am convinced the rise in PCOS, diabetes, and obesity represent an overlooked part of endocrine system damage caused by environmental pollutants and chemical additives in foods that affect us from the womb onward.

Polycystic Ovary Syndrome (PCOS): Hormonal Havoc That Devastates Health

Polycystic ovary syndrome (PCOS) has begun to get attention in women's magazines and physician's offices. In the past, it was viewed as "an infertility problem," meaning it is only an issue if you're trying to get pregnant. That label is woefully inadequate: PCOS is far more dangerous, and potentially deadly. And it is on the increase in young women today.

PCOS was first described in 1935 and called *Stein-Leventhal syndrome,* named for the doctors who first described the characteristic body changes and tiny cysts covering the ovaries. At that time, doctors thought it was a disorder that just affected the ovaries, causing excess body hair, irregular menses, infrequent ovulation, and follicles that don't develop but become multiple cysts. The name polycystic ovary syndrome, however, is seriously misleading. It is really a complex, multisystem endocrine disorder. In fact, PCOS is *the most common* endocrine disorder affecting young women in their childbearing years, affecting more than 6 percent of premenopausal women, including teenagers and prepubescent girls. Six percent of women may not sound like much. But stop for a moment: 6 percent means *millions* of women, or about one in every seventeen suffering from this serious endocrine disorder. And that statistic doesn't include prepubescent girls who have budding PCOS, not yet diagnosed.

The hormonal imbalance of PCOS leads to a *metabolic syndrome* with widespread effects that can wreak havoc throughout the brain and body. PCOS dramatically increases your risk of many serious health problems, beginning in your early teens. By age thirty, 50 percent of women with PCOS have either impaired glucose tolerance, significant insulin resistance, or overt diabetes. Women with PCOS have an *eleven*-fold increased risk of cardiovascular disease that can appear as early as the twenties and thirties. Newer studies report that women from thirty-nine to forty-nine years old with PCOS have a heart attack risk that is *four times* that of women without PCOS in this age group. Women with PCOS also have a higher risk, at younger ages, of uterine and breast cancers.

We know today that the diverse complications of PCOS are caused primarily by several critical hormone imbalances: elevated levels of androgens, higher-than-normal free testosterone, a high estrone-to-estradiol ratio, insulin resistance with elevated insulin levels, and abnormal cholesterol and triglyceride levels. The combination of elevated androgens and elevated insulin causes rapid waistline weight gain. The fatter you get, the more insulin resistant you become, and the more abnormal your hormone ratio becomes, the more fat you gain. This terrible vicious cycle puts young women with PCOS at an especially high risk for diabetes, which in turn causes damaging changes in the heart and the blood vessels throughout the body and increases the risk of premature heart attack or stroke. The excess insulin also increases risk of breast cancer later.

What Are the Symptoms of PCOS?

The most obvious ones are your body changes:

Marked weight gain. The pattern of weight gain holds clues about the presence of PCOS.

The weight gain is usually *rapid,* often without change in food intake. Many of my patients say it comes from nowhere and feels like the cookie monster running amuck inside your body. The pounds pack on faster than they can shop for new clothes. They are puzzled and frightened. They diet, they exercise, but nothing seems to halt this inexorable girth growth.

The excess fat is typically deposited around the waist, upper body, shoulders, and arms rather than the hips and thighs. Women tell me they feel like a fireplug or a barrel. Breasts get larger, fat sticks like glue under and around the arms and upper chest. Waistline? It disappears. The hormone imbalance creates the damaging apple-shaped body. Weight gain from overeating is usually more symmetrical for women.

The weight gain of PCOS is commonly accompanied by acne and excess face and body hair. Weight gain from simply overeating and underexercising usually doesn't come with these other problems.

A sixteen-year-old woman I saw recently had severe hormonal imbalance typical of PCOS, with a very high level of free testosterone and low estradiol. She had gained fifty pounds over six months despite a healthy diet and exercise regimen. She had PCOS, but her gynecologist had not recognized it. He saw her as simply a teenager obsessed with weight gain and complaining of PMS. His advice was to "just eat less, and you'll lose weight."

It is not that simple. The metabolic abnormalities of PCOS make it almost impossible for a woman to lose weight by simply eating less. The endocrine imbalances must be treated first.

PCOS can also occur in *thin* women. It doesn't always cause weight *gain*. So just because you are thin doesn't mean you can't have PCOS.

Excess facial and body hair. Hair that is often dark and coarse grows on the chin, cheeks, upper lip, chest, around the nipples, on the stomach and inner thigh, back, and buttocks. This excess hair growth is called *hirsutism*. Hirsutism itself is not a disease; it is a *symptom* of an underlying hormonal imbalance. In PCOS, excess hair is often caused by excess androgens (testosterone, DHEA, androstenedione). There is also overactivity of an enzyme called *5-alpha reductase* that converts testosterone to a more potent form called *dihydrotestosterone* (DHT) in the hair follicle, causing increased male-type hair growth.

Thinning scalp hair or hair loss. The changes in hair texture, thickness, and pattern of loss in PCOS are related to the excess androgens and are similar to menopausal women with higher androgens relative to their estradiol. Hair is thinner overall with loss of hair on the top and around the forehead. The PCOS pattern is similar to male-pattern baldness, again related to excess androgens.

Severe acne. The acne in PCOS is typically far worse than just simple adolescent "zits" the week before your period. The acne can be large, painful, inflamed cysts that look and feel like boils. In PCOS, the acne doesn't always confine itself to your face; you can have cystic acne outbreaks on your chest, back, arms, and legs. One young woman had become severely disfigured from the cystic acne, but had never been checked for possible PCOS despite the telltale signs. It took six months of aggressive hormonal management, but her acne resolved.

Irregular menstrual cycles. Sometimes women with PCOS go months without a period, other times periods are fairly regular. Some PCOS sufferers have very heavy bleeding; others have periods that are barely there. Some women may ovulate, others don't. The key point is that the menstrual cycle can be affected in many different ways.

Difficulty getting pregnant, or frequent miscarriages. The excess levels of male hormones combined with excess body fat lead to increased conversion of androstenedione, an androgen found in high concentration in body fat, to the estrone form of estrogen. Excess production of estrone feeds back to the brain and alters the pituitary secretion of FSH and LH, which in turn means the menstrual cycle progression gets disrupted. Ovulation is less likely. If there is no ovulation, progesterone isn't produced. High prolactin, found in about 60 percent of women with PCOS, also suppresses the normal menstrual cycle hormone production. There are several factors that combine to increase the problem of infertility: decreased ovulation, lower levels of both estradiol and progesterone, high levels of estrone and prolactin, excess androgens, and excess insulin and cortisol, to name a few. Miscarriages are more likely because the estradiol and progesterone levels are lower than needed to sustain early pregnancy before the placenta takes over making hormones.

The invisible changes *inside* the body, however, are even more ominous. These rob you of energy, fertility, mood stability, and health:

- *High androgen (male hormone) levels (testosterone, both free and total; DHEA-S; DHEA; androstenedione). This is the most consistent hormone abnormality in PCOS, seen in 70 to 80 percent or more.*
- *High estrone (E1) to estradiol (E2) ratio, also a consistent finding in the majority of PCOS sufferers, the same cause of many of the same symptoms of low estradiol seen in perimenopause.*
- *High LH to FSH ratio (the reverse of normal)—not always present*
- *Lower than normal SHBG, which means more male hormones are "free" and therefore more active, causing more of the external changes listed above*
- *Glucose intolerance, leading to "blood sugar swings" that affect memory, concentration, mood, sleep patterns, and weight gain*
- *Insulin resistance, usually with excess insulin production that makes you get fatter and fatter, even if you are eating less and exercising more*
- *High LDL ("bad") cholesterol and triglycerides with low HDL ("good") cholesterol*
- *Elevated prolactin, with or without nipple discharge* (galactorrhea)
- *High blood pressure*
- *Recurrent ovarian cysts; classic ultrasound findings are cysts around the ovary that appear like a "string of pearls." Not every woman with PCOS has cysts visible on ultrasound. The cysts can come and go,*

eluding the ultrasound. Or the cysts may be so tiny they aren't visible and are only found during laparoscopic surgery that is often done for other reasons.

PCOS is a master of disguise. Not all women with this disorder have all the symptoms or lab abnormalities. Some women with PCOS are quite thin. Not all will have irregular menstrual periods or difficulty getting pregnant. The variability in how the syndrome presents itself makes it difficult to create a specific criteria for diagnosis. This is different from, say, diabetes for which we have clear national standards for glucose levels that alert doctors to diabetes or the milder glucose intolerance. In a number of studies, women with abnormal ovaries on ultrasound overlapped with those who had abnormal hormone levels. Whether cysts are present on ultrasound does not, however, have much predictive value in determining who has the abnormal hormone levels characteristic of PCOS.

PCOS is both an elevated estrogen and an elevated androgen syndrome, but don't be misled. The terms *elevated estrogen, excess estrogen, estrogen dominance,* and *hyperestrogenic and hyperandrogenic* that some writers use about PCOS refer to the elevated estrone "estrogen" as a result of excess body fat. But it is estradiol, our most important and active form of estrogen, that is actually lower than expected in women with PCOS. My PCOS patients have a much lower than desirable estradiol level and have symptoms of estradiol decline, even with higher estrone levels. My research found only one report of polycystic ovarian disease with significantly elevated estradiol levels. In this case the plasma estradiol was so massively elevated, it suggested the presence of an estrogen-producing tumor, which is extremely rare.

The bottom line is that all estrogens are not alike. Estradiol has a dramatically different effect in your body from estrone. A thorough diagnostic evaluation, including detailed hormone testing of all ovarian hormones, is important because these hidden changes in metabolism and abnormal hormone ratios set you up for an increased risk of diabetes mellitus and heart disease at a young age.

Why PCOS Is Often Missed

Tragically, many physicians see PCOS as a "cosmetic" problem when young women complain of excess face or body hair and weight gain. Many physicians do not realize that PCOS has far-reaching and potentially devastating consequences.

Another reason PCOS is overlooked is that gynecologists have traditionally been taught that a hallmark of PCOS is a lack of menstruation (called *amenorrhea*). Therefore, if a woman is still having periods, "she could not have PCOS." We now know this is not correct. Many women with PCOS still have periods, they are just irregular and don't produce optimal levels or the normal balance of ovarian hormones. In addition, infertility is the most common reason women with undiagnosed PCOS see a physician. These women may go to a reproductive endocrinologist. But what if you are not trying to become pregnant? Especially if you still have menstrual periods, you are likely to be overlooked in our current, fragmented approach to women's health, even though you may have all the other metabolic changes of PCOS.

Another difficulty is that traditionally, endocrinologists in this country haven't focused on the ovary, since this endocrine organ is the "turf" of gynecologists. This "split" of a woman's endocrine system meant different doctors address different body parts, which obviously makes it hard for a woman with PCOS to get properly diagnosed. In the United States, endocrinologists focus on other endocrine disorders like thyroid and diabetes management. They rarely check ovarian hormones, especially estrogen levels. Gynecologists, on the other hand, are trained as surgeons, and don't routinely check hormone levels. They do not worry about women they perceive as having "just a cosmetic problem" of waistline weight gain and excess facial hair. The surgical training of gynecologists focuses on pregnancy and birth, on surgical approaches to correct gynecological problems like fibroids, endometriosis, and cancers. The problems caused by PCOS just haven't seemed as important in a busy obstetrical-surgical practice. PCOS also causes severe mood problems, typically evaluated and treated by psychiatrists. But in this country, psychiatrists are not taught much about the brain effects of ovarian hormones, and rarely check any hormone levels, much less the ovarian ones. The brain symptoms resulting from PCOS *hormone* imbalances are missed. Even worse, some of the "mood-stabilizer" medicines commonly used aggravate the hormone imbalances of PCOS.

So, what happens when all these specialty groups overlook the underlying metabolic changes in PCOS? Women with this very serious disorder are often discounted and simply told to "not worry, everybody misses periods sometimes," or "just go exercise and lose weight and your periods will come back. You'll be fine," or "just take this antidepressant or mood stabilizer and you'll get better." This happened to a thirty-five-year-old woman who then went on to have three heart attacks by the time she was thirty-eight, and almost died with the third one before her serious hormone imbalances from PCOS were diagnosed.

I have another concern about PCOS: The very treatment of PCOS-induced infertility may itself cause more problems. International specialists in the field of climacteric (menopause) medicine have studies showing that drug treatments such as clomiphene citrate (Clomid) that stimulate ovulation, as well as laparoscopic ovarian treatments to remove cysts, can cause premature menopause and a higher risk of ovarian cancer later. Women with PCOS have a double whammy: They often need specialized treatment to get pregnant, and some of those treatments can lead to serious problems later.

CAUSES OF PCOS

No one is certain what causes PCOS, but there are many proposed explanations, and we will likely find multiple causes that produce the same
metabolic syndrome and disruption of normal hormone production.

- Genetic factors
- Environmental factors, such as exposure to pesticides and other
  endocrine-disrupting chemicals
- Autoimmune disorders—ovarian, adrenal, pancreatic, and thyroid
- Excess insulin production related to obesity-induced insulin resistance
- Excess intake of substances such as excitatory amino acids
- Medications that increase prolactin

© Elizabeth Lee Vliet, M.D., 2003

Do I Have PCOS? Getting Tested

Doctors who specialize in researching and treating PCOS are the first to
tell you there is "no consensus" about tests and criteria to confirm the diagnosis.
But even if doctors can't agree on "diagnostic criteria," for the full-blown disorder, even having *some* of the abnormal findings can still wreak havoc on your
hormone balance and health. Even mild forms of PCOS can cause a lot of damage. Treatments that improve symptoms and help you feel better are similar,
regardless of whether you have all or some of the findings. I think sometimes in
medicine we get so hung up on "proof" of a diagnosis that we forget to focus on
the patient and what we can do to help alleviate her suffering no matter what
name it is given.

Taking a Look at Some Illustrative Results

Characteristic abnormal hormone levels in PCOS are illustrated by a sample
of results from the sixteen-year-old woman I mentioned earlier. Her doctor told
her to "just eat less and you'll lose weight." These are her hormone lab values,
with comments:

- *Total testosterone is 81 ng/dl. Optimal for women is the 40–60 ng/dl
  range, but some women start excess hair growth at levels over 50,
  especially if DHEA is also too high.*
- *Free testosterone is 20 ng/dl. Optimal is 4 to 6 if her total testosterone
  was in the desirable range.*
- *Free plus weakly bound testosterone is 37. Optimal is 10–15 if total
  testosterone is in the desirable range.*
- *DHEA 1093. Optimal is 300–500.*
- *Estradiol 32 (Day 19). At this point in the menstrual cycle, estradiol*

LABORATORY STUDIES TO CHECK FOR PCOS

- FSH, LH ratio (abnormal if shifted toward LH)
- Estradiol and estrone
- Free and total testosterone
- DHEA and DHEA-S
- Androstenedione (normal is up to 250 ng/dl)
- SHBG
- Eight A.M. cortisol, and if elevated, a twenty-four-hour urinary free cortisol or other tests of free cortisol
- 17-OH progesterone (to identify congenital adrenal hyperplasia [CAH] or 21-hydroxylase deficiency)
- Prolactin
- IGF-1
- Fasting, two- and three-hour postprandial glucose and insulin, or a five-hour insulin response to glucose test
- Thyroid profile, including thyroid antibodies
- Comprehensive metabolic profile that includes tests of liver and kidney function, lipids (cholesterol, HDL, LDL, TG), complete blood counts, calcium, magnesium, iron, and ferritin

© Elizabeth Lee Vliet, M.D., 2003

should be 200–250 pg/ml. This is seriously low, especially in the face of such high levels of her androgens.

- *Eight A.M. cortisol is high at 25. Healthy ranges at that time of day would be 10–18.*
- *NTx (N-telopeptide, a marker of bone breakdown) at 131 is high, even for an adolescent, and this reflects her very low estradiol. Her TSH, free T3, free T4, and thyroid antibodies are all in the optimal range.*

When you see how her androgen/estradiol ratio is severely out of balance, it isn't hard to understand why she had severe cystic acne (face, chest, back, arms), marked facial and body hair, severe mood swings, irritability (excess testosterone can do that!), and severe insomnia. She didn't have a "female" hormone profile. I started her on Ovcon 35, and spironolactone initially, since the BCPs suppress the ovaries' abnormal hormone production and also increases the SHBG that "binds up" excess free androgens. I also recommended a diet of 35 percent complex carbs, 35 percent protein, and 30 percent fat, emphasizing more of the vegetable oils instead of saturated fats.

Three months later, her total testosterone dropped to 25 ng/dl, free and weakly bound testosterone was 11, with a free testosterone of 6. Her DHEA had come down to 400, and her eight A.M. cortisol was now normal at 15. Since she was on the birth control pill that suppresses estradiol, I did not recheck estradiol at her first follow-up. I primarily wanted her androgens down to the normal ranges. Her acne cleared up nicely, her excess facial hair growth decreased, and she described her mood as more stable. Her weight was no longer on the up escalator, and she felt her body responding more normally to exercise and diet.

Getting Help for PCOS: What Are Some Treatments?

I see a lot of women with PCOS and they are of all ages, from menopausal women with complications from unrecognized PCOS when younger, to young girls already developing body changes that indicate risk of later problems. It is often quite a challenge to find the right combination of hormonal and nonhormonal approaches to restore balance. Most treatments are a process of fine-tuning various therapeutic approaches. Sometimes this is accomplished in a few months; for other women it takes a year or more to find the right combination.

The appropriate treatment depends on many variables, including age, whether you are trying to get pregnant now or want to preserve fertility for the future, whether you have other medical or gynecological problems, whether you have insulin resistance or diabetes, and if you have serious mood disturbances. Since the subject of infertility is quite complex, this chapter does not provide a detailed look at infertility. The focus is on integrated treatment for general management of PCOS to restore hormone balance, reduce health risks, and improve how you feel. PCOS is a medical problem where *individualization* is critical. There are, however, some general principles of treatment. Here are some ideas to explore with your own physicians.

Medication Approaches

Oral contraceptives, or birth control pills (BCPs). BCPs are one of the foundations of treatment helping with several problems in PCOS. They suppress the abnormal cycling of the ovaries and help prevent cysts from forming. They improve the balance of estrogen and androgens by increasing SHBG, which then keeps more of the androgens in the bound, less-active form and decreases hirsutism and acne. They provide daily progestin that prevents excess thickening of the lining of the uterus from the body fat estrogen (estrone) stimulation. Over time, such thickening, called *hyperplasia,* can lead to an increased risk of uterine cancer. Taking birth control pills helps preserve future fertility by preventing ovulation or loss of follicles at a time when you are not trying to get pregnant. BCP also prevent multiple cysts from forming and damaging the ovaries further. I find that patients with PCOS do better using BCPs that have higher estrogen to progestin ratios, such as Ovcon 35, Modicon, Orthocyclen, Yasmin, or Diane 35. In my experience, high-progestin pills with less estrogen (Loestrin, Alesse, Mircette) cause more of the negative progestin effects (weight gain, low libido, hair loss, acne, lethargy, headaches, depressed mood, abnormal glucose/insulin, high cholesterol, and high triglycerides) that are already common problems with PCOS. BCPs with a steady dose formula every day ("monophasic" pills) typically have fewer adverse effects, especially on moods, than triphasic pills with varying hormone content.

Ovarian hormone replacement therapy. There is more about this later, but generally I find the *bioidentical* forms of ovarian hormones, such as 17-beta estradiol or progesterone, cause fewer side effects and give more positive responses on the abnormal measures of PCOS. Women with PCOS already have higher than normal androgens so they do not generally need either DHEA or testosterone as part of their therapy. In fact, women with undiagnosed PCOS who take DHEA will commonly have more acne, facial and body hair, scalp hair loss, irritability, insomnia, and weight gain.

Insulin-sensitizing medication. In the last decade, a number of studies and clinical reports show that medicines which lower insulin and improve insulin response are effective in PCOS, both to address the metabolic imbalances and also to restore ovulatory cycles and fertility. Glucophage (metformin) and the glitazones Actos and Avandia, medicines approved for the treatment of diabetes, are common. Although none has yet been approved by the FDA for PCOS, studies are under way and physicians report success using these medications in an integrated treatment program.

In a 1998 study published in the *New England Journal of Medicine,* 90 percent of the women who took metformin either ovulated spontaneously or with help from the fertility drug Clomid. Only 12 percent of the women taking a placebo pill had ovulatory cycles, even if they also took Clomid. More studies on the safety of these medications on a developing fetus are needed, and women trying to get pregnant should discuss taking metformin with a fertility specialist. There was an encouraging study published in March 2002 in *Fertility and Sterility.* Researchers found a tenfold reduction in risk of gestational diabetes in women with PCOS who took metformin throughout pregnancy. This is a remarkable reduction in risk.

I use metformin successfully for many PCOS patients, and have found that it works well to reduce insulin resistance (and its complications) and facilitate weight loss in women not trying to become pregnant. Weight loss decreases many risk factors for both diabetes and heart disease.

Androgen-blocking medications. Excess androgens cause a lot of unwanted effects in PCOS, so if this hormone imbalance doesn't respond to the medicines above, there are a number of other effective androgen blockers: spironolactone (50–200 mg daily), flutamide (125–500 mg daily), finasteride (5 mg daily), and cyproterone acetate (2–50 mg daily). Sometimes leuprolide, dexamethasone, or ketoconazole may be necessary, all of which suppress androgen production in the ovaries and adrenal glands. These medicines have potentially serious side effects, so I generally use them only if a woman hasn't responded to any other options. Since leuprolide (Lupron) suppresses estrogen, you need to take estrogen replacement to avoid menopausal symptoms.

Mood-managing medicines: anxiolytics, antidepressants, anticonvulsants. The hormone imbalances of PCOS have many mood-disrupting effects, and can even mimic bipolar disorder, panic disorder, or major depression. Excess testosterone can cause anxiety and agitation that is often mistaken for a psychiatric disorder, and low estradiol can contribute to significant depression. Look at all the brain effects of the ovarian hormones that I discussed earlier (see Chapter 12), and you quickly see how the hormone problems in PCOS can cause such serious mood symptoms. If you have significant mood symptoms and think you have PCOS, have your hormones checked and the PCOS treated before concluding that you have a psychiatric disorder and need "mood managing" medicines.

A word of caution about Depakote (valproic acid). This medicine is being used more and more often as a "mood stabilizer" in younger women. I do not recommend this medication for women with possible PCOS; there have been reports that it can actually cause PCOS in 40 to 50 percent of female patients treated with it, primarily via its effect to increase prolactin production. It is not clear at this time whether other anticonvulsants (Tegretol, Dilantin, Neurontin, Lamictal, Topamax, etc.) have similar effects. I also do not recommend tricyclic antidepressants (Elavil, Pamelor, etc.) or Remeron for women with PCOS who are struggling with weight gain. These medicines stimulate appetite and increase the likelihood of insulin resistance.

Non-Medication Approaches

The best success for getting PCOS under control and feeling your best is to incorporate a number of strategies: dietary balance, physical activity, stress management, vitamins and supplements. These, working in concert with medications, restore hormonal balance, reduce long-term health risks, and improve energy level and mood. Exercise improves insulin sensitivity and glucose control, so it is a critical component to reverse hormone imbalances. For women with PCOS, reducing foods that quickly turn to glucose (sweets, simple carbs like pastas and breads, etc.) will minimize the adverse effects of excess insulin and glucose intolerance.

I don't recommend herbs for hormone-related symptoms if you have PCOS. First, they aren't adequate to restore hormone balance. Second, many herbs act as phytoestrogens and can further impair the function of ovaries and thyroid. Statistics show that women with PCOS often take multiple prescription medications, and most herbs have the potential for significant *drug-herb interactions* with oral contraceptives, prescription hormone medications, antidepressants, antianxiety medications, anticonvulsants, antibiotics, and others. For example, Saint-John's-wort can decrease the effectiveness of birth control pills by 50 percent because of the herb's ability to increase metabolic breakdown of the hormones in the liver. If you have PCOS and smoke cigarettes, stop. PCOS alone can cause early heart attacks. If you add the damage from cigarette smoking, it is like adding gasoline to a fire.

Adequate sleep and stress management are also important PCOS treatments.

If insomnia persists, talk to your doctor about sleep studies. Sleep apnea increases in women with PCOS because of the decline in estradiol levels and the increased body weight, especially in the upper abdomen, that impairs respiration at night.

Psychological support is also crucial. I find patients with PCOS have intense feelings of anger about being ignored and not diagnosed, and feelings of grief if pregnancy is desired but unfulfilled. Support groups and individual therapy are helpful in providing constructive release for intense feelings. Keep in mind, we are more than just body, we are also mind and spirit. PCOS can affect all dimensions of our lives, and your physical and emotional needs are important and valid. You are a *person*, not just a pelvis with reproductive problems.

Women with PCOS who express concern about weight, body hair, mood changes, and the other physical-psychological effects of PCOS are often not taken seriously in the usual health care settings. You need physicians and health professionals who are competent, and also empathic and caring. If you don't feel support from your current health professionals, seek new ones! You have the power, and right, to choose health partnerships that are mutually beneficial and helpful.

The Poignancy of PCOS: Women's Stories

Antonia illustrates overmedication when PCOS isn't diagnosed and treated as the metabolic-endocrine disorder it is. When she first came in she was twenty-seven years old, severely obese, with painful acne. She was so self-conscious that she rarely looked up when talking. For several years, she had been ballooning up and frightened by a body out of control. Her acne was impossible to control no matter what she tried. She had other troubling symptoms for someone so young: hot flashes, insomnia, fibromyalgia-type muscle pain, anxiety that became worse with her periods, daily tension headaches, migraine episodes, severe fatigue, daytime sleepiness—especially after meals—inability to concentrate, and shortness of breath that made her fear a lung problem.

She consulted multiple specialists, and when I saw her, she was being treated by a primary care physician, a neurologist for the migraines, a pain specialist for the daily headaches, a rheumatologist for the muscle pain, a psychiatrist for the anxiety, and she was scheduled to see a pulmonary specialist to check for asthma. Her gynecologist told her that her pelvic and Pap smears were normal, and she didn't have a hormone imbalance. She just needed to lose weight. No hormone levels were checked by the other physicians. When I checked the levels, the results were staggering. Her estradiol was markedly low; all of the androgens were seriously elevated, especially the free testosterone; her cortisol was elevated (another factor adding to her weight gain); her fasting and two-hour insulin and glucose levels were both elevated; and she had a high LH to FSH ratio. In short, she had all the classic indicators of PCOS. I felt sad that no one, out of all those doctors, had ever considered or checked her ovarian hormone levels, especially since her body shape and symptoms were such strong warning signals of PCOS.

By the time of her appointment with me, Antonia was taking *thirteen* medicines every day: a sleeping pill, two muscle relaxants, several pain meds, two mood stabilizers, Prozac and a tricyclic antidepressant, two antianxiety medicines, and a beta-blocker. Her medication costs were astronomical, but even more frightening, many of the medicines were making her weight gain and hormone imbalances *worse*. Tricyclics, with long-term use of SSRIs, can increase appetite, especially for carbs, which then increases insulin resistance. Beta-blockers made the insulin resistance worse as well, and can contribute to shortness of breath from effects on both lungs and heart. Beta-blockers also interfere with normal thyroid function, contributing to weight gain, low energy, and depressed mood. The Klonopin for anxiety and insomnia made her tired and sleepy during the day. It was a medication nightmare. She was trapped in the hormonal quicksand of PCOS and the quagmire of medication side effects that pulled her further into the PCOS hormone imbalances. Turning this around would be a long struggle, because it could take a year or more to improve the hormonal balance and gradually taper off the medications. Sadly, I only saw her a few times and never got to help her turn it around, because she was told by so many other professionals that her problems were not hormonal and that I was wrong.

My view has always been that ultimately it doesn't really matter who is "right" and who is "wrong" with a diagnostic label. Diagnoses are imperfect. What matters is whether the medicines make someone better or whether they aggravate underlying problems and make people worse. In Antonia's case, she *wasn't* getting better on all those medicines, and each had adverse effects that are well-documented in the medical literature. Her headaches weren't controlled, she still had trouble sleeping, and she was still gaining weight and suffering from acne and excess facial hair.

When I first saw *Georgia,* her hormone evaluation showed abnormal levels characteristic of PCOS. We worked with her over a number of months to restore a healthier hormone balance. But there is a part of her story before I saw her that gives me goose bumps every time I think about it. If you think people are silly to believe in God and guardian angels, her experience may convince you otherwise.

Her first heart attack was at age thirty-six. She was thirty-nine when I saw her and had already suffered *three* serious heart attacks and almost died during the third one. In fact, the cardiologist had told her husband she would not likely come out of the coma because her heart simply wasn't pumping enough blood, she wasn't responding to medications, and there was nothing else to try. What happened next was quite touching, and very meaningful to me. Two of Jodie's friends, one a patient of mine, took a copy of my previous book, which described the effects of estradiol on the heart, to Jodie's husband at the hospital where she was in ICU, in a coma. The doctors had told Jodie's family that it was "only a matter of time" before she died.

But Jodie and her friends had discussed something that no one thought important: Jodie's heart attacks always happened at the start of her menstrual period, a time when estradiol drops sharply, which can cause spasm and reduced blood flow in the coronary arteries to the heart. The two women showed the page in *Screaming to Be Heard* to Jodie's husband. He immediately said, "She always thought her heart attacks had something to do with her hormones, and asked many doctors about it, but they always told her it couldn't be. This is amazing." Right away, they went to the cardiologist and showed him the page describing estradiol's effect on the arteries and improved blood flow. They asked if he was willing to put an estradiol patch on Jodie. The cardiologist read the material and said, "Nothing else is working, we have nothing to lose. We may as well try it. It certainly won't hurt her."

To everyone's surprise, and relief, including the doctor's, Jodie's condition improved. Her "ejection fraction" (a measure of the blood being pumped by the heart) was at critically low values and wasn't coming up on the other medicines. Within a few hours after the Climara estradiol patch was put on, the ejection fraction began increasing significantly. Slowly she came out of the coma as her heart function improved. Her doctor continued the estradiol patch during the rest of her hospitalization, amazed at the changes. She was finally discharged, though she still had a long recovery from the damage to her heart.

She wrote her story to bring to her first consult with me. I was amazed at the progress after her near-death experience. I reviewed her serum hormone levels and showed her *why* the estradiol patch had helped so much. Her own menstrual Day 1 estradiol was barely detectable, and her free and total testosterone and DHEA were all quite high, as were her total and LDL cholesterol, triglycerides, and insulin. Low estradiol leads to coronary vasospasm that can seriously decrease blood flow to the heart muscle. The low estradiol, coupled with high androgens, high cholesterol with a high LDL and low HDL, and her high insulin had set her up for heart attacks. I explained that our goal was to keep her estradiol as steady as possible using an estradiol patch during bleeding days, and then decrease the androgens, improve her cholesterol profile, and decrease the excess insulin.

Four years later, she is doing well on her hormone and dietary plan that corrects these hormone imbalances. She is a more active mom, involved with her children and her life again. Through changes in her diet and a regular walking program, she has gradually lost the weight caused by PCOS. She is an avid spokesperson in Internet support groups for PCOS and said, "I want to help other women understand PCOS and get proper evaluation before someone else goes through what I did."

Body Fat Promoters: Glucose Intolerance/Hypoglycemia, Insulin Resistance, and Diabetes

If you have sudden, inexplicable weight gain or "creeping corpulence," feel so tired and draggy you can't get through the day, are overcome by sleep attacks after lunch, or have wicked mood swings, you may have one of the metabolic problems that often accompany ovarian hormone imbalances. *Syndrome X* is the name most often given to this cluster of insulin-glucose imbalances that occur in women with greater frequency as their estradiol declines. Syndrome X, also called Dysmetabolic Syndrome X, is a metabolic-endocrine syndrome with many similarities to PCOS, and may actually share some of the root causes. It's one of those "mysterious" women's disorders and today appears in younger and younger women, including prepubescent girls. Syndrome X–type findings in young girls is another ominous sign of environmental and dietary endocrine disruptors that are now more and more a problem for infants and children. These chemicals that I talked about earlier serve to set the stage for abnormal weight gain in childhood and then at puberty for girls, an increased production of androgens that make the metabolic effects even worse. What are these conditions, and what can you do about them? Let's explore these questions.

How Glucose Is Regulated: The Seesaw of Insulin and Glucagon

Glucose and oxygen are such critical fuels for the brain's survival that the body keeps tight control on levels. Since glucose changes have severe consequences, the body has ways to keep glucose from "swinging" to dangerous extremes, high or low. Insulin and glucagon are the two major regulators of the glucose in your bloodstream at any given time. They act in opposite ways, much like a seesaw, so they are called the *counterregulatory hormones*. When these two hormones work normally, insulin keeps blood glucose levels from rising too high, and glucagon prevents blood glucose from dropping too low. Insulin serves to lower glucose levels by moving it from the blood into muscle cells, where it burns to provide immediate energy, or by moving it into fat cells, where it is stored as fat for future energy needs. Glucagon has the opposite effect: It stimulates the liver and muscle cells to break down stored glycogen and send the glucose molecules rushing out of the cell into the bloodstream to raise blood sugar when levels drop too low. In addition to actual high or low blood glucose levels, the rate of rise and fall in glucose is a crucial factor that can also lead to the symptoms, and trigger insulin and glucagon release.

As we get fatter, however, insulin and glucagon don't work as well, so our body has difficulty keeping blood sugar in the healthy range. That's when we develop problems like hypoglycemia (low blood sugar), glucose intolerance (rapid rises and abrupt falls), insulin resistance (excess insulin and decreased sensitivity to insulin), and diabetes mellitus (sustained high blood glucose). Let's explore each, and how they relate to weight gain, middle spread, mood swings, and flagging energy for girls and women of any age.

Think of each of these "conditions" as being a series of steps along a path from being normal to becoming diabetic.

Hypoglycemia and Glucose Intolerance

Hypoglycemia, or "low blood sugar," usually goes hand in hand with something called *glucose intolerance,* the body's difficulty in handling glucose and other sugars normally. Both are common in early phase diabetes. Hypoglycemia is officially defined as a blood glucose level below 50 mg/dl, but you can have symptoms of hypoglycemia at higher levels if glucose falls rapidly. In fact, the *rate* of fall is more important in triggering symptoms than the actual blood level. It's similar to a smoke detector that doesn't distinguish between the serious smoke of a fire and the expected smoke of cooking. It sends out an alarm for both. If the steak on the stove sends up smoke faster, it will set off the alarm before a smoldering couch fire does.

Since glucose is so critical for brain cell survival, our brain has sensors that warn us at the slightest dip in adequate glucose supplies, whether from a rapidly *falling* glucose or an actual *low* level. This is why diabetics sometimes check blood sugar. They have likely experienced a high glucose level that falls and sets off the brain alarm, even though the actual level is still above normal. This is also the same way you experience symptoms of hypoglycemia only a short while after eating. Too much insulin, triggered by too much refined carbohydrate food, causes glucose levels to fall too fast, even though glucose may not drop below 50, the magic number for a hypoglycemia "diagnosis." Your brain and body haven't read textbook definitions, they just know what they need!

Sometimes it is hard to realize that the same trigger—rapidly falling glucose levels—can cause food cravings and anxious, panicky feelings. Many physicians don't realize that a rapidly falling glucose level can trigger a hypoglycemic fight-or-flight reaction, even though the glucose level doesn't drop below 50. So, in case you've been told you don't have these problems because your glucose is "normal," that's not necessarily the case. This problem is common in glucose intolerance and insulin resistance. Glucose intolerance simply means you have a tendency to "swing" between higher than desirable blood sugar levels after you eat, followed by rapidly falling or lower than desirable levels two to four hours later. It is an early warning of problems regulating glucose, and you could be on the way to developing diabetes. This situation should be a clue that you need to have glucose-insulin levels checked along with other hormones.

Insulin Resistance, or Syndrome X

Insulin is a major *anabolic* (tissue-building) hormone of metabolism, governing many aspects of glucose regulation, body fat storage, and other functions. Unlike the anabolic effects of testosterone, which builds muscle and bone, insulin is an anabolic hormone that *builds fat*. Insulin is a potent promoter of fat storage *(lipogenesis)* and a potent inhibitor of fat breakdown *(lipolysis)*. Insulin actually works to increase the ratio of fat to muscle, so the more insulin stimulation you have, the lower the ratio of the fat-burning muscle cells. *Excess* insulin is a serious problem, but lack of insulin can lead to death. You must have some insulin to get the glucose from the bloodstream to the cells that must have it for fuel to live. Glucose must also get to the fat cells to be stored as triglycerides for your body's later energy needs. This is why diabetics who don't make insulin must take it as shots, or in an insulin pump or nasal spray.

Excess insulin can happen no matter what your age. Some common triggers are (1) constant dieting with the wrong kind of foods, eating more high carbohydrate foods, and/or eating late in the day; (2) increased stress with high cortisol; (3) loss of estradiol; (4) high free testosterone relative to estradiol; (5) high levels of DHEA; (6) disrupted sleep and/or altered sleep-wake cycles, such as getting up at noon and staying up until two or three in the morning; (7) declining thyroid function; and (8) less physical activity—to name the most crucial for women.

Normally, when glucose is rising, insulin is produced in order to move the glucose out of the bloodstream for use by muscle or storage as fat. Insulin levels are supposed to then quickly drop back down to baseline after it has done its job. But as we gain body fat, the insulin receptors don't work as well. The cells become distorted in shape and size and this causes the "lock," or receptor site for insulin, to get out of proper alignment. As a result, the insulin molecule "key" no longer fits easily into the receptor. This impairs insulin responsiveness. When this happens, glucose levels remain high after you eat because the insulin, even though present, isn't working well. Your brain sensors detect continuing high glucose levels, and signal the pancreas to release even *more* insulin to bring glucose down. Your bloodstream and cells become flooded. Then suddenly, when all this insulin starts to work, the glucose rushes into the cells and your blood glucose level plummets.

We call this response "reactive hypoglycemia" (low blood sugar), and when it happens you feel ravenously hungry and also tend to feel shaky, sweaty, nauseous, light-headed, and experience fuzzy thinking and heart palpitations along with racing pulse. This drop in blood sugar creates intense food cravings, especially for sweets. As soon as you give in, however, the whole cycle starts all over again. A rapid rise in glucose makes you lethargic, sleepy, and unfocused. Then, when the glucose falls too fast from the excess insulin, you feel sweaty, anxious, irritable, and weepy.

Time and time again, I see this pattern accentuate menstrual cycle hormone changes. Pay attention to how you feel relative to when and what you eat, as well as where you are in your cycle. You can pick up clues that your normal insulin sensitivity isn't working, which means you are becoming insulin resistant. A waist measure greater than 33 inches is another clue that insulin resistance may be creeping up on you.

Insulin resistance refers to this entire pattern: high levels of both insulin and glucose in the bloodstream and excess insulin causing glucose to be stored as fat instead of used for immediate energy. Since the insulin isn't working properly to deliver a steady supply of glucose to working muscle cells, the effect is the same as not getting enough food. The cells are not getting their fuel, so you get hunger signals and eat more, even though plenty (of glucose) is circulating in the bloodstream. What's worse is that your fat cells are also screaming for more food. The excess insulin makes your body excel at storing excess fat, and less effective at allowing fat stores to convert to energy for muscles and the rest of the body. Each day this pattern repeats. You get fatter and fatter and fatter while you eat less and less and less.

Insulin resistance also causes a host of body-wrecking effects:

- *Impaired immune function making you susceptible to infections*
- *Increased buildup of the smooth muscle in artery walls that narrows the passage for blood flow, leading to reduced flow to critical organs*
- *Plaque buildup in the arteries also narrows the passage for blood flow, leading to strokes and heart attacks, even in younger women (as we saw in PCOS)*
- *More platelet stickiness leading to increased risk of clots*
- *Later, increased risk of breast cancer*

With all these damaging effects on the blood vessels, excess insulin, particularly when estradiol is too low, is now considered a risk factor for heart disease and early heart attacks. These may sound like problems for older women, but believe me, young women are not immune—I even see these problems in adolescent girls. In fact, the federal government is so concerned about the staggering rise in obesity and diabetes that the terms *glucose intolerance* and *impaired glucose tolerance* were changed to *prediabetes* to encourage people and doctors to test sooner, and prevent progression to diabetes.

With optimal levels of estradiol, we are less likely to have problems with insulin resistance because the estradiol improves insulin response in the cells. But estradiol loss is not the only way our ovaries are involved in this insulin pathway. Researchers have found insulin receptors in the ovary. Insulin acts at the ovarian receptors to change the enzymes so they make more androgens rather than the normal estradiol-estrone balance. Higher androgens then feed on the glucose regulating hormones and cause more insulin production; the higher insulin levels stimulate more androgen production in the ovary. It is a cycle that makes a woman grow fatter and fatter and fatter. This is a major cause of the marked weight gain in young women with PCOS or Syndrome X.

A milder form of this imbalance occurs in perimenopausal woman who are losing estradiol and "unmasking" the effects of their androgens (DHEA, testosterone, androstenedione). As you shift toward more androgen effects and away from the normal estradiol balance, more body fat builds around your waist and deep inside the abdomen (visceral fat), as it does in males. Low-fat, high-carbohydrate diets stimulate more insulin production by the pancreas and make this worse. More insulin pushes the body to store more abdominal fat. More abdominal fat then makes more insulin resistance. To correct the problems of excess insulin, four major areas have to balanced, as I describe in Chapters 16 and 17.

Diabetes Mellitus

Diabetes is a deadly disease. It kills twice as many women every year than does breast cancer. Most women don't know this, and are far more fearful of breast cancer. Diabetes is alarmingly more common as Americans get fatter, and is a woefully underrecognized medical problem, especially in younger women. Diabetes robs you of your energy, memory, sight, and kidney function. Diabetes attacks the tiny end arteries throughout the body that provide blood to cells. This is the reason complications of diabetes are diverse and affect many different organs. It can cause nerve damage, severe pain in the hands and feet, depression, dementia, amputation of limbs, early heart attacks, strokes, and premature death.

Diabetes is the third leading cause of death in the United States, as well as the third most expensive to treat. More important, diabetes disproportionately affects women in over 50 percent of the cases, with some 8 *million* women of all ages suffering its ravages. In the past, most diabetes began in adulthood as an outgrowth of obesity. That's why it was called *adult-onset diabetes* when I was in medical school. But that name is no longer valid. Today we see a truly alarming rise in "adult form" diabetes in children and teenagers. Now called *noninsulin dependent diabetes mellitus* (NIDDM), or Type II diabetes, to distinguish it from the insulin dependent, or Type I, diabetes, formerly called *juvenile-onset diabetes,* it must be treated early and aggressively.

Diabetes is a greater problem for women than men for two reasons: More women of all ages get diabetes, and women tend to have more severe and more frequent diabetic complications. Women have smaller arteries than men, so diabetes damages arteries throughout the body faster. Type II diabetes is the form caused by excess body fat, and is far more common in women. Depression is also more common in women, and in women with diabetes, depression occurs with a threefold greater frequency. Women get yet another hit: Certain antidepressants, such as tricyclics, can cause even higher blood sugars, memory loss, a marked increase in carbohydrate craving, and more weight gain—all making the diabetes worse.

The wrong choice of birth control pill (e.g., high-progestin pills) or the wrong type of hormone therapy can aggravate weight gain, hinder glucose control, and cause more yeast infections, already more prevalent in women with diabetes. Osteopenia and osteoporosis are also more common because high levels of glucose lead to decreased bone-building, decreased response to the parathyroid hormone, and decreased response to a type of vitamin D needed to build healthy bone.

Loss of optimal estradiol, for whatever cause, at whatever age, is one more factor that increases the risk of diabetes. Estradiol actually *improves* our sensitivity to insulin, and makes us less likely to become glucose intolerant and insulin resistant. Estradiol also prevents the excess androgen effects that aggravate insulin resistance and acts as an antioxidant to prevent the cell-damaging effects of excess glucose.

Optimal estradiol also counteracts the dangerous effects of excess glucose on blood platelets. Since excess glucose makes platelets stickier and more likely to clot, you are at greater risk for clots and stroke. Eating a high-carbohydrate diet makes this problem even worse: One Harvard study found that women aged thirty-eight to sixty-four who ate a diet high in refined carbohydrates had a 40 percent greater risk of heart attack or stroke than did women with a diet lower in refined carbohydrates. Diabetes complications can begin years before the disease is diagnosed, so you must watch for early signs of glucose intolerance and get tested and treated. In Chapter 17, I describe in detail how to get properly and thoroughly tested for glucose and insulin problems, using new guidelines from WHO and the American Diabetes Association.

In Summary
Insulin resistance, PCOS, Syndrome X, and diabetes all affect normal ovarian hormone balance, affect millions of women, causing untold pain and suffering, not to mention disability and early death. PCOS and Syndrome X desperately need careful attention by you and your physicians. These conditions must be recognized and treated when you are younger, before you have developed serious disease or permanent complications.

When women have irregular periods, 80 to 90 percent of the time they also have increased body/face hair, abnormal weight gain, and elevated androgens. These symptoms are often minimized by physicians, and PCOS rarely gets treated as early as it should. The good news is that PCOS and all the disorders in this chapter, *if recognized* early, can be treated with an integrated approach. You do not have to put up with feeling lousy and missing out on life.

If you suspect an imbalance in any of these hormone systems, get evaluated properly, as I describe in Chapter 17. Addressing these hormonal imbalances in young women can prevent many of the chronic weight and health problems commonly seen today. There are answers. There is no need to wait another ten or fifteen years to address the situation, as *Noel,* a twenty-eight-year-old patient with PCOS and insulin resistance happily found out. With a change in her birth control pill and the addition of Glucophage, spironolactone, and a higher protein meal plan, she exclaimed, "I didn't realize how messed up I was until I got better. I had adapted to all those symptoms and didn't realize how bad it was. I am eating better, I don't crave carbohydrates like I did, my body is reshaping, I am less heavy on top, I see my waist coming back, my headaches are almost gone, and I am not as depressed and foggy-brained as I was. I feel so encouraged . . . finally I have hope for a healthier future."

The Many Faces of Infertility:
Overlooked Factors

Introduction

There are few things more poignant and painful than a couple who fervently want a child only to learn that they cannot conceive. Today, many advances in assisted reproductive technologies can solve the problem of infertility for some. Yet it is an expensive, challenging, and emotional hormonal roller coaster for those who take this route. It has, unfortunately, a lower success rate than we would like. I am not a fertility specialist, and do not evaluate or treat infertility. Infertility is a huge, complex subject; an in-depth discussion of it is far beyond both the space available and my expertise (check Appendix II for a reading list and additional resources for infertility).

In the course of my hormone work over the years, however, I have identified subtle imbalances in thyroid, ovarian, and adrenal hormones that contribute to infertility. Once restored to healthy hormone levels, a number of my patients conceived without further treatments. From my clinical experiences with the hormone evaluations, I will share some common, often overlooked, causes of infertility that you can discuss with your physicians. Some are overlooked in traditional fertility centers because the standard medical school curriculum doesn't teach future physicians these connections. Others are lifestyle factors that doctors sometimes forget to address, or assume that most women know.

The three major areas that connect my hormone work with infertility are subclinical thyroid imbalances, subtle imbalances in ovarian hormones, and "endocrine disruptors" in herbs, supplements, our environment, lifestyles, and eating habits (see chapters in Section II for more information).

Keep in mind, just because you are given a "diagnosis" to explain your infertility that doesn't mean it's the only factor causing the problem. Since fertility declines significantly beginning about age twenty-seven, the older you are, the more important all of these other fertility "saboteurs" become. In dealing with something as complex as infertility, you must thoroughly eliminate or reduce as many "disruptors" as possible.

The factors discussed here, coupled with those identified by your physician or described in books on infertility, have an *additive* effect to lower your fertility. Identify as many as possible and remember that some of the same factors for women may also cause lower than normal testosterone levels, sperm counts, and/or sperm viability for men. This is particularly true of the chemicals discussed in Chapter 5, as well as the adverse effects of alcohol, cigarette, or marijuana use. If you have any fertility saboteurs, and the man's sperm is also less than optimal, the combined effect means your fertility as a couple is even lower than either one of you alone.

Subclinical Thyroid Fertility Saboteurs

The thyroid has a crucial role in regulating normal ovarian function and hormone production, so healthy thyroid function is critical to fertility. This section highlights key thyroid issues related specifically to infertility (see Chapters 9 and 17 for more information on the thyroid).

Undiagnosed Thyroiditis

Women have far higher rates of thyroiditis than men, and a telltale symptom is often "unexplained" infertility. Most fertility centers check for clinically evident hypothyroidism with a TSH and the standard tests of total T3 and T4 hormones. If the TSH is "normal," meaning anywhere between 0.5 to 5.0, testing for thyroid antibodies is rarely done. Therein lie two problems. One is that the "normal" TSH for women trying to conceive is actually between 0.5 and 2.0; women with TSH in the higher end of the normal range may have enough impairment of thyroid that they don't become pregnant. The second problem is that TSH can be normal, but the antibodies can be markedly elevated and interfere with thyroid function at the cellular level. Studies report elevated antibodies in the range of 10 to 50 percent in women with various "vague" clinical symptoms, including infertility, even though TSH is still normal.

For women, elevated thyroid antibodies lead to subclinical thyroid dysfunction—hypo or hyper—and can disrupt the extraordinary precision of the brain-ovarian pathways just enough to impair fertility, even before the TSH has reached the standard, arbitrary, cutoff points that "officially" diagnose hypo- or hyperthyroidism. You must have a test of the two primary thyroid antibodies, antithyroglobulin and antimicrosomal (also called *anti-thyroidperoxidase,* or *anti-TPO*), in order to detect the earliest subclinical stage of autoimmune thyroiditis. If these are elevated, low doses of thyroid hormone may help restore fertility.

Suboptimal Thyroid Hormone Replacement

A corollary of the first thyroid "saboteur" of fertility is diagnosing a hypothyroid condition and then not giving enough thyroid medication to return to an optimal range for fertility. Recent studies from a variety of countries find that TSH levels above 2.0 indicate less than optimal thyroid replacement for fertility in women. But also keep in mind that excess thyroid hormone can impair fertility, too. When treating thyroid conditions in women who are trying to conceive, I adjust the dose until TSH is in the range of 0.5 to 2.0 for optimal, safe thyroid hormone replacement (see Chapter 17 for further discussion).

Foods and Medicines That Diminish Thyroid Function

There are a number of medications commonly prescribed for women that can decrease T4 conversion to T3, the more active form of thyroid hormone. Examples are glucocorticoids (such as prednisone), used for asthma or autoimmune disorders, and beta-blockers (such as Inderal or propanolol), used in younger women for migraine headache prevention or to treat palpitations from mitral valve prolapse. Another disruptor of this T4 to T3 pathway is soy isoflavones, the current darling of supplements for women with all kinds of menstrual, PMS, or menopause problems. Red clover isoflavones, such as found in Promensil and other over-the-counter products, have similar effects, as do foods high in phytates. Coumestrol, a phytoestrogen found in many fruits, grains, and coffee, is associated with reduced ovulation and increased early pregnancy loss of the embryos in mice when fed amounts even as low as 100 parts per billion. High phytoestrogen exposure in sheep caused cycle abnormalities, infertility, and early embryo loss; phytoestrogens also cause reproductive abnormalities in rats. Vegetarians with a high intake of phytoestrogens have more irregular menstrual cycles, lower ovarian hormone levels, and decreased frequency of ovulation. Don't overdo the soy or phytoestrogens if you are trying to get pregnant.

Some medications increase the amount of thyroid binding globulin (TBG), the thyroid hormone carrier protein in the bloodstream, which in turn means less thyroid hormone in the free, and therefore active, portion. If you are taking thyroid hormones, these factors must be taken into account in adjusting the dose up or down as needed. For example, birth control pills increase TBG and decrease the free active hormone, which means you might need a slight dose increase of thyroid hormones to stop hypothyroid symptoms. Heroin or methadone also increase TBG and may aggravate hypothyroidism as well as impair fertility in other ways. TBG is also increased by Tamoxifen, 5-flurouracil, clofibrate, and perphenazine. If you take any of these, talk with your doctor about checking the free T3 and T4 to see if they are optimal.

Excess androgens (such as testosterone or DHEA) and high cortisol (stress, remember?) both decrease TBG, as do corticosteroids such as prednisone. When taking these hormones, you may actually become a little hyperthyroid from the increase in free thyroid hormones, and your doctor may need to slightly decrease your dose to stay in the desirable range. Salicylates (found in aspirin and many foods) and nonsteroidal anti-inflammatory medicines (Advil, Aleve, Motrin, among many others) may decrease the binding of T4 to thyroid binding globulin, which also means more T4 in the free, active phase. Other common, often overlooked, factors can affect thyroid balance, which in turn affects ovaries, so pay close attention to all of these if you are trying to conceive (see Chapters 9 and 17 for more information).

Dieting Disruptors of Your Thyroid

Diets either too low in proteins or too low in carbohydrates, as well as too low in total calories, also impair the thyroid gland's ability to make T3 from T4. Dieting causes the body to prepare for famine rather than pregnancy, so it shifts more of the active, free thyroid hormones into the "stored," inactive protein-bound form. This shift makes you functionally hypothyroid, even if all the tests appear "normal." These changes are the body's protective responses against having too little fuel to run its systems (see Chapter 7 for more detail).

Iodine deficiency is another dietary contributor to subtle thyroid dysfunction. We are taught that iodine deficiency doesn't exist in the United States any longer, since the advent of iodized salt. But let's look closer at this statement. More and more women today completely cut out added salt in their diet and eat more low-salt foods, especially women in their reproductive years who are watching their weight or making dietary changes to relieve PMS.

In addition, most of the Midwestern states make up the "goiter belt," so-called because of high rates of hypothyroidism due to iodine-deficient soils. If the soil doesn't contain enough iodine, that means vegetables grown in the soil can't absorb adequate iodine either. The thyroid gland is critically dependent upon the right balance of iodine to function normally. This is true even if you take thyroid medication. Many good multivitamins contain iodine, but far too many women in their reproductive years still don't take a multivitamin every day. And if you are significantly deficient, even a multivitamin may not be adequate. If your TSH is in the target range and you still have symptoms of hypothyroidism, this is another factor to check.

Ovarian Hormone Imbalances

Premature Decline in Estradiol

Once again, young women can have less than optimal estradiol due to many causes, even when progesterone levels are still in the healthy, normal range. As it relates to infertility, optimal levels of estradiol are needed in the first half of the menstrual cycle to "prime" the ovary for a healthy "egg" at ovulation in the second half of the cycle. Optimal estradiol is needed to prime the endometrial lining of the uterus to create a receptive "nest" for the fertilized egg to implant and grow. Estradiol is also needed to produce enough, and the right type, of cervical mucus around ovulation, creating a favorable environment for sperm. With the optimal rise in estradiol in the first half of your cycle, cervical mucus increases over tenfold, and changes to a clear, stretchy, more liquid, and alkaline makeup so the sperm survive during their journey from vagina to fallopian tube to penetrate the egg. "Hostile" mucus is caused by a number of factors, but insufficient estradiol is a fairly simple one to correct. Some fertility specialists suggest that if follicular phase estradiol levels are too low, women can wear a low-dose estradiol patch (usually 0.025–0.05 mg) for Days 10 to 14 to improve cervical mucus and growth of the uterine lining. This approach depends on knowing your serum hormone levels to determine treatments.

After ovulation, the rise in progesterone once again changes the cervical mucus to become thicker and more viscous, which provides a barrier to bacteria that might harm a developing fertilized egg. Once pregnant, you need optimal levels of both estradiol and progesterone to maintain the early stage of gestation before the placenta forms and takes over the hormone-producing role.

Overlooking PCOS and Excess Androgens

PCOS is the number one cause of infertility in women who do not ovulate and is the most common endocrine disorder in women of reproductive age. It is also the most overlooked, underdiagnosed endocrine disorder in younger women (see Chapter 13 for detailed information). PCOS wreaks havoc with your entire endocrine system, causing excess production of testosterone, DHEA, and estrone along with lower than optimal levels of estradiol and progesterone. These imbalances lead to erratic or nonexistent ovulation and irregular cycles. Women with PCOS have excess insulin and cortisol levels that further interfere with fertility by many different pathways, including adverse effects on the thyroid. About 60 percent of PCOS patients also have elevated prolactin, which suppresses fertility. If women's hormone levels aren't checked completely, PCOS is often missed, along with other causes of excess androgens that impair fertility.

Progesterone Excess, Use of OTC Progesterone Creams

This may surprise you. After all, doesn't progesterone help pregnancy? Yes, but there's a catch. Progesterone helps pregnancy only if it's *in the right balance* with estradiol. If you use over-the-counter progesterone cream for fertility and you haven't had reliable serum hormone measures first, you may be treating the wrong problem. *Many* other types of hormone imbalances create symptoms similar to those often listed in popular media as caused by "progesterone-deficiency/estrogen dominance," a syndrome that is far less common than the reverse—low estradiol with normal progesterone levels.

Some progesterone creams available over the counter actually have so much progesterone that regular use can actually suppress ovaries, inhibit ovulation, and lead to even less production of estradiol. Don't self-medicate with these widely touted creams if you are trying to get pregnant. If you need hormone boosting, do it under the guidance of a reputable specialist who can oversee an integrated approach to your infertility.

Endocrine Disruptors in Your Lifestyle and Habits

Dieting—Especially Extremely Low-Fat Diets, High-Soy Diets

Overly restrictive dieting is so basic, and yet it is so often overlooked as a factor contributing to ovarian suppression and infertility. Keep in mind that all ovarian sex hormones and adrenal steroid hormones are made from the building block cholesterol. If you cut back fat to below about 20 percent of your total daily calories, there is not enough for the liver to make cholesterol to then be turned into critical hormones. If you are trying to get pregnant, you need 25 to 30 percent of your daily calories from fat, preferably the healthy, unsaturated vegetable oils.

You'd have to be a hermit to miss all the ads proclaiming soy's fabulous phytoestrogen load, but did you realize that all of these phytoestrogens compete with your own ovarian hormones at receptor sites and prevent your own hormones from working properly? A number of current studies have shown that a diet high in soy caused decreases from 20 to 50 percent in ovarian production of both estradiol and progesterone. This is a critical, overlooked point in all the media hype about soy. This effect of soy on hormone production explains why vegetarians have a higher frequency of irregular menstrual cycles than women who eat animal sources of protein. Suffice it to say, you can easily control these fertility disruptors in your diet (see Chapters 4 and 18 for more detail).

Excessive Thinness

You have heard the saying that you can never be too rich or too thin. When it comes to fertility, you can definitely be too thin. The rail-thin bodies of today's celebrities are emulated by young women, yet worldwide studies in various ethnic groups show that women's fertility is impaired when body fat drops below 20 to 22 percent of total body mass. Mother Nature meant for women to have extra fat as fuel stores to support a pregnancy in case of food scarcity, so our fertility suffers if we lose too much fat.

Obesity

Obesity also impairs fertility, in part from insulin resistance and in part from increased production of androgens and estrone in the body fat, as well as other pathways. The more obese a woman, the less likely she will become pregnant and the higher her chances of miscarriage. Although I certainly empathize with the difficulties of losing excess weight, it is worth the time, energy, and effort to invest in a healthy weight-loss program if you're trying to get pregnant. Weight loss provides a more optimal hormonal environment of the body to sustain a pregnancy (see Chapter 13 for more detail).

Too Much Exercise

Excess exercise suppresses ovarian cycles and hormone production and can impair fertility (see Chapter 8). If you have trouble getting pregnant, talk with your physician or exercise physiologist about decreasing the frequency and intensity of your workouts to a lower level, such as three to four days a week. Try walking briskly for twenty to forty minutes rather than high-intensity stair-climbing for ninety minutes or jogging five or more miles a day six days a week!

Excess Stress and Sleep Deprivation

Women burn the candle at both ends today, living hectic lives that cause increased cortisol, reduced ovarian function, decreased deep sleep at night, and decreased growth hormone production at night. And these are just a few of the adverse metabolic effects. Reread Chapter 7 for in-depth explanations about the effects of stress and how to avoid it.

Herbs That Sabotage Your Fertility

There are many herbs that cause infertility, miscarriages, abortions, birth defects, and premature labor. In fact, long before the development of modern contraceptives, women in ancient cultures used plant medicines to control their fertility. Women healers around the world knew which herbs prevented pregnancy and which ones could induce abortions. But since the healers' use of herbs as contraceptives was in violation of church doctrine, many were burned at the stake as "witches" in Europe during the Middle Ages. In all the extensive marketing of herbs as "more natural" and "safer" options than prescription medicines, we have lost sight of our ancestors' knowledge of how powerful herbs are. If you are in your reproductive years, avoid using herbs when you are trying to conceive. You don't want to inadvertently have a miscarriage or cause birth defects in your baby just because some ad tells you herbs are "natural" and "safe."

Some of the herbs that can cause infertility, abortions, birth defects, or premature labor are actually in common use today. A few that have been found to have adverse effects on fertility and pregnancy are: *black cohosh, blue cohosh, cat's claw, chaste tree, dong quai, feverfew, ginseng, gotu kola, ma huang (ephedra), passionflower, evening primrose, red clover, Saint-John's-wort, Vitex, and wild yam.*

Women are not the only ones who should use caution with herbs. Men's sperm can be affected, too. A March 1999 study published in *Fertility and Sterility*, described adverse effects on male sperm viability and ability to fertilize an egg from four commonly used herbs: Saint-John's-wort, echinacea purpura, gingko biloba, and saw palmetto. Saw palmetto made sperm less viable, while the other three decreased viability *and* affected the sperm's ability to penetrate the egg for fertilization. More ominous, sperm exposed to Saint-John's-wort developed a mutation of the tumor-suppressor gene, BRCA1, a shocking finding. As you have probably seen in the news, mutations in this gene significantly increase the risk of both breast and ovarian cancers in women who inherit the altered gene.

Manufacturers of many vitamin and mineral supplements today add a variety of herbs to sell more products to consumers enthusiastic about "natural medicines." Read labels carefully. If you are trying to conceive, avoid using products with any of the herbs listed above.

Excitotoxins in Soft Drinks, Snacks, and Convenience Foods

Excitatory amino acids, like glutamate and aspartate, are ubiquitous in our foods and soft drinks today. They can disrupt the pituitary pathways that regulate ovarian function. This is a factor not addressed in most medical settings that treat infertility. Even if excitatory amino acids have not been found to cause obvious birth defects, there is some evidence that they can adversely affect subtle neurobehavioral and neuroendocrine pathways in a developing baby. You can control what you eat and drink. Clean up your diet, and get rid of these fertility saboteurs. Even if there are other "diagnoses" for your infertility, you will further help the situation if you eliminate these endocrine disruptors (see Chapter 4 for more details).

Cigarettes, Alcohol, Marijuana, Excess Caffeine, and Stimulant Use

There are many pathways where these substances disrupt ovary hormone production in women (and testicular function in men). A *teratogen* is a drug or chemical that causes damage to the fetus ("birth defects"). Caffeine, cigarette smoking, cocaine, and marijuana are *suspected* environmental teratogens, while alcohol and ionizing radiation (in the atmosphere) are *confirmed* teratogens. Teratogen exposure is another factor contributing to early pregnancy loss before you are even sure you are pregnant, as well as causing recurrent miscarriages later on.

Each one of these "endocrine disruptors" alone can interfere with fertility; using more than one on a regular basis has even more adverse impact. Do a basic "housecleaning" and get rid of these fertility robbers before you spend thousands of dollars on infertility testing and treatment, especially if you *are* in such a program now. Your efforts will give *you* a healthier body, a better chance of becoming pregnant, and are definitely better for your baby (see Chapter 6).

Chemical Exposure at Home or Work

Serious endocrine disruptors such as pesticides, PCBs, bisphenol-A, organic solvents, and others described in Chapter 5 have far more damaging effects on fertility—for men and women—than most consumers and physicians realize. Heavy metals such as lead and mercury, organic solvents, alcohol, and ionizing radiation are confirmed environmental teratogens for a developing embryo. They can cause both early and later miscarriages. Several thousand animal and human studies show truly alarming effects on reproductive pathways, as well as ways these same chemicals disrupt important thyroid pathways. And as mentioned earlier, if your thyroid isn't working right, there's a high probability that your ovaries aren't either. (See Appendix II for some of these studies.)

There are some practical steps you can take to reduce your exposure to these chemicals. Keep in mind, however, if you question most physicians, they may not answer definitively, because past studies on the toxicity of these compounds have primarily focused on cancer-causing effects rather than effects on fertility, sustaining a pregnancy, or the impact on a developing embryo. Doctors simply may not know the possible future effects with some of these hormonally active agents. It was not long ago that DES was given to pregnant women in the mistaken belief that it helped sustain a healthy pregnancy; we now know otherwise. DES and similar hormone-disruptors taken during pregnancy can cause serious abnormalities in both male and female embryos, as well as increased miscarriage rates in DES daughters and diminished quality of sperm in DES sons.

Remember, medicine is slow to accept new connections and even slower to change. Doctors want scientific proof before they act. While that's a plus in many ways, physicians need to heed the warnings from biologists reporting serious reproductive and neurological problems in animals. If you are struggling with infertility, this is a crucial issue for you. Just in case the environmental scientists are really right, I encourage you to take the time to eliminate these endocrine disruptors from your home and work environment (see Chapters 5 and 18 for more information).

In Summary

Fertility is a delicate balance of many interconnected factors: age, hormone levels, body fat, what you eat, what you drink, how much you exercise, what medicines you take, what supplements you take, what's present in your environment, your vitamins and minerals, your genetic makeup, your immune function, your mental outlook, how much stress you live with—just to name some major ones. Problems in one of these *add* to problems in others. The more fertility robbers you have, the less likely you are to be able to conceive. Follow the recommendations of your fertility specialist, but also work on getting rid of these other fertility disruptors I have described in this chapter.

15

The Ovaries and Your Other Body Systems

Introduction

Our ovaries are marvelous, magnificent organs that month after month, year after year, produce hormones that permeate every cell, tissue, and organ in our body, providing metabolic power for our cellular engines. Ovarian hormones have major effects on the function of all our systems, not just our ability to become pregnant, carry a child, nurse, and menstruate. Eyes, hair, skin, bones, muscles, joints, heart, lungs, brain and nerves, ears and hearing, vocal cords, digestive tract, kidney, pancreas, bladder, and immune system. There isn't a single part of the body that isn't affected by estradiol, and to a lesser degree testosterone. In our reproductive years, progesterone also affects many of these systems, helping our body prepare for pregnancy, but also often blocking estradiol actions and producing effects that we may not always like, such as PMS and insulin resistance.

Your Ovaries Are Connected to Your Eyes, Skin, Hair, Voice, and More

Estrogen and Your Eyes

So you hit thirty and your eyes feel dry and scratchy. Your contact lenses aren't as comfortable. Or maybe you started birth control pills and can't wear contacts at all. Your skin is dry and itchy, your hair thinner. As one thirty-four-year-old mother of three said, "I'm getting pimples again like a teenager, my hair is falling out, and I have all these wrinkles. What is going on?"

Remember, estrogen is Mother Nature's moisturizer. That means everything from skin, scalp, eyes, mouth, and nose to intestinal tract, bladder, and vagina are all affected by increasing dryness as estradiol declines and we are left with an excess of estrone and androgens. Dry eyes result from loss of optimal estradiol effects that moisturize the tissue on the eyeball. Testosterone is also involved in maintaining secretions to moisturize the eye. To fit properly, contact lenses "float" over the eye on a thin film of water. If the surface isn't moist, contact lenses don't have their "floating pad," and so they feel scratchy or burning.

Other eye problems are triggered by low estradiol: age-related macular degeneration (ARMD), glaucoma, cataracts, decreased visual sharpness, and decreased visual coordination. Research shows that estrogen replacement therapy helps reverse all of these adverse changes to the eyes. For example, one study of perimenopausal women with eye problems found that one third had dryness, tearing, decreased visual acuity, decreased visual coordination, red and swollen lids, or a sensation of a foreign object in the eye. The authors reported that all improved with estradiol therapy, including a topical ophthalmic solution applied directly to the eye. Objective tests by eye specialists confirmed the improvement.

Other studies support these positive effects of hormones on the eye. Some studies go back many years, making it surprising that this information is not more widely used in medical settings when women describe these symptoms. A 1971 study showed better hydration of the cornea during the highest estrogen phase of the menstrual cycle. Another group reported in 1981 that corneal sensitivity decreased toward the end of pregnancy and during the preovulatory peak of estradiol in the menstrual cycle, both normal times of high estradiol levels. Recent research has confirmed these findings. Specialists think that low estrogen makes the eyes more susceptible to deficiencies in aqueous formation and decreases the formation of the lipid layer of the eye. Both changes make us vulnerable to "dry eye," or keratoconjunctivitis sicca (KCS). Testosterone adds to estradiol effects on eye moisture by improving function of the meibomian glands in the eyelid. Testosterone and estradiol ophthalmic solutions are already being studied by eye specialists in Europe as an effective treatment of "dry-eye syndrome."

Progesterone, on the other hand, has a number of effects that make your vision less sharp, or even blurred. Progesterone rises during the second half of the cycle, and during pregnancy causes the meibomian glands to increase production of a fatty material that creates an oily film and deposits on the eye's surface, leading to blurred vision and reduced wearing time with contact lenses. Rising progesterone also affects how the brain processes visual information. During a woman's PMS week, visual perception skills are decreased, and research shows *less* visual sensitivity as well as diminished detection and discrimination abilities. You aren't imagining it if your vision seems less "sharp" the week before your period, or if you started Depo-Provera or high-progestin birth control pills!

Estrogen and Your Skin

You can tell dry skin by its look and feel. Just looking at the skin, however, doesn't readily reveal the loss of *collagen,* which gives skin its elasticity and firmness. As estradiol declines, so does collagen formation. Dry skin plus the loss of collagen gives the leathery, wrinkled, sagging appearance associated with aging. Skin collagen decreases markedly after age forty in most women as estradiol declines. It decreases in younger women who lose estradiol for other reasons. The decrease in collagen is greater in women who have a surgical menopause. No one dies of "old age of the skin," so it isn't surprising estradiol effects on skin aging haven't been studied as much as effects on more critical body systems, such as heart, bone, and brain. A 1992 study from Spain evaluating the effects of different estrogen regimens on skin collagen content shows that estrogen replacement prevented decrease in skin collagen. The amount of collagen benefit varied depending on type of therapy used. Transdermal patches using 17-beta estradiol show the greatest degree of collagen preservation. Oral conjugated equine estrogens (Premarin) with a low amount of 17-beta estradiol were not as effective.

Other changes in the skin related to loss of optimal estradiol are more unusual. Dermatographism refers to an atypical type of allergic reaction in the skin that causes a reddened, raised line where you "write" or draw a shape on the skin with a fingernail or other sharp object. It occurs more frequently with low estradiol levels. One thirty-one-year-old woman I treated developed a severe form of this after being on Loestrin for three years, with its high progestin–low estradiol content. Even touching her skin caused raised red welts that persisted for hours. The dermatographism resolved with a birth control pill containing a higher amount of estrogen and less progestin.

Formication, a sensation of something crawling inside or on the skin, is another unusual skin change caused by low estradiol. It may itch or feel like constant little twitches just under the skin. It's an unpleasant feeling; rather like hordes of ants traveling in your skin. Women say they think they are going crazy. This feeling is exacerbated by doctors who say they've never heard of such a thing. This "crawly, itchy feeling" has been described for decades as part of the menopausal changes, and is likely due to nerves endings that are hypersensitive from loss of estradiol. Many doctors don't recognize that it can occur in younger women who have low estradiol levels. Formication resolves quickly when the right balance of estradiol is restored.

Hormones and Your Hair

Thinning, brittle, dry hair is not life-threatening, but it is certainly a source of major distress to many women. I'm not talking about the occasional "bad hair" day. When your hormones are out of kilter your hair shows it. Losing hair *(alopecia)* is one of the more common problems women report, right up there with insomnia, fatigue, mood swings, and loss of sex drive. Declining estradiol, excess testosterone as well as low testosterone, excess DHEA, hypo- and hyperthyroidism, low or excess cortisol, several vitamin or mineral deficiencies, vitamin A excess, and low ferritin are a few common causes for women to lose hair. Dermatologists often tell my patients they have "menopausal alopecia," which certainly implies a hormone cause. Then they usually prescribe Rogaine without even suggesting hormone levels be checked. Before you get expensive medical evaluations, supplements, medications, or beauty products, at least get a careful and reliable blood test of your ovarian and thyroid hormone levels, including thyroid antibodies. Saliva hormone levels do not give you an accurate picture of actual hormone delivery to the hair follicle.

Estrogen and Your Sinuses

Some of you may have suddenly begun having "chronic sinusitis," "sinus headaches," or "sinus infections." Hormone changes play a role here, too. The nose and sinus cavities of the face and forehead are lined with mucus membranes sensitive to the loss of estradiol. Just as the loss causes dryness of the lining of the vagina, it also causes moisture loss and diminished mucus production by the tissues lining the nose and sinuses. Mucus helps to trap viruses, allergens, and bacteria from the air you breathe. When the mucus membrane becomes drier, it can't clear out all these invaders. Small arteries become constricted when estradiol levels fall, decreasing blood flow. Immune cells and proteins carried by the blood aren't as available to tissues to ward off or destroy the invader particles. Taking antihistamines and decongestants daily just makes this worse, since these medicines cause more drying and constriction of the blood vessels. Get your hormone levels checked. Boosting your hormone levels may be more appropriate than taking decongestants and antihistamines every day. Use natural saline nose sprays, or a steam bath for your face several times a week, as a helpful solution for sinus congestion, especially if you put a few drops of eucalyptus or peppermint oil in the hot water.

If you notice marked changes in your hair, skin, and eyes along with other hormone-related symptoms, it is time to check your hormone levels and your bone density as well. The visible changes in hair and skin can be a clue to damaging, invisible bone changes inside your body.

Hormones and Your Voice

Josie is a professional opera singer. She had a hysterectomy and removal of the ovaries for endometriosis and ovarian cysts in her early forties. Her gynecologist initially prescribed Premarin, but it caused migraines and increased blood pressure. Then he tried Estratest, a combination of estrogen and testosterone, to see if this would relieve her headaches and improve libido. By the time I saw her, a year later, she had completely lost her soprano voice and could not perform in concerts. She was losing her career and livelihood. She had also gained a great deal of weight despite careful attention to diet. Her blood pressure had skyrocketed, and she still had frequent migraine headaches, both problems she had not experienced prior to the initial hormone therapy.

Her hormone evaluation explained why she lost her soprano voice: Her estradiol was far too low at less than 30 pg/ml, and her total testosterone was significantly elevated at 176 ng/dl (normal for women is about 50 ng/dl). Her free testosterone level was also markedly elevated. The excess total and free testosterone, along with very low estradiol, causes a women's voice to become very deep. The fixed hormone combinations in products like Estratest make it impossible to regulate each hormone for the optimal amounts each individual woman needs. Too much testosterone made her ravenously hungry, contributing to weight gain. In combination with low estradiol, excess testosterone also raises blood pressure and causes headaches.

I recommended she change to 17-beta estradiol and stop the Estratest. Because of her high blood pressure, I prescribed a transdermal patch because it lowers blood pressure more effectively than oral estrogen. Headaches can be caused by the rapid rise and fall in estradiol. The patch form gives gradual absorption and reduces the fluctuations in blood level. The steadier estradiol delivery decreased her migraines as she learned to recognize signs that the patch was wearing off. When she felt irritable, foggy, headachy, or could not sleep, she would put on a new patch. Since her testosterone was too high, I suggested she let the levels fall gradually after stopping the Estratest, which would help her voice return to normal.

Three months later, she was exuberant. "I feel so much better now! My voice is completely clear and back to normal. I am so grateful that my vocal cords weren't permanently damaged by all that testosterone. My headaches are much less frequent, and my blood pressure is back to normal." Her estradiol had risen to 120 pg/ml and testosterone dropped to 13 ng/dl, quite a dramatic difference from Estratest levels. Six months later, she headed to Italy for a series of concerts, her voice completely restored. A year later, she says, "We got the voice fixed and I am really pleased with that part. I haven't had a migraine headache since the change to estradiol. My energy level is great. My primary care physician was pleased that my blood pressure is staying normal, and he agrees to work with all the things I learned from you." She uses one Climara transdermal estradiol patch every five days, and occasionally adds another patch when under a lot of stress and metabolizing estrogen faster.

The title of a 1998 French medical article says it all: "The Voice and Menopause: The Twilight of the Divas." The larynx is a hormonal target. The tone of the voice depends on the balance of estrogen and androgens. With hysterectomy and surgical menopause, or the decrease in estradiol from natural menopause, the balance changes toward androgen dominance. Loss of estradiol also leads to loss of elasticity in the vocal cords, making it harder to hold notes, particularly high notes in the soprano range. The French researchers found that a significant percentage of menopausal women had a "menopausal voice syndrome," manifested by lack of power and intensity, voice fatigue, and a narrower range of notes. Their conclusion is similar to observations from my practice. I find that with optimal hormonal replacement, the singing and speaking voice typically recover. Women also tend to develop more vocal cord nodules with the menopausal hormone changes.

Voice changes are not just a problem at menopause. Young women with PCOS, endometriosis, thyroid, or other hormone problems can also have adverse voice effects from excess androgenic hormones. For example, Danazol, an androgenlike treatment for endometriosis, has the potential to cause significant voice deepening. If treatment with androgenic hormones continues too long, the changes in vocal cord structure, elasticity, and voice quality are often irreversible.

Ovaries and Your Gut: A Panoply of Problems

Irritable Bowel Syndrome (IBS)

"Irritable" bowel syndrome affects far more women than men, but no one seems to know what causes it. IBS causes chronic, recurrent, crampy, colicky abdominal pain, and bouts of severe diarrhea, often alternating with constipation. In spite of intensive research, no one has found a single structural or biochemical "lesion" to define IBS. A variety of factors trigger these painful symptoms, including interactions between the gut and the brain, and between the gut and hormone fluctuations. Women with IBS typically say their symptoms get significantly worse around menstruation, suggesting ovarian hormones play a role in the gut.

Progesterone slows down the smooth muscle action in the walls of the intestine, leading to a slower transit time of food through the intestine. Women typically describe feeling abdominal fullness, bloating, and mild constipation during the ten days or so in the cycle when progesterone is high, even if they don't have IBS. If you are experiencing a decline in estradiol and you still have normal levels of progesterone in this cycle phase, constipation can be a major problem, especially if you do not get enough magnesium. Estradiol improves the muscular contractions of the intestinal smooth muscle, and prevents constipation when levels are in balance. This is usually the week after your period when estradiol rises and progesterone is not produced. When estradiol levels fall sharply, either with ovulation or just prior to bleeding, the falling estrogen triggers firing of the brain's alarm center, causing a burst of fight-or-flight chemicals that in turn cause spasm and hyperactivity in the gut wall muscles that can lead to diarrhea. Even women without IBS notice that bowel movements are easier, and looser, during menstrual days than the week before menstruation, when progesterone is high. Imagine how a decrease in estradiol and the surge of fight-or-flight hormones, plus a loss of ovulation that produces progesterone to slow the gut, can cause significant problems for women who suffer from IBS!

The vagus nerve helps regulate normal gut function and motility. Vagal tone has to be normal for food and wastes to move properly through the intestinal tract. The neurotransmitter serotonin also plays a critical role in normal gut function. Women with the constipation-dominate form of IBS appear to have abnormal stimulation from the vagus nerve to the intestine. Women with diarrhea-dominant IBS often improve when they take a serotonin "booster" such as Prozac, Paxil, Luvox, or Zoloft. We know also that excess serotonin activity from these same medicines can also *cause* diarrhea, so the right balance of serotonin and other chemical messengers is crucial. Estradiol has direct effects on the intestinal muscle and nerves to maintain gut motility and function, but it also enhances serotonin levels. Low estradiol levels decrease serotonin production—another way low estradiol aggravates IBS. If estradiol is restored to healthy levels, many women with IBS improve enough that they do not need the serotonin-booster medicines.

Women with IBS also tend to have backaches, headaches, painful menses (*dysmenorrhea*), painful sex (*dyspareunia*), fibromyalgia, and sleep disturbances (multiple awakenings, fragmented sleep). Many of these other problems are influenced by abnormal serotonin activity as women lose optimal estradiol, and some are triggered by release of other chemical messengers called *prostaglandins*. We know that a rise in progesterone increases the production of several prostaglandins, increases the breakdown of serotonin, and blocks estradiol binding at a number of different estrogen receptors. All of these patterns lead me to focus on the estradiol-progesterone *balance* in young women with these problems, in addition to the actual levels of these critical hormones, and incorporate estradiol into my treatment approaches.

Chronic Constipation

There are many causes for chronic constipation. Some are simple and straightforward, such as lack of dietary fiber, low magnesium, or too much fat. Some are due to treatable medical disorders like hypothyroidism or diabetes. Some are due to more serious medical conditions, such as toxic megacolon. You just read the ways that estradiol and progesterone affect the smooth gut muscle and motility of the intestinal tract, so you can see how too little estradiol with too much progesterone can cause constipation.

Estradiol improves intestinal function and motility in another way: It aids calcium and magnesium absorption in the gut, and uptake from the blood into the cells. Both functions have to occur properly in order for these critical minerals to do their jobs. Calcium and magnesium must be in the right balance for the bowels to work smoothly and not get "stuck" in slow gear. When your estradiol is too low, it leads to decreased stomach acid production, which means you don't absorb calcium, magnesium, and other minerals from food or supplements as well as you should. Estradiol also enhances magnesium use by our muscles and bone. If you don't have sufficient estradiol, you won't absorb magnesium into the bloodstream as well *and* magnesium won't be able to move from the blood into the gut smooth muscles for normal bowel movements. Constipation gets worse.

Women today have much lower magnesium intake than women of earlier generations. We consume large amounts of soft drinks that contain phosphates (sometimes called *phosphoric acid*) that attach to magnesium and calcium from foods and supplements, thereby diminishing absorption. At the same time, glutamate (MSG) and aspartate (Nutrasweet) in soft drinks *increase* the body's need for magnesium. Magnesium is depleted in other ways: high coffee consumption, stimulant medications (decongestants used in cold and allergy products, some antidepressants, many asthma medicines, over-the-counter diet pills, the herb ephedra, to name a few), cortisone medications used to treat asthma and arthritis, and the ever-present stress in our lives. If you are a Type-A woman leading a high-stress life and drinking lots of soft drinks, you are depleting your magnesium stores rapidly.

Add all these hormone effects to the typical American diet, about one quarter of the fiber and twice the fat we need, along with low magnesium, and you can see why the bowels rebel, become sluggish, or stop working properly.

Ovaries and Your Heart: Hormone Effects on Palpitations, Flutters, and Arrhythmias

Remember *Georgia*? She is the young woman who had three serious heart attacks, each with falling estradiol at the beginning of her bleeding days. She had severe PCOS causing low estradiol and excess androgens that triggered spasms of the coronary arteries leading to heart attacks. Hormone imbalances can cause other heart-related problems as well.

You may have experienced mild versions of heart symptoms, even in your teens or twenties. Now you are in your thirties, and all of a sudden there are horrendous palpitations, flutters, and pounding sensations. You feel anxious; your stomach is upset; your skin cool and clammy. What's going on? You're healthy, and have never had these problems before. Is it a panic attack? A heart attack? You see your family doctor, who checks you over, says you're too young for heart problems, you're fine. He tells you to relax more and reduce your stress. With a deep sigh of relief, you go on about your daily routine. But a few weeks later, it happens again. *What is this?*

Kerry is thirty-four and works as a respiratory therapist at a large urban hospital. She had been diagnosed with *ventricular tachycardia* (VT), an abnormal heart rhythm manifested by extremely rapid heartbeat that causes dizziness, light-headedness, and fainting. These symptoms happen when the heart is beating too fast and the ventricles don't have time to fill with enough blood to pump with each beat. As a result, the brain doesn't get enough blood flow, causing fainting episodes *(syncope)*. It is quite frightening, but the primary danger of VT occurs if it degenerates into more serious arrhythmias, such as ventricular fibrillation (or *V-fib*, as you have probably heard many times on *ER*) that can lead to death. Consequently, when these episodes hit, or she has fainting spells, she is admitted to the hospital for cardiac monitoring until stable.

She had been in the ICU on three separate occasions for particularly bad attacks. Her doctors were puzzled. The cardiologist could not find an underlying disease. Nor did she have evidence of plaque buildup in the arteries of the heart causing a blockage that contributes to rhythm disturbances. She was diagnosed as "anxious and stressed," and her doctors prescribed Xanax. But with her medical background, Kerry was trained to think about patterns and connections. Her observations about the timing of VT episodes led her to the consult with me.

This is her story, in her own words, from her first appointment: "I have had a miserable year with three hospitalizations for arrhythmias. First time, it was hot and I was taking care of my horse, and I got so dizzy I couldn't stand up. It passed and I didn't think much about it. Then it happened again while I was at work at the hospital. I had a run of V-tach [ventricular tachycardia]; they called a code [medical term for emergency treatment of cardiac arrest], did all kinds of tests, and found nothing wrong. I was put on Tenormin, and that really affected me badly. Now I know what low blood pressure feels like. I could hardly get off the couch! I was tapered off it, but I still had very low BP, and then I had another episode of those horrible arrhythmias. I remember it was right before my period was supposed to start, and it struck me as odd, because that's when it happened the last two times. They checked me out and sent me home, but this time with meds for anxiety. My doctor just told me I was stressed and anxious. I took Buspar, but it kept me up all night, so I weaned myself off. Then they recommended Xanax to take as I needed it, and that seemed to at least help some.

"The next time it happened, I was palping [having palpitations] really bad, so I put myself on the monitor, and found I had an irregular heartbeat. [Remember, she works in a hospital and deals with abnormal heart rhythms, so she knew how to read her own EKG strip!] I showed the cardiologist, and they put me back in the hospital, but then another physician said there was nothing wrong, I was just anxious. I suffered a lot of humiliation and I was really upset; they should have known I was an intelligent woman and a medically trained person. I *knew* there was really something wrong. I was having my period when it happened each time. It was getting so that it happened like clockwork every month right before my period. [Do you see a major clue here?] Right before my period starts, I have these feelings like I am going to pass out. This is a miserable way to live; I only have two weeks of feeling good. I'm an outdoors person, I love riding, and I want to be active, but I can't do what I want to do when I feel so lousy. I do everything right, I drink very little alcohol, I don't drink caffeine, I don't smoke, I eat well, and my stress is no different from what it has always been. I need something to help this."

All her episodes happened with the onset of menstrual bleeding, an important clue to a potential hormone change setting off a heart rhythm change. I sometimes find it hard to understand why this isn't more obvious to health professionals, particularly when an educated, medically trained patient gives such a descriptive history of the repeated association with menses. Remember, too, that she was carefully checked for all the "usual" causes of heart problems and nothing abnormal was found. But hormone changes can trigger such disruptions in heart rhythm. When your period starts, the drop in blood levels of estradiol affects the brain's center that regulates heart rate and blood pressure in several ways. The diagram on page 284 shows the sequence of events whenever estradiol falls abruptly, whether during your monthly cycle, or after a baby is born, or leading up to menopause.

So there you are, a cascade of responses affecting heart rate and rhythm from a hormone-triggered release of the brain's alarm chemicals. When we don't understand what is happening, our psychological fear response intensifies the body's physical responses from the drop in estradiol. This is such a common occurrence that many women don't notice it until the hormone drops are so marked that the body's responses are more intense. If your estradiol declines for any reason, then the fall in estradiol before menses triggers a much more pronounced physical response, and suddenly, you are aware of it and perhaps even frightened.

Most doctors don't ask you *when* in the menstrual cycle you have palpitations; panicky episodes; heart flutters, racing, or pounding; queasy or nauseous feelings; sweating; or anxiety for no apparent reason. That's because physicians are not

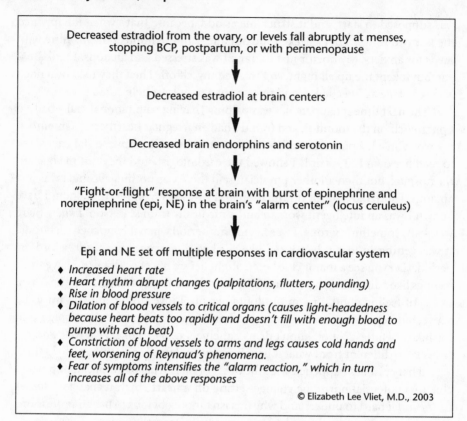

Decreased estradiol from the ovary, or levels fall abruptly at menses, stopping BCP, postpartum, or with perimenopause

↓

Decreased estradiol at brain centers

↓

Decreased brain endorphins and serotonin

↓

"Fight-or-flight" response at brain with burst of epinephrine and norepinephrine (epi, NE) in the brain's "alarm center" (locus ceruleus)

↓

Epi and NE set off multiple responses in cardiovascular system

- *Increased heart rate*
- *Heart rhythm abrupt changes (palpitations, flutters, pounding)*
- *Rise in blood pressure*
- *Dilation of blood vessels to critical organs (causes light-headedness because heart beats too rapidly and doesn't fill with enough blood to pump with each beat)*
- *Constriction of blood vessels to arms and legs causes cold hands and feet, worsening of Reynaud's phenomenon.*
- *Fear of symptoms intensifies the "alarm reaction," which in turn increases all of the above responses*

© Elizabeth Lee Vliet, M.D., 2003

taught to think that women's unique hormone shifts are that important, even though we know that estradiol, testosterone, and progesterone have diverse effects throughout the brain and body. Doctors who are not taught to think about these hormone connections don't realize that women's observations of menstrual cycle timing are clues to physical changes triggering symptoms.

Other than reproduction, I wasn't taught about ovarian hormone connections in medical school or during my formal specialty training. When I first started out, it didn't occur to me to ask when in the menstrual cycle a symptom appeared. It was not until I had been in practice for a few years, listening carefully to women's vivid descriptions, that I realized I was hearing the same patterns and connections from many different patients. I started asking *why* these similarities? Women say they know "its a physical, chemical kind of thing." They describe it well, but are told that "it can't be" or "it's caused by stress," so their body knowledge is written off and lost, connections between the dots aren't made, and women suffer. In Kerry's situation, her doctors had ruled out the more serious causes of arrhythmias, but had not considered the known heart effects from the physical hormone changes of menses. Her treatment with Xanax or beta-blockers did not correct the underlying cause.

When working with patients like Kerry, I want to know why a recurring pattern happens. I research the medical literature to see what I can find to explain it. The more I do this, the more information I find that has been in the peer-reviewed, published menopause and endocrine literature, sometimes for decades. It is sad, and costly, that such information is overlooked and not incorporated into treatment plans to help prevent overuse of other medications and needless expensive testing. Women's descriptions are "on target" more times than not. Doctors need to *listen* to what they say, and *value* their input to arrive at treatment options that work, that make sense.

Falling estradiol was the likely cause of Kerry's problems, so it made sense to try an estradiol patch applied two days before her next period to keep her estradiol steadier. I could test this theory easily. If Kerry didn't like how she felt, she could simply take the patch off, and the added estradiol would metabolize quickly and be gone in about twenty-four hours. She was thrilled, and quick to understand the concept of stabilizing estradiol because of her training in cardiac function. She used the estradiol patch during bleeding days for her next several cycles and did not have any cardiac episodes. It worked so well we began a trial on a combined estrogen-progestin low-dose birth control pill. A constant daily dose of estrogen and progestin effectively suppressed the ovarian cycles so that she didn't experience the normal ups and downs of a menstrual cycle. I recommended she take the active hormone pills daily without stopping to have a period each month. This prevents the "destabilization" of the brain centers that regulate heart rate and rhythm, and stops the fall in estradiol from triggering arrhythmias.

Six months later, she said, "I am doing wonderfully, absolutely fine! I sleep better, my skin and hair are better, I am not having any palpitations. I am not on any other medications—I was on a ton of stuff before to control the arrhythmias. I was able to wean off everything else. I don't have any runs of PVCs the way I did before. I am feeling really well now."

Cardiovascular Symptoms or Disease? How Do You Tell the Difference?

Symptoms are changes and sensations you experience, such as headaches, racing heart, clammy skin, pain, flushing, and tingling, among many others. These changes can indicate a normal body response to environmental stimuli or even to your own thoughts. These sensations can also be a potential warning of disease. Not all symptoms indicate disease, and not all diseases (especially in the early stages) produce symptoms. Hypertension and osteoporosis are classic examples of diseases that do not produce symptoms until the damage is already done. As a physician, my role is to help patients sort out symptoms, identify links to possible diseases, and determine what disease could explain the entire cluster of symptoms, as well as what disease could be present but may be silent and symptomless.

Palpitations, fluttering or pounding sensations in the chest, can be disturbing. They can occur when we are frightened as part of the normal fight-or-flight response, a natural response to a fearful situation. They can occur in certain types of benign heart disease such as mitral valve prolapse, or in potentially serious heart disease such as atrial fibrillation. They can occur from something as simple as falling blood glucose. Most doctors evaluate possible heart disease causes thoroughly; they often just forget to explore other metabolic causes, such as the heart's response to brain effects from declining estradiol, as we saw with Kerry.

Palpitations become more frequent, and more intense, as women move into the perimenopause hormonal declines. But palpitations can occur at any age if dieting, illness, surgery, or stress has pushed estradiol too low. In numerous studies, palpitations occur in 40 to 60 percent of women during the menstrual cycle when estradiol levels drop (bleeding days and around ovulation). For 15 to 20 percent of women, palpitations are the *only* symptom of declining estradiol. The brain senses the drop in estradiol, and sends an alarm signal that something is changing rapidly and out of balance. The increase in heart rate is a normal response to the release of chemical messengers in the fight-or-flight reaction. The heart rhythm changes and palpitations occur as a response to that alarm signal, but this doesn't necessarily mean that you have heart disease.

Diverse diseases such as anemia and hyperthyroidism can also produce palpitations by other mechanisms. Irregular heartbeats can be a side effect of many medications, herbs, allergy and cold products (see Chapter 8). Panic disorder is a biological condition of excess, erratic production of adrenaline-type compounds in the brain that can cause palpitations. So keep in mind that palpitations have many causes. The treatments will be different, depending on the specific cause identified by a careful, comprehensive evaluation that should include a test of your hormones.

Ovaries and Your Lungs: Asthma and Your Menstrual Cycle

Asthma is another illness that hits men and women, and doctors have traditionally thought treatment is the same for either sex. But the more we study differences in body chemistry and disease patterns in women and men, the more we find that women's unique hormonal makeup governs body chemistry, response to medicines, and also affects *when* flare-ups are likely.

In ancient Greece, Hippocrates, the father of modern medicine, observed that the wheezing and difficulty breathing (now called *asthma*) became worse in women around their menses. His astute observations about women's health, like his observations about muscle and joint pain and its relationship to menses and menopause, lay gathering dust in libraries for the last 2,500 years. In the early twentieth century, other observant physicians published a classic paper describing asthma in the premenstrual and menstrual phases of a woman's cycle. Again, these observations were overlooked until the last two decades of the twentieth century when several other studies documented the association between menstrual cycle phase and increased asthma attacks. Interesting data from Finland show that hospital admission rates for treatment of asthma were about the same for young girls and boys, but rates were much higher for women age twenty-five

SUMMARY OF KEY ESTRADIOL (E2) BENEFITS ON OUR HEART AND BLOOD VESSELS

- E2 lowers blood pressure by dilating blood vessels
- E2 increases HDL ("good") cholesterol
- E2 decreases total cholesterol and ("bad") LDL
- E2 improves carbohydrate metabolism, decreasing risk of diabetes, a risk factor for heart disease
- E2 reduces platelet stickiness and clumping that causes clots, artery-clogging plaque, strokes
- E2 reduces risk of blood clots by several mechanisms, such as lower fibrinogen levels
- E2 has antioxidant effects on artery walls, thereby helping to reduce plaque build-up
- E2 reverses the impaired blood vessel response to the chemical messenger acetylcholine in plaque-filled coronary arteries—a gender-specific effect
- E2 increases release of endothelium-derived NO (nitric oxide), a potent vasodilator, that helps to open blood vessels and increase blood flow
- E2 acts as a calcium-channel blocker, which also helps blood vessels dilate, improving blood flow, and also lowering blood pressure
- E2 alters synthesis, release, and response to peptides (e.g., endothelin-I and angiotensin-II) that constrict blood vessels, raise blood pressure, and reduce blood flow to tissues
- E2 increases transport of oxygen in the blood across the cells (endothelium) lining arteries so that more oxygen is delivered to the tissues

© Elizabeth Lee Vliet, M.D., 2003

to fifty-five (the reproductive and perimenopausal years) than for men the same age. Finnish researchers also looked at occupational asthma rates, and found alarming trends in the gender differences. From 1986 to 1993, the annual incidence of persistent asthma among people age fifteen to sixty-four years was stable in men but *increased 43 percent* in women. During that same period occupational asthma *increased 70 percent* in women. In the twenty-first century, physicians are beginning to pay "official" attention to these issues.

The majority of studies that track menstrual cycle relationships to asthma episodes find that about one third of women with asthma experience more intense asthma attacks in the few days before, and during, menses as both estradiol and progesterone fall. That's a significant percent of patients with obvious evidence of hormone changes being a trigger, yet most physicians still overlook the connection. Another interesting finding is that women with these menstrual asthma flare-ups do not respond as well to corticosteroid treatment. Women with increased asthma attacks in the days just prior to and during bleeding report significantly *greater* use of their inhalers and other medicines, yet still have a much *lower* peak expiratory flow rate (PEFR), longer asthma episodes, and more severe attacks than those without menstrual exacerbation. Ovarian hormones clearly *must* play a role.

These are times in the cycle when estradiol and progesterone fall to their lowest levels. This means that women whose asthma is worse with falling hormones do not respond as well to the usual medications for asthma. This observation shouldn't be surprising. If a fall in hormones is causing the constricted airways and changes in the immune system, it makes intuitive sense that standard asthma medications might not work as well as at other times. It also makes sense to use treatment approaches that better correct and stabilize hormone levels.

One hormone-based theory explains the link between asthma and menses based on the changes in airways that occur with the drop in progesterone the two or three days before menses. Progesterone relaxes smooth muscle tissue. In the gut, this action causes constipation, but in the lung, smooth muscle relaxation acts to dilate the bronchioles, increasing air flow, which is a good thing. But progesterone also acts as an immunosuppressant hormone, so when levels fall, the immune system is *more* reactive, making asthmatics more sensitive to environmental allergens. The drop in both progesterone and estradiol before menses can also destabilize the walls of tiny capillaries, leading to fluid leakage in the airways, which causes edema of the mucosa lining the airways, making it harder to breathe.

When I work with women whose asthma is worse around their periods, I find it effective to prescribe daily birth control pills with no break for menses. The daily progestin keeps the uterine lining from building up, so it is not necessary to stop for bleeding to occur. I typically use pills with a higher estrogen-to-progestin ratio. Other physicians who have tried birth control pills to prevent asthma flares describe mixed results. This happens, in part, because most physicians still tell women to stop the pills for a period each month, and also use pills too high in progestin relative to the estrogen, which can cause more constriction of airways because of progestin effects that are different from our natural progesterone.

Intramuscular injections of progesterone are also used to prevent severe menstrual asthma attacks, but some women report a depressed mood and more fluid retention with this approach. This happens because their estradiol balance isn't addressed at the same time. If progesterone is injected to prevent asthma without following the usual menstrual cycle, it changes your cycle and actually contributes to heavier, more irregular bleeding. In some severe cases of menstrual asthma attacks, some physicians try medications such as Lupron, which suppresses ovarian cycles and reduces the menstrual asthma attacks. But women then develop menopausal symptoms if estradiol is not added back. Women who have Lupron treatment with no estrogen replacement often tell me the "cure" is far worse than the original problem!

For most women whose asthma is worse around menstrual days, episodes are typically relatively mild. Some have such a mild increase in asthma symptoms, they do not even recognize deterioration in their breathing during menstruation. Then there are a few women who have such severe asthmatic attacks with menses that they require hospitalization and need ventilators. In June 2001, Dr. Yue Chen and coinvestigators from the University of Ottawa in Canada reported that obese women have almost double the risk of developing asthma compared to women of normal weight, and a greater risk of asthma than obese men.

We must pay close attention to gender differences and to ways the menstrual cycle and its changes alter the responses that trigger asthma. We must include hormonal evaluations, and possibly hormonal treatments in our management options for women's asthma. If you have asthma, speak up and ask your doctors about these connections.

Asthma Triggers in Your Medicines and Foods

During specialty training at Johns Hopkins, I became aware of potentially serious, and bizarre, patients' reactions to things as seemingly innocuous as the coloring agents in medicines. Even vitamins and herbal products have coloring agents that cause these problems. One patient with asthma was admitted for another problem. In treating that illness, the asthma was getting worse. I could not figure out what was happening, since asthma medications were stable and blood levels therapeutic. My mother, a research scientist at the time, was studying the role of tartrazine-based dyes in allergic reactions. After talking with her, I raised the possibility that the orange-colored tablets we used to treat the other illness affected this patient's asthma. We changed medication to a white, dye-free tablet, and within a short period the asthma cleared. Since the patient was curious about the orange dye, she took the pill one more time. The wheezing returned rapidly. She was convinced.

This happened over twenty years ago, and remains a lesson I share with patients and other physicians. Asthma is a complex disease, with many causes and triggers. Obviously, colorings on medicines is not a primary cause for most people, but we learn from situations like this. If you have asthma, watch out for any food colorings that could be a hidden trigger of your attacks.

Immune System Goes Awry: Allergies, Food, and Chemical Sensitivities

In my practice, I see a striking number of women with ovarian hormone imbalances, well-documented in laboratory studies, who also have an increase in allergies, chemical sensitivities, intolerance to perfumes, and a variety of adverse reactions to environmental chemicals. Ovarian hormones play crucial roles in regulating immune function. Progesterone, for example, is the hormone that suppresses a mother's immune system so she won't destroy the foreign tissue of a developing baby. Without progesterone to thwart her immune response, the mother's body would attack the fetus like the body attacks transplants. Estradiol revs up the immune response, and when estradiol is too low, we are more easily "overloaded" by common chemicals, fragrances, and allergens that we tolerated just fine when hormones were in balance. It is amazing to hear so many women say that after their estradiol balance is restored to healthier levels, not only do they sleep better and have more energy, they also notice their allergies are less severe. They aren't as bothered by chemicals or strong smells, and need less allergy medication.

Ovaries and Your Bones: Osteoporosis Isn't Just for Older Women

Over the last twenty years, I have diagnosed many young women in their twenties and thirties with osteopenia or osteoporosis. Such significant bone loss happens to young women because of the environmental, dietary, autoimmune, and other factors that disrupt the ovaries' optimal production of estradiol, and often testosterone. The body can't build healthy new bone in a normal fashion. And then there is the damage to ovaries from cigarette smoking, chronic dieting, or excessive exercise—all of which can stop or decrease normal menstruation and hormone production.

While the cause may vary, the result of too little estradiol is poor absorption of calcium and magnesium, poor deposition of these crucial minerals into bone, and an increase in bone breakdown compared to the rate of building new bone. Low calcium and magnesium intake, or loss of these minerals from drinking too many soft drinks or too much alcohol or coffee, rob bone from young women. If you are one of these young women, you won't reach menopause with a normal bone level, and are at even greater risk of debilitating fractures.

Fredricka was twenty-five and already had many symptoms of ovarian decline and low estradiol. Her doctor would not check her actual serum hormone levels, even though she had marked insomnia, fatigue, loss of sex drive, weight gain, PMS, and a depressed mood the second half of her cycle. Her doctor told her she was too young for a bone density test, and said, "Besides, you look too healthy to have any bone loss."

I tested her hormone levels, and the results indicated the need for a bone density test. She was shocked to find that, compared to a healthy peak bone mass for a woman her age, she was already 2.5 standard deviations below the desirable level at *both* spine and hip. This is the cut-off used by the World Health Organization to define osteoporosis. Fredricka had osteoporosis at age twenty-five! Her serum estradiol level on Day 2 of her cycle was only 15 pg/ml, instead of the normal 80–90 pg/ml at this cycle phase, and her testosterone was 10 ng/dl instead of 40–50 ng/dl. For Day 20, her estradiol was 74 pg/ml when it should have been in the 200–250 pg/ml range. Even with such low levels of estradiol and testosterone, her progesterone was still at the upper end of a healthy ovulatory range level at 18 ng/ml. Her NTx, a marker of bone breakdown products in the urine, was 65, much higher than the 35 or lower considered standard for her age.

What caused this young woman's osteoporosis? She was very thin, and pushed herself with dieting to keep her weight "ideal." In reality, she was underweight. She smokes two packs of cigarettes a day, and has done so since she was fifteen years old; and on weekends, she often has eight to ten beers, as well as one or two after work each evening. She often skipped lunch, and drank four to six Cokes a day for energy. Her mother had developed severe osteoporosis about ten years earlier than average, which further increased Fredricka's risk.

I checked her for other causes of early bone loss and did not find evidence of other underlying diseases. She unknowingly depleted her "bone bank account" with the soft drinks, alcohol, cigarettes, and dieting. Fredricka was an attractive woman by society's standards, and looked healthy in spite of her significantly abnormal ovarian hormone levels, poor nutrition, and lifestyle habits. But you can't tell from the outside how healthy a woman is on the inside. Her doctor fell into that trap, and as a result, missed crucial problems.

Female hormones play a critical role in bone growth. Estradiol and testosterone both facilitate calcium and magnesium deposits into bone for strength. These two hormones also regulate the rate of bone breakdown carried out by bone cells called *osteoclasts* so that breakdown doesn't occur faster than new bone is made. Estradiol "primes" the bone cells called *osteoblasts* that stimulate new bone formation. Progesterone has a slight effect on the bone-building cells (osteoblasts) and assists in stimulating new bone growth, but progesterone is only a "helper" that can carry out its job *only if* adequate estradiol is present to prime the osteoblasts. Testosterone has a much greater bone-building effect than progesterone, and it not only stimulates new bone *growth* to build bone density, it also enhances bone *strength*. Studies on bone metabolism worldwide show women need a certain minimum level of estradiol, usually 80–90 pg/ml, to prevent excess bone breakdown. Similar bone metabolism studies in men, interestingly enough, find that men also need a minimum level of estradiol, 50–60 pg/ml, working *with* their testosterone, to prevent bone loss.

You may not need to add hormones from an outside source for enough circulating hormones to prevent bone loss. Fredricka could help her ovaries return to producing the hormones she needs to improve her bones if she cleaned up her lifestyle. Cutting out the soft drinks and alcohol would help her body use the calcium and magnesium from foods or supplements. The problem is, if you are a younger woman, no one thinks you are losing bone. Until you actually measure bone density and hormone levels with reliable tests, you just can't know. Obviously, the bone density and hormone tests were crucial for Fredricka's evaluation because she and I had no other way to know this information in time to reverse the loss.

National statistics for young women's use of alcohol and cigarettes are alarming. This doesn't include the staggering numbers of women who are dieting and have deficiencies of calcium and magnesium. We are sitting on a time bomb of bone loss in young women today. It is too late to wait until menopause to check your bone density, since osteopenia (early, less severe bone loss) and osteoporosis are highly preventable and treatable if caught early. I check NTx, a marker of bone breakdown, on all new patients regardless of age. If it is too high, and there is low estradiol and/or testosterone levels, I definitely recommend a bone density test, and tests for other causes of bone loss if appropriate.

Other Risk Factors for Bone Loss in Young Women

There are several medications that increase the risk of bone loss in younger women: corticosteroids, gonadotrophin releasing hormone (GnRH) antagonists such as Lupron or Synarel, anticonvulsants such as Dilantin, beta-blockers, and high doses of thyroid medication. Medical conditions such as hyperthyroidism, malabsorption, prolactinoma, hyperparathyroidism, or immobilization due to trauma are also situations that can lead to bone loss in younger women. Young women with asthma, Lupus, or early-onset arthritis syndromes taking daily corticosteroids are at especially high risk for developing premenopausal osteoporosis.

Corticosteroids cause more rapid bone breakdown. They also cause the bone that remains to become increasingly brittle. If you have one of these illnesses and are on corticosteroid therapy long-term, you must urge your doctor to order both the NTx and DEXA tests. You can work with your physicians to prevent bone breakdown and rebuild what you lost. Both Actonel and Fosamax are excellent medications approved for prevention and treatment of bone loss. These medicines prevent the breakdown process, called *resorption*, and also aid development of new, strong bone. New medicines that stimulate the parathyroid hormone are in clinical trials and show much promise.

Excess cortisol in all of its forms hastens bone breakdown, even in young women. Many women are advised to take adrenal glandulars as a treatment for "chronic fatigue" on the theory that they are tired because of "adrenal insufficiency" or "adrenal exhaustion." Alternative medicine practitioners commonly misuse these two terms, and patients are given "diagnoses" without the proper medical evaluation to accurately determine adrenal function. Using the "adrenal glandulars" or "adrenal support" products sold in health food, naturopath, and chiropractic offices can cause excess corticosteroid effects leading to bone loss over time, even if these products are milder than the prescription forms of these hormones. Avoid taking medicines like Cortef for "chronic fatigue" unless you have a well-documented deficiency of cortisol (adrenal insufficiency). This must be diagnosed using the standard, reliable laboratory measures (see Chapter 17), not the highly touted, but inaccurate, saliva tests.

On the other hand, if you truly do have adrenal insufficiency (AI, also called *Addison's disease*), adrenal glandulars sold over the counter are *not adequate* treatment. AI is a serious medical disorder and can be life-threatening. It must be treated appropriately with prescription-grade medication monitored by an endocrinologist experienced in the treatment of adrenal insufficiency.

Testing for Bone Loss

Until 1985, the only way to diagnose osteoporosis was to wait for fractures, rather like waiting for a stroke as the sign of high blood pressure. Bone mineral

TECHNIQUES FOR MEASURING BONE DENSITY

Each of these techniques offers advantages and disadvantages in accuracy, precision, radiation exposure, cost, and information obtained

- *Dual-energy X-ray absorptiometry (DEXA)*—measures bones in the hip, lumbar spine, total body, or wrist; indicated for diagnosis, evaluation of fracture risk, and monitoring therapy. DEXA is the diagnostic tool of choice because it measures multiple sites with the least amount of radiation exposure, about one tenth that from a chest X ray according to 1998 guidelines from the National Osteoporosis Foundation. It is noninvasive, quick, and precise. Younger women need to have the BMD tests done on the hip and spine because tests of heel and wrist are not reliable in women under age sixty-five. DEXA is the tool used to measure bone density in most of the clinical trials of osteoporosis medications. Cost ranges from $125 to $350. Most states now require insurance carriers to pay for this test in women with multiple risk factors for osteoporosis.

Definitions based on World Health Organization (WHO) criteria:
   T-score less than or equal to -1 means normal BMD
   T-score between -1 and -2.5 is osteopenia, or low bone mass
   T-score greater than or equal to 2.5 is osteoporosis

- *Quantitative computerized tomography (QCT)*—measure bones in the hip, lumbar spine, or total body (but most common site is the spine); indicated for diagnosis, evaluation of fracture risk, and monitoring therapy. This is much more expensive, often costing around $1,000, and it exposes you to much more radiation than DEXA. It is not the preferred test.
- *Single-energy X-ray absorptiometry (SXA)*—measures bones of the forearm, finger, or heel; precise but not able to detect sufficient change in bone mass required to monitor effectiveness of therapy. Especially in younger women, there are very high rates of *false negatives* that make you think you are fine, but you can actually still have significant bone loss in the hip or spine.
- *Quantitative ultrasound (QUS)*—measures bones of the heel, proximal tibia, wrist, or finger; precise, but not able to detect sufficient change in bone mass required to monitor effectiveness of therapy. This test is not useful for women under age sixty-five due to high rates of false negatives. Heel measurements are of little value if you have had previous ankle trauma or a fracture requiring immobilization of the lower leg.

density (BMD) testing, primarily with dual-energy X-ray absorptiometry (DEXA) of the hip and spine now gives an accurate and precise diagnosis of osteopenia or osteoporosis before a fracture. In terms of value to identify early disease so that effective treatment can be started, development of DEXA testing is the equivalent of the blood pressure cuff to identify high blood pressure. You may have read about bone density tests using the heel or wrist scans; research shows these are not reliable for women under age sixty-five. If you are a younger woman with risk factors for bone loss, you need to have the DEXA hip and spine test.

Oh, My Aching Muscles: Hormone Connections in Aches and Pains

Muscle aches *(myalgias)* and joint pain *(arthralgias)* are common complaints in women with low levels of ovarian hormones. Hippocrates first described the connection 2,500 years ago in menopausal women and "women with scant menses." Modern research confirms that low estradiol levels play a role in these symptoms. But what about younger women? Is it possible for hormone changes to cause stiff, sore muscles and aching joints?

At different times in the lives of younger women, hormones can be out of balance and lead to arthralgias and myalgias when 17-beta estradiol is low or falls sharply, or when progesterone, testosterone, or DHEA are too high relative to estradiol. Unfortunately, these potential hormonal connections are simply "off the radar screen" for most doctors, so young women usually get pain medicines rather than testing of hormone levels to identify a cause of the pain.

COMMON HORMONE SHIFTS CAUSING MUSCLE AND JOINT PAIN PROBLEMS IN WOMEN

- Postpartum (particularly if the pregnancy is after age thirty-five)
- Women with PCOS who have high androgens, low estradiol
- Two to four years after tubal ligation
- Two to four years after hysterectomy if ovaries are not removed
- Two months to one year after hysterectomy if ovaries are removed and hormone therapy either is not prescribed or hormones are not optimally restored to healthy levels
- Women with premature ovarian decline (POD), particularly following viral illnesses
- Women with autoimmune ovarian disorders, particularly if severe enough to cause premature ovarian failure (POF)
- During times of loss of menses and optimal hormone levels: dieting, prolonged stress, prolonged illness; during active alcohol and drug abuse
- Perimenopause, associated with sleep changes
- After menopause, particularly if not on ERT/HRT or if hormone therapy is giving suboptimal replacement

© Elizabeth Lee Vliet, M.D., 2003

Mechanisms of Hormone Effects on Muscles and Joints

How does a decline in 17-beta estradiol cause joint and muscle pain? There are a variety of pathways by which estradiol has positive effects on the health of muscles and joints, via effects on serotonin, endorphins, pain threshold, muscle tissue, cartilage formation, and blood flow to joints and muscles, to name a few. Loss of estradiol means decreased blood flow to muscles and joints, less elasticity of connective tissue such as the cartilage supporting joints, lower levels of serotonin to modulate pain, and nerve endings more sensitive to pain. Loss of estradiol also makes you less sensitive to the effects of pain medicines.

Declining estradiol disrupts the brain centers that regulate sleep. Sleep disruption decreases Stage 4 deep sleep, reducing growth hormone secretion, so muscles can't repair normally at night and you wake up stiff and sore. Other sleep-disrupting factors with lower estradiol: Nerve endings are more susceptible to pain and this disrupts sleep; muscle and joint pain disrupts sleep; then the stress to the body of continued sleep loss increases imbalance in cortisol, norepinephrine, serotonin, and endorphins. All of these lead to more pain and more sleep disruption, further decreasing your ovary hormone production. The diagram on page 296 summarizes these connections.

In Summary

There is so much confusing media coverage about estrogen. Problems are overblown; important functions and benefits are minimized or ignored. Health writers, and physicians as well, overlook crucial and essential differences between the 17-beta estradiol our body makes and the foreign, mixed estrogens in Premarin, the product given to about 85 percent of women in the United States. There is little awareness of FDA-approved bioidentical hormone options that have been available since the 1970s. Media stories never point out that most of the studies in this country are based on use of Premarin or PremPro, estrogens significantly different from that which your body produces naturally. These vital sources of information for the general public in this country consider all estrogens and estrogen formulations to be the same! No wonder you get confused reading the headlines.

Few talk about 17-beta estradiol and what it does to keep you healthy and feeling well. Every system in your body uses this hormone to help the cells work properly. You need to know such information to make choices that will help you maintain your health, energy, and vitality, as well as choices that help reduce your risk of diseases later in life. For example, if a study like HERS only measures hormone effects *after* cardiovascular disease has already blocked the heart's arteries, it isn't surprising that they found no significant benefit. It's too late. The horse is already out of the barn, so to speak. All estrogen preparations are not the same, and should not be confused. Articles in women's magazines, newspapers, and TV medical news spots don't address these points either, omitting crucial information that could help you understand what research findings really mean.

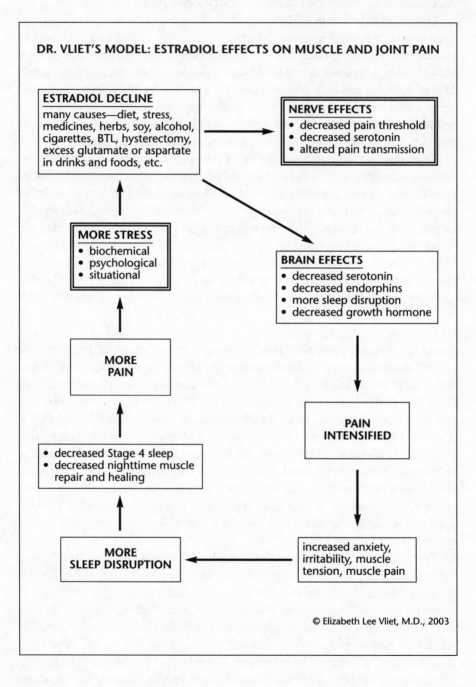

DR. VLIET'S MODEL: ESTRADIOL EFFECTS ON MUSCLE AND JOINT PAIN

ESTRADIOL DECLINE
many causes—diet, stress, medicines, herbs, soy, alcohol, cigarettes, BTL, hysterectomy, excess glutamate or aspartate in drinks and foods, etc.

NERVE EFFECTS
• decreased pain threshold
• decreased serotonin
• altered pain transmission

MORE STRESS
• biochemical
• psychological
• situational

BRAIN EFFECTS
• decreased serotonin
• decreased endorphins
• more sleep disruption
• decreased growth hormone

MORE PAIN

• decreased Stage 4 sleep
• decreased nighttime muscle repair and healing

PAIN INTENSIFIED

MORE SLEEP DISRUPTION

increased anxiety, irritability, muscle tension, muscle pain

© Elizabeth Lee Vliet, M.D., 2003

Our ovaries really are at the "hub" of a wheel symbolizing our entire body. With the many connections via the "spokes" of hormone pathways and receptors touching all the tissues and organs of our body, estradiol, progesterone, testosterone, and DHEA have profound effects. Today, most doctors practice specialties based on organ systems around the rim of the wheel, and they typically don't follow the "spokes" of hormone connections back to the hub. That's why they commonly miss the many effects of ovarian hormones. Your menstrual cycle pattern of changes in symptoms, however, can give you a clue to this hormone connection between your ovaries at the hub and other body systems around the rim of your "wheel." You are not imagining it. *Nothing* is impossible when it comes to the diverse ways the body expresses imbalance. Younger women, whom nature designed to have higher optimal levels during reproductive years, can and do have serious medical complications when ovarian hormones are adversely affected by lifestyle, dietary, environmental, or medical factors. Pay attention. Trust your observations. Find a physician who will be responsive to your concerns. Have your ovarian hormones properly checked.

SECTION IV

Getting Well—
Your Action Plan

16

Balancing Ovarian Hormones for Optimal Health

Finding Your Hormone Balance

Getting anything just right takes time, patience, and work. Balancing hormones is no different. There are many hormone treatment options available to you, both FDA-approved prescription forms and individually compounded ones. What should you use? How do you start? What tests should you ask your physician about? How do you interpret the results? What are the optimal hormone levels for most women to feel their best? What are the critical levels to prevent disease? How do you identify risk factors? What are the best hormone approaches? This chapter takes you step by step through this sometimes bewildering maze.

Step 1: Get Tested

If you scored high on the self-test at the beginning of the book or have any of the symptoms of ovarian decline described throughout, the first step is a comprehensive hormone evaluation. This is important; don't skip this step. Reliable hormone levels can validate your suspicions about a connection between hormones and symptoms. Proper testing also indicates which hormones need adjusting, since symptoms are often similar, due to many different causes. For example, symptoms of low thyroid can mimic those of low estrogen and vice versa.

What is the best method of testing hormones?

I have explored many ways to test hormones but have found that serum (blood) tests are the most reliable and accurately correlate with the symptoms patients describe. Saliva, hair analysis, or urine tests of hormone levels are not reliable or complete and generally don't correlate with symptoms. And they aren't even always less expensive. Saliva and urine hormone tests are widely touted through newsletters, direct mail, and the Internet by "experts" because they are available without a physician's order. You wind up wasting money because blood tests must be done before exploring treatment choices with your physician. Serum (blood) tests have been, and still are, the *gold standard* for researchers and physicians in need of reliable measurements to successfully make treatment decisions. Serum hormone levels are the ones used by fertility specialists. If the blood tests of ovarian hormones are reliable and widely used to help women get pregnant, they should certainly be the method of measurement for women with other types of hormone-related problems.

The reason serum tests better reflect hormone levels is that your ovarian hormones are transported in the blood *three* ways: *bound,* attached to sex hormone binding globulin (SHBG), a carrier protein; *weakly bound,* attached to albumin; and *free,* not bound to carrier protein. The free amount is typically only 1 to 2 percent of the total circulating hormone.

Current research shows that for the ovary's hormones, *both* the free portion and the portions weakly bound to albumin are biologically active at the receptors. The portion bound to sex hormone binding globulin (SHBG) is your reserve, like a savings account, ready for use the instant the body needs it. Serum tests for ovarian hormones measure *all* of these circulating forms: total, weakly bound, and free, to give you a complete picture of the steroid hormones available to act at tissues of the body, much like looking at all of your bank accounts to figure your total assets.

Kits that measure saliva levels of ovarian and other hormones only show the small part in the free fraction, and the amount of the free fraction excreted into the saliva from serum. To continue the analogy, this only counts the money in your hand, not what is in your pocket (free), checking account (weakly bound), or savings account (bound). Urine hormone assays only measure the metabolic breakdown products of the various forms of the hormones, not the active forms. These tests are *indirect* and give only a partial picture, similar to only looking at the sum of money you have already spent. They are less useful in measuring the circulating levels of the active forms of the ovarian hormones, the important information for treatment decisions.

What serum blood tests should I request?

Ovarian hormones. Estradiol, progesterone, testosterone (free and weakly bound, and total), DHEA (conjugated and unconjugated), along with FSH and LH, drawn on Day 1 to Day 3 of your menstrual cycle. Measure the estradiol and progesterone levels again on Day 20. If you no longer menstruate, have had a hysterectomy, or take birth control pills, then measure all the ovarian hormones once during the placebo week of BCP, or at any time if you are not taking BCP. Have the tests done in the morning before any hormone medication, or just before a new patch, if you are currently using hormones. Recheck these levels two or three months after you start hormone therapy, change medications, or have a surgical procedure such as a tubal ligation or hysterectomy. Checking levels confirms that your therapy meets currently accepted minimum thresholds for preserving bone, brain, and other benefits of your hormone therapy. I recommend these tests in addition to those listed above:

Thyroid. For women, this should include TSH, free T4, free T3, and thyroid antibodies (antithyroglobulin and antimicrosomal). Together, these are more sensitive indicators of subtle (subclinical) thyroid disorders, long before the TSH moves out of the normal range. See Chapter 17 for more information.

Prolactin. This test measures the hormone produced by the pituitary. An elevated prolactin level can indicate a pituitary hormone–producing tumor. These are usually benign, but the hormone production from a small tumor (*microadenoma*) can be enough to disrupt ovarian cycles, cause loss of menstrual periods, and contribute to headaches, depression, and weight problems. Elevated prolactin is also a side effect of many medicines (see Chapter 8). Have your prolactin level checked between seven and eight in the morning for the most accurate results.

Ca 125. This is a cancer antigen that can be elevated by ovarian cancer. Benign conditions such as endometriosis, fibroids, ovarian cysts, or even an early pregnancy can also elevate Ca 125, which can also be useful information to help decide the best treatment. We do not use this test to *diagnose* ovarian cancer, but it is the best early warning at this time. If it is elevated, you need further evaluation, such as a pelvic ultrasound. I encourage doing a Ca 125 for all patients, especially if there is a family history of ovarian cancer, or if you have vague abdominal symptoms (gas, bloating, distension, change in bowel movements, or pain) that do not respond to other treatment.

What are the "optimal" hormone levels for well-being that also reduce risk of later problems, such as osteoporosis and adverse cardiovascular changes?

When you don't feel well it is disappointing to be told, "Good news, everything is normal!" It is not that you want to be sick, but the fact is you don't feel well and want to know why. First, have the right tests, and review how to interpret the results correlated with your symptoms. Accurate interpretation of the test results can actually show something *is* wrong with your hormone levels. Instead of having your physician interpret the results based on *lab* "normals," consider what your body needs to function best. I find many physicians do not realize the dramatic impact that declining ovarian hormones can have on how you feel, particularly if the doctor is not experienced with ovarian hormone levels or the nonreproductive problems triggered by suboptimal hormone balance. Test results can fall within the lab reference range considered "normal," even though this range is too broad to be meaningful. Besides, a lab "normal" is not necessarily the "optimal" number for you to feel your best.

For **estradiol,** women generally say they feel their best when serum levels of estradiol are above 90–100 pg/ml. This is actually the *lower* end of the range for healthy menstrual cycle levels. Patients literally drag themselves into my office with estradiol levels of 10–30 pg/ml, yet they had been told it was "normal" because it fell within the reference range on the lab report. No wonder they feel miserable! Levels up to about 200 or so are the *normal* estradiol levels of the first half of the menstrual cycle in premenopausal women. Around ovulation, estradiol levels typically peak in the 300–500 pg/ml range, and then in the luteal phase a healthy level of estradiol is generally in the 200–300 pg/ml range. International research finds that estradiol levels should be above 80–90 pg/ml to prevent bone loss, maintain brain function, and provide cardiovascular benefits.

For **testosterone,** I find women typically feel best when serum levels of total testosterone are between 40 and 60 ng/dl (400–600 pg/ml), with the percent of free testosterone at 1 to 2 percent of the total. Levels below 30 ng/dl are generally too low to maintain your usual libido, intensity of orgasm, energy level, and bone mass. The majority of menopausal women I evaluate, particularly those with surgical removal of the ovaries in their thirties and forties, have total testosterone levels of less than 10, and barely detectable amounts of free testosterone. No wonder they don't have any sexual desire! This is also a significant factor in fatigue, as well as loss of muscle and bone.

Progesterone, the dominant hormone in the second half of the menstrual cycle, is measured and compared with the amount of estrogen present to decide which hormone is too low and causing symptoms. If you have ovulated, your luteal phase progesterone level rises greater than 5, up to about 25 ng/dl, while follicular levels will be less than 1, or about 0.1–0.4 ng/dl.

Follicle stimulating hormone (FSH) is produced by the pituitary gland, and its main function is to stimulate the ovary to produce new follicles every month. The follicles produce estradiol and progesterone. When estradiol levels drop, the FSH rises as the brain works to stimulate the ovaries to continue hormone production. High FSH (above 20 mIU/ml) indicates estradiol is too low and is one marker used to define menopause.

Thyroid stimulating hormone (TSH) is the hormone that stimulates the thyroid gland to produce more T3 and T4. If your thyroid is failing *(hypothyroidism),* TSH is high (i.e., greater than 4 or 5 on most lab ranges), although some women can have symptoms of low thyroid when the TSH is over about 3. If there is excess of thyroid hormone *(hyperthyroidism),* the TSH is less than 0.3. An optimal range of TSH for most women is generally between 0.5 and 2.0, especially if you are trying to conceive.

DHEA. Levels of this androgen vary greatly, depending on the type of assay and reference ranges used by the lab, so I can't give specific numbers here. DHEA is produced by both the ovaries and adrenal glands, so both forms should be checked. Significantly elevated DHEA is typically seen in PCOS, Syndrome X, and adrenal adenomas and is a major cause of the adverse physical and metabolic changes.

What other tests are important in a comprehensive hormone evaluation?

The goal of a comprehensive hormone evaluation is to determine whether any hormones are too low or too high and whether your problems are a result of a hormone imbalance. The goal is to avoid the common mistake of misdiagnosing hormonal imbalance as psychiatric disorders—somatization, manic-depressive illness, major depressive disorder, anxiety, stress, chronic fatigue, or chronic candidiasis. Reliable, objective measures identify the cause more accurately than simply relying on the symptoms, since many different disorders have similar symptoms.

In addition to the serum hormone levels, have a mammogram and bone density test if you are thirty-five or over. You also need a breast and pelvic exam with a Pap smear, which can be done either by your primary care physician, gynecologist, or nurse practitioner. He or she can also look for other clues to hormone imbalance, such as excess body hair (hirsutism), loss of body hair (alopecia), changes in skin pigmentation, enlarged or painful thyroid, patterns in body fat distribution, atrophic changes of breast and vagina, loss of height, and abnormal pulses, to name a few.

With all the tests, it is important to integrate the numbers with symptoms to correlate the pattern of body changes with the fluctuations in blood levels. The findings may lie at any point in the "normal" range and still not be right for your body's needs. Sometimes your results may be *slightly* outside the "normal" range, but not medically significant. Insist doctors treat *you*, not just your lab numbers.

I RECOMMEND THE FOLLOWING TESTS AS AN OVERALL HEALTH ASSESSMENT

Comprehensive metabolic profile: Includes tests for liver, kidney, adrenal function, electrolytes, and complete blood counts. It helps to screen for serious metabolic disorders that may cause similar symptoms to those seen with decline in estradiol or thyroid hormones (see my book *Women, Weight and Hormones* for more detail).

Fasting lipid profile: This includes cholesterol, HDL, LDL, triglycerides to help check your risk of later heart disease. Elevated triglycerides are a risk factor for both diabetes and heart disease, and are also a reason to use the patch form of estradiol instead of oral.

Fasting glucose and insulin: This checks for diabetes or insulin resistance (both are risk factors for heart disease). Fasting glucose should be between 70 and 110. Low blood glucose, or hypoglycemia, is a fasting glucose less than 60. Glucose intolerance is now considered to be a fasting glucose of 111–125; above 126 is the new ADA cut-off to indicate diabetes.

Eight A.M. cortisol: This is the "stress" hormone produced by the adrenal glands. Levels that are too high can indicate a stress response to physical factors, benign effects on binding proteins from birth control pills, or could mean the presence of a disease like Cushing's syndrome. Eight A.M. cortisol levels less than 5 to 7 can indicate chronic stress effects (sometimes called *adrenal exhaustion*), or the serious adrenal insufficiency Addison's disease.

Ferritin: This is a measure of iron stores. If too low (more common in women who still bleed monthly), it is associated with fatigue, hair loss, "restless legs," insomnia, and muscle aches; if too high, ferritin is associated with increased risk of cardiovascular disease as well as fatigue, aching muscles or joints, and headaches. A healthy range for women is approximately 60–90 ng/ml.

Bone density of the hip and spine: DEXA—dual-energy X ray—is the most reliable test for women under age sixty-five. Heel and wrist bone density tests do not correlate well with degree of bone loss at hip and spine, which are the really critical areas. Heel or wrist tests may be cheaper, quicker, and easier but may give you false reassurance. DEXA tests of hip and spine are now covered by most insurance plans. Costs vary widely; shop around for the best price.

Urine or serum test of N-telopeptide: This measures the rate of bone building versus bone breakdown. If this number is higher than 35, it indicates that you are already beginning the process of excessive bone breakdown and are at higher risk for osteoporosis and fractures later. You should begin to take aggressive steps now to build and preserve bone.

Glucose tolerance test (GTT) with insulin levels: If you have this test, you need to do the full five-hour version; a three-hour test misses important symptom information from *falling* glucose in the fourth and fifth hours. A GTT should be done in the luteal phase of the menstrual cycle (three to five days before the start of your period) if you have risk factors for PCOS, Syndrome X, or insulin resistance risk factors (see Chapters 13 and 17). This allows for early identification of women at high risk for developing diabetes and heart disease. A patient symptom log should be coordinated throughout the test.

Waist-to-hip ratio: This ratio gives an idea of your health risks based on *where* the fat is located as well as by *how much fat* you have. As women get older, the ratio of testosterone to estradiol increases, and there is more gain in fat around the waist and upper body. *Waist-to-hip ratios of more than 0.8 for women or 1.0 for men means you have become an "apple,"* and you are at increased health risk of diabetes or heart disease. To calculate waist-to-hip ratio, measure your waist at its narrowest point, then measure your hips at the widest point. Divide the waist measure by the hip measure. Example: A woman with a 35-inch waist and 46-inch hip has a WH ratio of 0.76 (35 divided by 46).

Step 2: Evaluating Your Risks and Identifying Your Needs

Once you identify your hormone status and other baseline measures with reliable tests, the next step is to determine how the results clarify your symptoms and your individual risks. Compare your test results with the information on optimal hormone levels. Do your symptoms coincide with times of hormone fluctuation in your cycle? Do you exhibit signs of decreasing ovarian hormone levels or hormone imbalance? You and your physician should review this information, assess your individual disease risk, and discuss hormone options to help you make an educated decision about treatment.

1. *Evaluate your lifestyle habits (diet, exercise, sleep, and work; whether or not you take the right vitamins and minerals, smoke, use alcohol or drugs, or take OTC and prescription medications) and work to eliminate the unhealthy ones.*

2. *Examine your own health risks, illness patterns, and any diseases that can be helped by hormone therapy, such as high cholesterol, high blood pressure, memory loss, depression, diabetes, osteoporosis or osteopenia, to mention a few.*

3. *Check your family history, especially first-degree relatives (parents and siblings) for common problems that can affect symptoms and future disease risks, such as diabetes, PCOS, elevated cholesterol, heart disease, high blood pressure, thyroid disease, obesity, depression, cancers, osteoporosis, and dementias. All can have a bearing on the importance of optimal estradiol balance as you get older.*

Based upon your risk assessment, weigh the potential benefits of hormone therapy against the risks. This risk-benefit analysis should be based on medically sound, up-to-date information and not on fear from an Internet or news-magazine piece or a friend's opinion. Then take your own "values inventory" to determine what quality-of-life aspects are important to you and how hormone therapy can help.

You need to ask yourself questions specific to *you:* What are *my* health risks? Will they be helped by hormones? Which of *my* health risks can be made worse? Are hormones appropriate for me? Which type of hormone therapy, and route of taking hormones, is best suited to my needs? What options do I have? The following sections will help answer these questions, but first, let's set the record straight about some of the common myths and misunderstandings about hormones.

Do hormones cause cancer?

Hormones don't *cause* cancer. There are many risk factors for cancer including genetics, exposure to environmental chemicals and radiation, diet, smoking, and other lifestyle-related habits. The highest breast, endometrial, and colon cancer rates occur in postmenopausal women who are obese, which means they have an excess of estrone. Estrogen and progesterone may both facilitate the growth of an *existing* cancer, but there is no data that shows either hormone *causes* cancers.

What about the studies that show taking estrogen after menopause increases your risk of breast cancer?

The studies showing increased risk are those in which women were primarily using Premarin, the horse-derived mixture of estrogens that are chemically very different from the human 17-beta estradiol. With all the extra horse-derived estrogens, this product delivers a high total load of foreign estrogens that you don't get from either the patch or the pill form of 17-beta estradiol. This is a critical point that most media articles do not tell you, and many physicians overlook.

All women, whether they take hormones or not, have an increased risk of breast cancer just by getting older. In addition, multiple worldwide studies also show that women who *do* develop breast cancer while taking estrogen develop cancers that are the less aggressive types and have better survival rates than do women who develop breast cancer when *not* taking hormones.

Are all estrogens the same?

No. The estrogens made by your body differ from estrogenic compounds found in plants (phytoestrogens), synthetic estrogens as in birth control pills, and the mixed, animal-derived estrogens such as Premarin. All are chemically quite different. These nonhuman forms are different molecular "keys" and don't quite fit the "locks" of the estrogen receptors in your body to cause the same responses as your own 17-beta estradiol. These chemical differences can be helpful, as in BCPs providing contraception, or the differences can lead to unwanted side effects.

Are all birth control pills the same?

No, they are definitely not. Different pills contain different ratios of estrogen and progestin, as well as different chemical types of progestins. The lower the estrogen (E) relative to the progestin (P), the more likely you will have increased appetite, acne, weight gain, low sex drive, fatigue, headaches, and negative moods (irritability, depression). The better the E:P ratio, the less likely you are to have these side effects. The *type* of progestin, as well as the amount, plays a role in the kinds of side effects you may have. If one pill causes problems, try one with a better balance of estrogen, or a different chemical class of progestin. The new non-oral vaginal ring, Nuvaring, has even lower amounts of both hormones, and can be a good option if you don't feel well on oral BCPs.

Does the estrogen and/or progestin in birth control pills cause blood clots?

The data on this issue is based on oral estrogen, primarily Premarin, or older high-dose forms of birth control pills. Newer data on the patch (transdermal) form of estradiol, our bioidentical premenopausal estrogen, shows that estradiol actually decreases the risk of thrombophlebitis (blood clots) by lowering fibrinogen and decreasing platelet "stickiness." Older data that suggests birth control pills (BCPs) caused blood clots was based on BCP use by cigarette smokers and on high-dose pills no longer available today. Cigarette smoking was determined to be the causative factor in the strokes that occurred in women taking BCPs.

Does taking hormones make you fat?

No, taking the proper type of hormones does not make you fat. Loss of healthy, premenopausal hormonal *balance* does. The right hormones, in the right balance, actually helps you lose excess body fat more readily, provided you follow a balanced meal plan and increase physical activity.

I am concerned about taking birth control pills because of previous bad experiences. Have they changed?

Yes, there are many new options available today. The older pills had much higher doses of both hormones—for example, 100 mcg estrogen versus today's 20–35 mcg pills. None of the older, high-dose pills are even available today. Today's BCP formulas are also much less in the progestin content compared to the pills that first came on the market. About 1990, birth control pills were also recommended by the FDA for nonsmoking women over age forty because of the many potential health benefits and reduction in rates of ovarian and uterine cancers. The FDA concluded benefits far outweighed the slight risks. In addition, some women also find they have fewer side effects with the new contraceptive patch, vaginal ring, or intrauterine device.

My doctor prescribed PremPro. Why are you telling me to take something different?

Everyone is different. PremPro contains a fixed-dose combination of the horse-derived mixture of estrogens, Premarin, with a synthetic progestin called Provera. The fixed dose of each is not necessarily the right one for every woman, and many women have problems with weight gain and breast enlargement or tenderness with this combination. There are newer, FDA-approved options available, such as Activella, that give lower doses of the progestin and also have 17-beta estradiol identical to that made by the ovary. There are FDA-approved patches and tablets of 17-beta estradiol, as well as pills and vaginal creams with natural progesterone available. I suggest that you talk with your physician about the more natural options available today.

Premarin just happened to be the *first* estrogen preparation available to be given orally and has been in use a long time. That doesn't mean it is the *best* option for everyone. The Model T Ford was the first mass-produced automobile, but it certainly isn't the best option for use on today's high-speed interstates. Why should you take an estrogen produced before technology and science could duplicate the estrogen made by your body? Your body will do better with your own kind of "hormone power" rather than one Mother Nature gave horses!

Many doctors still use Premarin and PremPro because of habit and the convenience of using a one-prescription-fits-all approach to women's hormones. It takes time and effort to fine-tune hormones on an individual basis. If you have symptoms or side effects on Premarin or PremPro, demand a different option.

A recent study showed hormone replacement therapy doesn't prevent heart disease. Is this true?

The study that made the headlines in 2000 was the Heart, Estrogen-Progestin Replacement Study (HERS), and then the 2002 preliminary findings for the PremPro group in the Women's Health Initiative (WHI). The newspapers didn't tell you, however, about these studies' serious short-comings. Here are a few critical ones: (1) this wasn't really a "prevention" study, since we use the term to refer to ways of preventing disease. In HERS, women were older and *already had* heart disease with major blockage of the coronary arteries before taking hormones; (2) we really would not expect to see a *reversal of existing disease* in the short time frame of the study; (3) the hormone therapy was PremPro, a combined product of horse-derived estrogens and a potent synthetic progestin (MPA) that is not the best type to improve lipids and other heart disease risk factors; (4) none of the women were given natural progesterone instead of the synthetic progestin, even though we already have a number of studies, including the 1995 PEPI trial, showing better effects on lipids with natural progesterone; (5) the WHI participants were also fifteen years older, on average, than is customary for starting hormones, and a significant percentage were obese and had high blood pressure and other types of CVD. Again, this is not the best type of person to use PremPro. This is another example of headlines, researchers, and many physicians missing the point about crucial differences among types of hormones.

Are hormones for everyone? Not necessarily. If you have no health risks, great bone density, and no symptoms, you probably don't need hormones. Just monitor your health with objective tests and evaluate hormone options later if your situation changes.

Are there nonhormonal alternatives to reduce symptoms? Yes, but many are not as effective as you may need, and most (including herbs) have side effects you must consider. Many medicines, as well as other therapies, can relieve or treat *symptoms*. The more important issue to address with your doctor is the underlying cause of your problems. The *cause* should then be treated. Don't just use herbal Band-Aids to treat symptoms. Keep in mind that many women take multiple medications and still don't feel well. If this is true for you, and tests show a hormonally based problem, then it makes sense to try hormones and treat the cause.

Step 3: Choosing a Hormone Approach

Although many physicians think all the estrogens for ERT are essentially the same, and the manufacturers of the leading products want you to think that, too, *they are not*. There are many differences and different effects with various hormone preparations, as many studies of the past decade, and my own clinical experience, prove. Understand the different types of hormone approaches available. Choose the best one for you. But why start with hormones, and not diet, exercise, and reduction of stress, as is often suggested first? Your hormones are the metabolic fuel that power cells. You may not have the energy to exercise if your hormone fuel tank is empty. Improving your hormone balance provides an important biochemical foundation upon which to build an integrated approach to your overall mind-body-spirit health. I think it is crucial to address underlying hormonal imbalances first, so that you are better able to incorporate healthy lifestyle choices (see Chapters 13 and 15). It is hard to make significant lifestyle changes if you are too tired to get out of bed in the morning because your hormones are out of kilter and you aren't sleeping!

Natural vs. Synthetic. A lot of women want to only take natural hormones. This is why many use the "wild yam" skin creams advertised as a source of progesterone, or dong quai (an herb that supposedly has estrogenic compounds), or estriol (weakest of the three primary human estrogens) instead of "drugs," which are "synthetic." The words *natural* and *synthetic* are confusing. Don't be misled by clever marketing.

Actually, something *synthetic* can also be *natural,* while something *natural* can be *foreign or "supernatural"* for the human body. Premarin is a "natural" mixture of estrogens because a biological organism, a horse, makes it. But Premarin is not natural for the human body. Genistein found in soy and red clover, among others, is a "natural" substance because it comes from a biological source, the soy plant. But it is "unnatural" for our bodies. We don't make these same compounds and don't have the enzymes to change the genistein or clover isoflavones into our own 17-beta estradiol, or progesterone, or testosterone.

Making "natural" hormones bioidentical to those in the human body is a process that must be done in the laboratory. We call it "synthesizing," from the Greek word meaning "a putting together, composition; to make something." Synthetic simply means "produced by synthesis." In common usage today, *synthetic* has come to mean "artificial," which is not always correct. Unithroid and Estrace are "synthetic" in that they have been made in the laboratory, rather than within a biological organism. Yet they are "natural" because they are the exact same molecular structure as the hormones made by the thyroid and ovary, respectively.

"Natural," Bioidentical Human Estrogens. The sources for the bioidentical human forms of ovarian hormones are actually precursor molecules called *sterols* found in plants such as soybeans and yams. The plant sterols are purified and chemically converted in the laboratory to produce chemical molecules identical to those made in the human body. Our body does not have the enzymes to make this conversion. The resulting 17-beta estradiol, progesterone, or testosterone is then compounded into standardized tablets that regulate the amount of hormone given. The standardization of dose in each tablet allows a physician to know exactly the amount given so that the prescription can be tailored to each individual woman's needs. This method is better than using health food store mixtures from plant/herbal sources, *because it is difficult to determine the correct dose of plant compounds,* or their unwanted effects in your body. Women buy these over-the-counter products because they are touted as more natural and

"safer" than prescription hormones. Neither claim is accurate. Purity isn't regulated, there may be heavy-metal contamination, and you also get additional chemicals native to plants that your body does not need.

I recommend using prescription-grade *17-beta estradiol,* which is what keeps your body's cellular machinery working at optimal effectiveness. There are several FDA-approved brands of 17-beta estradiol commercially available in this country, and all contain estradiol derived from soybean or wild-yam precursor molecules. Doctors have said in the media recently: "We don't have studies on bioidentical hormones." This is not correct. Obviously, in order to obtain FDA approval, studies were done and accepted as showing safety and effectiveness of these other products. These are (as of this writing): Estrace tablets and vaginal cream (FDA-approved in 1976), Gynediol tablets, transdermal patches (Alora, Climara, Vivelle, Vivelle DOT, Estraderm, Esclim), combination estradiol-progestin products (Activella, Ortho-Prefest, CombiPatch), and vaginal preparations such as Estrace creams, Vagifem tablets, and Estring vaginal ring.

I do not recommend using estriol, the weaker placenta-derived form of estrogen, because extensive studies over the last thirty to forty years have shown that it doesn't provide the necessary protective effects on bone, heart, brain, and nerves as does premenopausal 17-beta estradiol. In addition, use skepticism about the marketing hype that estriol is "safer" or "prevents breast cancer." Many studies have addressed this issue, and there is no reputable scientific data to support these claims.

Synthetic Estrogens: Not Native to the Human Body. All of these estrogens have slightly different chemical structures from the three human forms (estradiol, estrone, estriol) and are therefore more potent, and have somewhat different effects and side effects on the body. There are appropriate uses for each, such as contraception.

- **Ethinyl estradiol (EE):** *This is the most common form of estrogen found in the birth control pill. Birth control pills are widely used in perimenopausal women who need control of irregular cycles and erratic bleeding. I recommend BCP for this purpose. EE is not widely used in the United States for postmenopausal ERT because it is more potent than we need after reaching menopause and contraception is no longer needed.*
- **Estradiol valerate:** *Estradiol valerate is a synthetic estrogen commonly used for menopause therapy in Europe and other countries, but less so in the United States. It is available for oral or intramuscular delivery and is more potent and typically lasts longer than 17-beta estradiol. Once in the body, however, estradiol valerate separates into its two components and provides the same estradiol your ovaries made. Estradiol valerate was the estradiol used in the 1979 Swedish study that initially reported a higher risk of breast cancer in estrogen users. Follow-up analysis of the same data from the Swedish researchers published in 1992, showed no*

increase in breast cancer risk in users of any types of estrogen, including estradiol valerate. This update, however, did not get press attention or make headlines.

Phytoestrogens. Phytoestrogens are estrogenic compounds such as isoflavones found in several hundred different plants, including soybeans, red clover, and grains. These are biologically weaker than the native human estrogens, but there is another issue to consider: concentration in the bloodstream. Isoflavone supplements can quickly give high serum concentrations of the phytoestrogens that overwhelm the miniscule amounts of estradiol and wind up competing with and inhibiting the action of your own hormone. This makes your body's estradiol less effective. Health articles and product ads don't tell you this part of the picture.

Although the phytoestrogens are less potent than 17-beta estradiol, herbalists often recommend them as a "natural" source of estrogen. These products are heavily marketed for PMS and menopausal remedies, with claims that they are "safer" than our own hormones. But several recent double-blind, placebo-controlled, prospective studies in the international menopause literature have found that phytoestrogen products were no more effective than placebo even for controlling hot flashes, much less all the other functions of our own ovarian estradiol. There can also be adverse effects. Ginseng, for example, is often recommended, but it can cause high blood pressure, insomnia, anxiety, and agitation if taken in the currently recommended doses, and studies clearly show it does not have measurable estrogenic effect. These findings make sense when you consider that plant sterols are all chemically different molecular "keys" from our own estradiol.

At the Fork in the Road: Deciding What to Take

Premenopausal women who are still menstruating but experiencing ovarian decline and health risks like bone loss, or menopausal symptoms such as hot flashes or fragmented sleep, have two roads to consider: One is to use birth control pills; the other is to use natural hormonal supplementation with estradiol, progesterone, and testosterone as appropriate. There are advantages and disadvantages to each approach. If you decide on one, you haven't locked yourself in for the rest of your life. At any time, you can change your mind, stop what you are doing, and try another option.

Option I: Using Birth Control Pills to Put Your Ovaries at Rest

Birth control pills deliver hormones constantly. The steady dose of both estrogen and progestin mimics early pregnancy, telling the brain not to send out the FSH and LH signals to stimulate the ovaries for a menstrual cycle. The Pill suppresses your cycles and ovulation, preventing the roller-coaster ride of monthly hormone ups and downs, and effectively puts the ovaries "at rest." As a result of the steadier hormone levels, my patients tell me their PMS symptoms are often markedly diminished, and they feel more even.

You hear reports of unpleasant side effects with BCPs, or you may have tried them and felt terrible. In my experience, this usually happens when the progestin dose is too high and the estrogen too low. The key is to choose the pill with the right estrogen-to-progestin ratio for your body, which can help you feel better, calm the turbulence of your cycles, and minimize side effects. There are many new and more effective options available than even a decade ago. If you had a bad experience in the past, you may be pleasantly surprised with modern BCPs, or the patch, ring, or IUD.

Newer low-dose BCPs provide other health benefits beyond contraception and hormonal stability. In fact, in a medical article in *Ob. Gyn. News* in 1999, Dr. Patricia J. Sulak of the Scott and White Clinic in Temple, Texas, said, *"BCP are one of the most important preventive health measures in all of medicine. There's no medicine that offers reproductive-age women more benefits; there's nothing out there that even touches OCs [oral contraceptives]."*

Many studies show that women who *don't* stay on the pill have heavy periods and irregular periods, premenstrual syndrome, functional ovarian cysts, and a higher likelihood of endometriosis and fibroids. BCPs work especially well for women over thirty whose ovaries often start acting up with the beginning of ovarian decline. Since 80 to 90 percent of all women develop irregular bleeding before menopause, BCPs can help reduce the amount of menstrual flow as well as the common erratic bleeding. Women with PCOS can actually help preserve future fertility by starting BCPs at a younger age, and staying on them except when attempting pregnancy, and when breast-feeding.

There is other good news about the protective effects of oral contraceptives: Studies show they reduce the ovarian cancer risk by 50 to 60 percent, and endometrial cancer risk by more than 75 percent if taken five years or more. In addition, 1994 studies from Italy, along with others since, show a significant protective effect on maintaining bone density in women taking OCs during perimenopause. Other health benefits of birth control pills are listed in the box on page 315.

In my practice, I find patients gain additional benefits from BCPs, including

- *Better preservation of bone mass*
- *Reduced menstrual migraine frequency by continuous pill use, with no break for periods*
- *Reduced excess androgen effects in PCOS*
- *Improved muscle and joint pain*
- *Improved cyclic mood swings, decreased cyclic anxiety*
- *Improved energy, decreased fatigue*
- *Improved vulvar and vulvodynia pain (if low-progestin pills are used)*
- *Improved vaginal lubrication and interest in sex*

BENEFICIAL EFFECTS OF ORAL CONTRACEPTIVES

Condition or Disease	Decrease Compared to Nonpill Users
1. Menstrual Disorders	**DECREASE:**
Dysmenorrhea	63%
Menopausal symptoms	72%
Menorrhagia	48%
Irregular menstruation	35%
Intermenstrual bleeding	28%
Premenstrual tension (PMS)	29% [reduction in symptoms is better than this with low progestin–higher estrogen pill]
2. Reproductive Organ Tumors	**DECREASE:**
Breast: fibrocystic/fibroadenomas	60–75%
Breast biopsies	50%
Benign ovarian cysts	65% [using monophasic, steady-dose pills]
Uterine fibroids (fibroma)	59%
Ovarian cancer	40%
Endometrial cancer	50%
3. Other Reproductive Disorders	**DECREASE:**
Endometriosis	50–60%
Pelvic inflammatory disease	10–70%
Toxic shock syndrome	60%
Uterine retroversion	24%
4. Other Health Problems	**DECREASE:**
Rheumatoid arthritis	50%
Iron deficiency anemia	45%
Duodenal ulcer	40%
Sebaceous cysts	24% [better decrease with some progestins than others]
Acne	20% [better response rate with low-progestin dose and androgen-blocking progestins]

Richard P. Dickey, M.D., Ph.D. *Managing Contraceptive Pill Patients,* 11th edition, (Essential Medical Information Systems, 2002).

Comments in brackets by Dr. Vliet.

So how do you choose a birth control pill?

If you are using BCPs to decrease symptoms of PMS, PCOS, endometriosis, fibroids, heavy bleeding, or migraines, I recommend a BCP formula with a low progestin content relative to the estrogen to reduce typical progestin side effects like depression, weight gain, headaches, fatigue, acne, low sex drive, vaginal dryness, and other unwanted side effects. A pill that contains a steady dose *(monophasic)* of both estrogen and progestin gives better suppression of ovarian cycling and keeps you on a more even keel than does a triphasic pill that has varying hormone levels.

BCPs with better estrogen content (30–35 mcg of ethinyl estradiol), such as Ovcon 35, Modicon, Orthocyclen, Ortho-Cept, Yasmin, or Diane 35 are important for maintaining bone mass, improving mood/sleep/hot flashes, maintaining normal libido and orgasm ability, and so on. Pills with high progestin and low estrogen ratios (such as Alesse, Mircette, Loestrin) have more unwanted side effects of weight gain, bloating, constipation, acne, fatigue, depression, low sex drive, difficulty having an orgasm, and vaginal dryness, as well as erratic bleeding.

You need a certain amount of progestin to suppress ovary cycles and prevent hormone fluctuations that trigger symptoms and to protect the lining of the uterus from becoming too thick (hyperplasia) as it would if you took estrogen alone. A low-progestin pill still accomplishes both of these goals. The disadvantage is that with less progestin you might initially have more breakthrough bleeding and spotting, which can be annoying. This is temporary and should resolve after three to six months on the BCPs. If bleeding remains a problem, a straightforward way to manage it is to increase the progestin content for just a few months. You aren't likely to become depressed on the higher progestin if you just take it for a short time. Taking a higher progestin pill for two or three cycles usually stops the bleeding problems effectively. You can even do this every few months if needed.

When you stop the active hormone pills in the birth control pill pack, it is the drop in progestin that triggers a period, while the drop in estrogen causes headaches, muscle aches, insomnia, pain flares, or mood symptoms. To keep the estrogen level steady, to prevent headaches or other symptoms between BCP packs, I recommend the use of an estradiol pill or estradiol patch for the days off BCPs to prevent the drop in estrogen between pill packs. This low dose of estrogen doesn't typically alter bleeding, and can do a lot to decrease symptoms between pill packs.

If you prefer *not* having periods every month, you can take the active hormone pills every day, with no break between packs. Yes, you can be in control of when you have a period! This option seems to be a well-hidden secret. You simply throw away the placebo pills and go right into your next pill pack. You can do this for three to six packs and then stop for three or four days to have a period, if you wish. If you are taking the pills continuously and start to have bothersome breakthrough bleeding, stop them at any time for four to five days to have a period, which should typically alleviate that problem. Talk with your doctor about the suggestions above and also ask your doctor about supplemental estradiol whenever you stop the active BCPs if you have headaches or other symptoms from the drop in estrogen during your period.

Common side effects with BCPs. Whenever you increase the female hormones estrogen and progesterone (or the progestin in birth control pills), you can expect some breast tenderness and fullness, mild feelings of fluid retention or bloating, headaches, cramps, feelings of tiredness, and possibly "queasiness" or nausea like in early pregnancy. Initial weight gain of a few pounds is typically due to *fluid* balance changes, not increased body *fat*. These are usually temporary side effects and commonly resolve by about the third pill pack.

Breakthrough bleeding and spotting are also quite common in the early months of using any birth control pills. This usually stops after three to six months on the pill. Be patient. Most women tell me they feel much better overall with the pill, so it can be worth the inconvenience of some spotting for a while to achieve these other benefits.

Most studies to date show no increased risk of breast cancer in women who use the birth control pill. Check the National Cancer Institute graphs for the last forty years. You will see that over the time that BCPs exponentially increased in use, the graph for breast cancer has remained steady, and even began decreasing slightly in 1996. These graphs are available from the American Cancer Society (see Appendix II).

Please read your pill package insert for possible serious reactions. Notify your gynecologist or primary care physician promptly if you have any of these problems. And remember, *do not smoke cigarettes while taking birth control pills*, as smoking may increase your risk of stroke.

Transitioning: BCP to menopause HRT options. By using an oral contraceptive in the years of hormone decline, you typically do not experience the hot flashes and other symptoms that mark the endocrine transition to actual menopause. So how do you decide when to change to postmenopausal hormone options? This is best done with the assistance of a knowledgeable health professional so that you don't experience any unwanted effects from stopping oral contraceptives abruptly or from differences in potency of the birth control pills and the natural hormones.

I recommend that you have an annual blood test to measure FSH, beginning at age fifty or so. Take this test on the fifth to seventh days off the active birth control pills, during the "placebo" week when you menstruate. If the FSH is checked at the end of the week of placebo pills, you are off hormones long enough for FSH to rise into the menopausal range, if you are menopausal. If you have not yet reached menopause, the FSH will still be low on these days. If you check FSH while taking the hormone-containing BCPs, it is suppressed to a level usually less than 3 or 4 and will not give an accurate determination of your menopausal status.

You *do not* have to stop the oral contraceptives for several months in order to check the FSH, as many women are told. Your physician may not yet be aware of how and when to check FSH, since it is still relatively new to use oral contraceptives for perimenopausal women into their early fifties. If your FSH is greater than 20 mIU/ml on the days off the hormone-containing birth control pills, then you have reached the endocrine stage of menopause and it's time to consider a switch to the postmenopausal hormone options. If the FSH is still less than 20, you could possibly still become pregnant (although it is uncommon), and you may want to stay on the oral contraceptives until your FSH is higher than 20.

Option II: The Other Fork in the Road

What if you are still premenopausal and need a hormone "boost" but do not want to take birth control pills? There are options. You can choose to follow your cycle and supplement with 17-beta estradiol pills, patches, or creams to compensate for ovarian decline. This is a bit more complicated and unpredictable to manage, but it can work well for many women. You still experience the ups and downs of your cycle, but you ease the symptoms of low estradiol, as well as have its other benefits. When your own ovaries stop making progesterone, you need to add it to trigger a regular shedding of the uterine lining and prevent bleeding problems or excess buildup of the uterine lining (hyperplasia). There are several FDA-approved options available, as I explain below. For women with a normal cycle who have regular bleeding, body markers of ovulation with a rise in progesterone from the ovaries, you may ask your doctor about adding supplemental progesterone later, after regular cycles stop, you start skipping periods, can no longer feel yourself ovulating, or you have erratic bleeding.

Forms of estradiol. Typically, I find that 17-beta estradiol options give better relief of symptoms than conjugated equine estrogens (Premarin and PremPro) or esterified estrogens (Estratab and Estratest). You and your physician must work together to adjust your dose to give you levels closer to the healthy menstrual cycle range described earlier. For optimal benefits on pain, mood, and sleep pathways in particular, the dose may need to be adjusted because traditional HRT doses are based on the *minimally* effective dose.

Options include: (a) transdermal estradiol (Climara, Vivelle DOT, Esclim, and generics); (b) oral micronized estradiol (Estrace and Gynediol brands) or generic 17-beta estradiol ("estradiol"); (c) if the transdermal route is preferable, but you have rashes with patches, try a compounded prescription estradiol cream that can be absorbed through the skin; (d) the vaginal ring (Estring), vaginal cream (Estrace), or vaginal tablets (Vagifem) are all very good options for topical vaginal and urinary urogenital effects, but these doses are too low for significant systemic benefits (i.e., to relieve hot flashes, improve sleep, etc.); (e) injectable estrogens, or pellets and implants, are an option as well. These deliver higher levels initially, with an unpredictable fall in levels prior to next injection or implant. I use injectable forms occasionally if a particular woman does better with this route, but they are more difficult to regulate and fine-tune, especially if your own ovaries still make any measurable estradiol. I don't use estradiol implants because they are hard to regulate, and unlike patches and pills, a woman can't "stop" an implant herself if she's having problems.

Patch or pill? The brands of transdermal estrogen patches listed earlier are recent innovations. Their delivery of the human 17-beta estradiol is the most "natural" of all. The estradiol is absorbed through the skin, directly into the blood, much like the ovary delivers hormones to the bloodstream before menopause, without going through the stomach and liver first. The "first pass" metabolism in the liver breaks down some of the estradiol into estrone, making it less effective for estradiol's normal functions and adding some potential side effects. The estradiol patches all look like a circular, oval, or rectangular Band-Aid that sticks to the skin and stays in place for several days as the hormones are slowly absorbed. As the hormone delivery falls, the patch is replaced. Each brand of patch lasts for a slightly different time, and women metabolize the hormones at different rates, not necessarily at the rate specified by the manufacturer. Different brands also have very different adhesives, so it can take some experimentation to find the right brand and change schedule and dose strength for you. The patch has several advantages over oral delivery, as summarized below.

ADVANTAGES OF TRANSDERMAL ESTRADIOL OVER ORAL

- Patches keep blood levels of estradiol fairly steady, similar to ovarian hormone production.
- Bypassing the liver's first-pass metabolism can *decrease* triglycerides (TG). Oral estrogen in some women increases TG, which is not desirable because high TG is an independent risk factor for heart disease and diabetes in women.
- Transdermal delivery of estradiol improves glucose-insulin pathways, an important benefit for women with insulin resistance or diabetes.
- Patches provide better relief of hormonally triggered migraines due to slower rise and fall in blood levels.
- Patches typically have better dilating effects on blood vessels and help lower blood pressure more effectively than oral estrogen does.
- Patches typically *decrease* clotting factors like fibrinogen and blood pressure–raising factors (such as rennin substrate) better than oral estrogen does.
- Patches deliver much less estrone than oral forms, an advantage for overweight women whose body fat makes excess estrone, which is considered a risk factor for breast cancer.

© Elizabeth Lee Vliet, M.D., 2003

Patches are a very good option for estrogen therapy, with only two primary drawbacks: (1) the skin irritation from the adhesive bothers some women, and (2) if you have a low level of HDL, you may need the extra boost provided by oral estrogen stimulating the liver to make more HDL. The patch (as well as skin gels available in Europe) gives the beneficial *physiological* (normal) effect of estrogen to maintain the normal level of HDL cholesterol, but not the *pharmacologic* (greater than normal) effect of extra liver stimulation to make more HDL as seen with the oral estrogens. If you have a normal cholesterol profile, the patch should be all you need for the physiologic benefits. If you have *high* total cholesterol and *low* HDL, an *oral* form of estradiol typically provides greater *decrease* in total cholesterol and *increase* in HDL for desirable cardiovascular effects.

Progesterone. I frequently use compounded natural progesterone for my patients, as well as the FDA-approved products, Prometrium and Crinone. For many women, the natural hormone progesterone causes fewer side effects than the synthetic progestins (Provera, Cycrin, MPA, norethindrone, levonorgestrel, etc.), but there are also times when the potency of the synthetics provides better control of medical problems such as heavy bleeding or endometriosis. Furthermore, some women just feel better on one of the synthetics than they do with natural progesterone. There is a great deal of individual variation, so ignore the sweeping generalizations that one is always better than another. Find out which option helps you feel your best.

Current accepted doses for progesterone to provide therapeutic effects on the uterine lining (endometrium) without excess buildup (hyperplasia) are as follows:

1. *For a **cyclic regimen**, the usual dose is 200 mg of oral micronized progesterone (i.e., Prometrium) for ten to fourteen days a month. If you are allergic to peanut oil and can't use Prometrium, compounded forms are available. Crinone is a vaginal gel in sustained release form, and the 4 percent strength is given every other night for six doses a month. The FDA-approved dose schedule gives 40 mg every other day, or an average daily dose of 20 mg. If Crinone isn't readily available, a similar preparation can be made up by a compounding pharmacist.*
2. *For a **continuous daily regimen**, the accepted dose is 100 mg oral progesterone every day, usually best given at bedtime because it is sedating for most women.*

Note: Progestins are more potent than natural progesterone, and are therefore used in much lower doses. For example, Provera (MPA) or Aygestin (norethindrone) 2.5 mg is usually given for a daily schedule, or 5 mg is used for ten to fourteen days in a cyclic regimen. For women using lower doses of estradiol, Micronor or Nor QD (0.35 mg norethindrone) may be sufficient to prevent hyperplasia, and the lower dose has fewer side effects.

Caution: Progesterone doses in excess of 300 mg a day orally (or creams containing more than 20–30 mg per day) cause blood levels of progesterone that are as high as those found in the third trimester of pregnancy. I see women getting prescriptions for 100 mg per gram of progesterone creams, to be applied twice daily. Such a dose is excessive, particularly since the FDA-approved dosing for transdermal versus oral is usually for transdermal forms to be about one tenth of the typical oral dose. If you do the math, you can quickly see that 100 mg/gm cream is roughly equivalent to about 1,000 mg oral progesterone. Two applications of such a cream each day would give you roughly the equivalent of taking 2,000 mg in a pill or tablet! Compare this with the dose of Crinone approved by the FDA and you see the difference. No wonder women using this feel fat, bloated, and depressed!

Higher doses of progesterone are often recommended for PMS treatment, but can cause or aggravate many other problems: marked weight gain similar to pregnancy; high blood glucose and decreased glucose control in diabetics or women with insulin resistance; high triglycerides; high cholesterol; higher than normal insulin production; more backaches, due to ligaments becoming lax or "loose" from progesterone effects; headaches, or intensified migraines; decreased sex drive; and depressed, lethargic mood.

One problem is that many health specialists who recommend such high doses of natural progesterone do not check serum levels of progesterone, do not monitor the cholesterol-triglyceride profile, and do not check for changes in fasting glucose and insulin. They miss these developing problems. In addition, excess progesterone often causes lethargy and fatigue. Be careful about too much progesterone, especially if you are overweight, have diabetes, hypertension, elevated cholesterol or triglycerides, or a history of depression.

If you think progesterone is a "wonder" hormone and doubt the potential for serious side effects with it, simply recall two common pregnancy-related problems most women know: pregnancy-induced ("gestational") diabetes, and toxemia or preeclampsia, a severe form of high blood pressure that occurs in the latter part of pregnancy. These two problems often occur in the last stages of pregnancy when progesterone levels are at their highest. If you use natural progesterone for hormone therapy, stick with the FDA-approved and medically accepted dose ranges.

Testosterone or DHEA. Consider adding androgen if you have documented low serum levels, but do not base a treatment decision on the highly variable and unreliable saliva test for testosterone and DHEA. Serious side effects can occur with too much of either. Pain, headaches, acne, hair loss, insomnia, anxiety, and irritability are worse if androgens are given before optimal estradiol is restored. In addition, it is far better to restore testosterone directly than to try DHEA, since the conversion of DHEA to testosterone is fairly unpredictable, especially if your ovaries are declining or have been surgically removed.

Women's testosterone levels are obviously not the same as those of men. For some time the only synthetic testosterone available was methyl testosterone, the one associated with causing liver damage, and a few others not natural to the human body. Until more recently doctors were not aware that women needed considerably lower doses of testosterone. This is the root of horror stories about testosterone causing mustaches and beards, voice changes, and liver damage. It isn't that the hormone is bad; it is that we haven't had the native form available, commercial doses have been too high, and it hasn't been used with much finesse for women!

Through the miracle of the laboratory, soybeans are turned into *boy*beans, now that scientists can synthesize exact molecular replicas of women's own testosterone. Using the micronization process, we now have a form of natural testosterone that is not lost to the digestive process when taken orally, just like we have for progesterone and estradiol. Prescription-grade (USP) testosterone is standardized, so I know exactly how much of the hormone I prescribe and can fine-tune it for each individual. Testosterone is made up, by compounding pharmacists, as skin cream, skin gel, sublingual tablets, injections, and vaginal suppositories. The method of delivery determines the amount absorbed, how it metabolizes into other forms, and the effects—desirable or undesirable. Gels and troches are often touted as "best," but I find that the slower absorption forms cause fewer problems because a rapid rise in blood level of testosterone can cause aggressiveness, pounding headaches, insomnia, and irritability.

Currently, commercial brands of testosterone don't have doses low enough for women on a daily basis. Compounded prescriptions allow a fine-tuning of the dose. I use a sustained-release tablet or capsule, or a slow-release cream form. Oral doses generally are 1–4 mg daily. Transdermal cream doses need to be lower, since non-oral routes (transdermal, vaginal, sublingual) have more rapid and more complete absorption as a result of bypassing the first-pass metabolism in the liver that increases breakdown. You and your health professionals need to understand this, because many women get excessive doses of testosterone creams or sublingual troches, which can create horrible side effects. For example, a 2 percent testosterone cream (widely recommended in a number of women's health books) contains *20 mg/gram* of cream delivering about **20 times** the dose most women need in this readily absorbed form. By comparison, most of my testosterone prescriptions are for 0.125 mg/gram up to about 1 mg/gram (0.1 percent) of cream (1 gram = ¼ teaspoon of cream).

Most women need only very small amounts of testosterone to achieve desired benefits. I usually start patients on 1.00–1.25 mg of oral sustained-release micronized testosterone and gradually increase based on the woman's description of symptoms and her serum levels. Most women achieve the desirable response at an oral dose between 1 and 4 mg a day. Recheck the testosterone level in the morning before your next dose, to be sure it isn't remaining too high twenty-four hours after you take it. If you want to be sure the dose is providing enough testosterone, check a blood level about 4 hours after a dose.

Sometimes oral doses are not absorbed adequately for desirable blood levels or cause adverse changes in cholesterol. Changing to a gradually absorbed transdermal cream often improves the overall response. The transdermal cream form of testosterone (and DHEA, when appropriate) is less likely to have negative effects on the good HDL cholesterol, since absorption into the bloodstream through the skin bypasses the liver first-pass metabolism. Cream forms are an option for testosterone therapy for women with high cholesterol or low HDL who need the other benefits of testosterone. A testosterone patch for women is in clinical trials, but not yet available.

To help you make the important decisions about what is best for you and your health needs, I have summarized the benefits of adding testosterone to a hormone therapy regimen (see below). I also give you some pointers on what to look for as effects of too little or too much testosterone or DHEA.

Summary of Testosterone and DHEA Effects

TOO LITTLE	JUST RIGHT	TOO MUCH
low energy	normal energy	hyper feelings
loss of sex drive	normal libido	increased libido
slowed down	alert, interested	"scattered" thoughts, similar to ADHD
depressed mood	positive mood	irritable, anxious, edgy, tense, aggressive
fewer dreams	normal dreams	intense dreaming, aggressive dreams, violent dreams, disrupted sleep
thin, fine hair	hair thicker	increased facial hair
hair loss (alopecia)	normal hair growth	hair loss (alopecia)
dry, thin skin	normal skin	acne, oily skin
loss of muscle mass and strength	healthy muscle mass	muscle spasms and tenseness, aching

Step 4: Monitor Effectiveness and Adjust as Needed

The importance of checking estradiol levels to monitor progress and effectiveness of treatment was dramatically shown in a 1998 study by Drs. Vihtamaki and Tuimala. They evaluated whether women and their doctors correctly judged estrogen dose solely based on the degree of improvement in symptoms. Interestingly, they found that as many as 45 percent of women who had reported their symptoms completely relieved still had serum estradiol levels below the currently accepted thresholds for protective estradiol effects on the brain, bone, and other target tissues. These physicians concluded that we cannot tell by symptom relief alone that women are getting the right amount of estradiol. They stated definitively that follow-up blood tests are necessary for proper monitoring, just as physicians do with other hormones like thyroid.

How often do you need to recheck levels? Generally, about every two or three months after the start or change of medication, or when new symptoms appear or grow worse. Treatment decisions should be based on *both* clinical symptoms *and* objective laboratory results.

If You Are Sensitive to Progestins, What Else Is Available?

There is a new contraceptive patch, **Ortho Evra**, that contains ethinyl estradiol and the progestin norelgestromin. Ortho Evra is worn on the abdomen, and a new patch is applied once a week. It is designed to release 20 mcg ethinyl estradiol and 150 mcg of norelgestromin per twenty-four hours, in a steady, gradual absorption. Since it is a non-oral combination contraceptive, it should have fewer of the typical side effects such as nausea and headaches that can occur with an oral BCP. This is also a better option for women who have elevated triglycerides, since the non-oral form doesn't typically aggravate this problem. Another plus is that you don't have to remember to take a pill every day.

Nuvaring is a new contraceptive in the form of a soft vaginal ring, containing both ethinyl estradiol (15 mcg or 0.015 mg) and a new progestin called etonogestrel (0.120 mg). This product allows both hormones to be slowly released into the vaginal tissue and then absorbed directly into the bloodstream, bypassing the "first-pass" effect through the liver. This means lower doses of both hormones can be used, which in turn helps to minimize the typical side effects that often occur with oral BCPs. The ring is pliable and easy to insert by a woman herself. It is removed at the end of three weeks if you want to have your usual period. If you want to skip a menstrual period, you may leave the ring in place for four weeks, which keeps the hormone delivery steady and prevents the drop in progestin that triggers a period. Nuvaring has worked very well for many of our patients who had bothersome side effects with the oral pills, so it may be an option to discuss with your physician. To read more about it, check the website *www.nuvaring.com*.

Mirena and **Progestasert** are two intrauterine progestin-delivery systems approved as contraceptives rather than as progestin therapy in peri- or menopausal women, but they are options for women who have side effects with oral progestins. Both release a small amount of progestin daily directly into the lining of the uterus, and very little progestin is absorbed into the total body circulation. This reduces the likelihood of the unpleasant side effects—headaches, depression, low libido, weight gain, and vaginal dryness—often associated with progestins in hormone therapy and birth control pills. Some women use these intrauterine delivery systems successfully if they cannot tolerate any other form. A number of recent studies show that these products deliver enough progestin to effectively suppress the buildup of the uterine lining. There are some drawbacks, however, so it is important to discuss these issues with your health professional.

Possible problems with either Mirena or Progestasert include increase in ovarian cysts, increased risk of pelvic inflammatory disease if there are multiple sexual partners, increased risk of ectopic pregnancy, erratic bleeding, and menstrual changes. If you need a progestin and nothing else has worked, ask your doctor about these products. Pregnancy rates are less than 0.02 percent, and the IUD (Mirena or Progestasert) also reduces the amount of monthly bleeding for most women after the initial three- to six-month adjustment. After a year, about 20 percent of women have no further bleeding. Mirena can be changed every five years, and Progestasert is changed annually.

In Summary

If you decide to use hormone approaches to correct health problems and relieve troublesome symptoms, there is a systematic way to achieve your goals and minimize unwanted effects. There are many options to try. Work with a knowledgeable health professional to create a hormone supplement program fine-tuned to your body's needs to restore the balance of your natural levels. It can be done.

Don't expect quick solutions to complex problems, however. It takes time, persistence, and patience. If you have complex problems and many different symptoms, or are sensitive to medications, it could take six to twelve months to find exactly the right combination for your needs so that your body can heal and repair for overall improvement. There are reliable, objective measures that will help you track your progress, in addition to your observations and feelings. Don't settle for feeling lousy every day. Don't continue what doesn't work. There are a variety of ways to rekindle your sexual spark, energy level, and vitality.

17

Test-and-Treat Strategies for Optimal Thyroid, Adrenal, and Glucose-Insulin Balance

Introduction

Although this is an "ovary" book, we certainly can't take the isolationist approach of talking about one body part or one hormone system separate from all the rest. You have seen the many ways that the ovaries interact with other body systems and how the ovarian hormones affect many other pathways and functions of the body beyond reproduction. Here I highlight how to get checked for other common hormone imbalances, describe some pitfalls to avoid with treatment and techniques I use to help women restore optimal hormone balance.

Keep in mind as you read this chapter, many women have the mistaken idea that if their basal body temperature is lower than 98.6 in the mornings, it automatically means they have hypothyroidism, even if other thyroid tests are in the desirable ranges. There are many causes of lower than normal body temperature, including ovarian hormone decline. There is a great deal of overlap in the symptoms that occur with imbalances of your thyroid, ovarian, adrenal, glucose-insulin pathways. If you want a clear picture of *what* is out of balance and how to fix it, you must have a careful, complete, systematic hormone evaluation that looks at all these pieces of the puzzle, rather than just rely on a list of symptoms to make a "diagnosis."

Thyroid Tests: What to Have Checked and How to Interpret Your Results

Thyroid disorders can be a significant cause of infertility, menstrual irregularity, and abnormal ovarian hormone production. Too often, thyroid symptoms like fatigue or low energy or memory loss are dismissed as "stress." Young women can and do experience thyroid problems even when TSH is normal. We see a lot of women in their forties and fifties who have had hypothyroid symptoms for years, going back to their twenties and thirties, and have been unable to have them properly diagnosed even though their quality of life was eroded away. I want you to understand some basics about thyroid testing and treatment approaches. Then find a physician who will work with you to get it done right. My message: Don't let a potential thyroid problem go untreated; if you do, you will have more serious and chronic health problems later.

Complete thyroid testing (including antibodies) is crucial if there are any of the mood or fatigue symptoms described earlier, particularly during the postpartum period. You also need complete tests of thyroid function if you have developed other problems, such as high blood pressure, heart arrhythmias, high cholesterol, marked weight gain, diabetes, depression, anxiety, or memory, attention, and concentration difficulties.

Most standard thyroid panels, particularly in HMO settings, only check TSH and *total* thyroid hormones because this standard profile is cheaper and saves the insurance company money. For women with infertility or menstrual irregularities and symptoms that may be caused by thyroid disorders, however, I find these standard profiles inadequate to diagnose early phases of thyroid imbalance. Thyroid antibodies, even though not checked in the standard profile, may be significantly elevated and cause thyroid dysfunction and infertility, although the TSH is still within the normal range. In addition, it is really the amount of thyroid hormones present in the bloodstream in the free, active form that determines how effectively your thyroid hormones are working. This is especially the case for women taking birth control pills, since they affect thyroid binding globulin.

I always check *free* T3 and *free* T4 as well as *both* types of thyroid antibodies in my patients. I suggest you ask your doctor to do the same. There isn't a major difference in cost, and the information is far more helpful in sorting out the cause of your problems, as well as fine-tuning any thyroid medicines. The following thyroid tests are the ones I think are important for women. These tests can be done on any day of your menstrual cycle:

- *Ultra-sensitive thyroid stimulating hormone (TSH)*
- *Free T4 (levothyroxine)*
- *Free T3 (triiodothyronine)*
- *Antimicrosomal antibody (antithyroid peroxidase antibody, or anti-TPO), an antibody to the thyroid gland tissue*
- *Antithyroglobulin antibody, an antibody to the T4 thyroid hormone itself*
- *Thyroid binding globulin, a measure of the carrier protein level in the bloodstream. It can be increased or decreased by a variety of medicines and dietary factors, so checking the level may help sort out a puzzling thyroid problem.*
- *The thyroid releasing hormone (TRH) stimulation test is also available, but I generally don't find it necessary if the ones above are done. Ideally, this test should be done by an endocrinologist, since it requires awareness of pitfalls and special considerations to interpret it properly.*

Go for What's Optimal, Not Just What's "Normal"

If a health professional tells you that your thyroid tests are "normal," that doesn't mean you still could not have a subtle thyroid dysfunction contributing to your menstrual disturbances, infertility, fatigue, or mood or weight problems. In fact, for women, these symptoms commonly occur before TSH goes up into an obviously abnormal range. It's a little like waiting for the lake to go bone dry before you call it a water shortage, instead of taking conservation steps when you see the water level is down. In our practice, we find that women are often told that their thyroid is "normal," without having the complete thyroid tests done. When I do the more complete testing procedure, I often find elevated antibodies or low free fractions of T3 and T4 hormones to explain puzzling symptoms.

Another key point is that many women, and too many physicians, don't take into account that a "normal range" on a laboratory report is just that: a range. Each one of you will feel your best at a somewhat different point along that range. Some of you will require higher than "normal"—or lower—levels in order to feel well and to function optimally. We must look at the lab results in conjunction with the symptoms described by each individual. After all, as a physician, I am treating *people,* not lab values.

It is also possible that one or more lab measures may fall in the normal range while other, more subtle measures—such as thyroid antibodies—are abnormal. This is when it is very important to listen with an open mind to each woman, and her descriptions of what is wrong, and trust in what she says and knows about her body. As a general rule of thumb, I like to see women's TSH between 0.5 and about 2.0 to indicate *optimal* thyroid function. I can't easily give you actual numbers for optimal levels of free T3 and free T4 because these will vary depending on what lab you use, what test they do, and what units of measure they are using, all of which affect the reference range.

The Dangers of "Wilson's Syndrome" Protocols and Relying on Basal Body Temperature Tests

Women ask about a condition of impaired conversion of T4 to T3 that Dr. Denis Wilson purportedly "discovered" and named for himself ("Wilson's syndrome"). This condition has actually been in thyroid medical textbooks for many years, and was not newly discovered by Dr. Wilson. It is one of the many defects in the thyroid pathways that come under the larger heading of "thyroid resistance syndromes." Failure to adequately convert T4 to T3 can have many causes.

Difficulty making sufficient T3 clearly exists and is more common in women than men, particularly in the early stages of an autoimmune thyroiditis. In women with disturbed menstrual cycles, a test of free T3 is actually more critical than the standard T4 measures, since T3 is vital to brain regulatory pathways, ovarian interactions, and muscle and fat metabolism. The blood test for free T3 is accurate and helps answer the question of whether the body converts T4 to T3 or not.

Ignoring the advances in blood testing methods in the last two decades, proponents of Wilson's syndrome tell you that blood tests are not reliable and recommend checking your morning basal body temperature orally or under your arm (axillary temperature) to see if you have low free T3. The publications further direct you to increase the amount of T3 you take until your morning body temperature is back to normal at 98.6 degrees. This has led to many women having the mistaken idea that if their basal body temperature is lower than 98.6 in the mornings, it automatically means hypothyroidism, even if other thyroid tests are in the desirable ranges. There are *many* causes of lower than normal body temperature, including ovarian hormone decline.

Doctors who recommend the basal body temperature method, like Wilson, Broda Barnes, and many fibromyalgia specialists, have ignored basic female biology. Women's ovarian hormones are also important body temperature regulators. Most women know this from their own experiences each month. If low estradiol is the cause of body temperature problems, you can't get your body temperature back to "normal" just by taking T3 hormone. In fact, you may wind up hospitalized, because the combination of low estradiol and excess T3 can cause potentially lethal heart rhythm disturbances, dangerously high blood pressure, and sudden death. Excess T3 and low estradiol can also accelerate bone loss and cause severe anxiety and insomnia.

Excess T3 alone can also cause high blood pressure, severe palpitations, and shortness of breath, nervousness, panic attacks, agitation, irritability, increased sweating, and fatigue from overstimulation throughout the body. All of these problems are intensified by low estradiol. (Remember, excess thyroid will suppress normal ovarian function, which then makes the estradiol even lower.) Even with excess T3, however, basal body temperatures typically remain low unless you also restore estradiol levels to optimal ranges.

Today, with the sensitivity of current test methods, we can get a reliable answer to the T3 issue to determine a thyroid problem, along with reliable blood tests of estradiol and cortisol. Your physician needs to use thyroid medication carefully to avoid serious problems from too much. And, *you* should not change your thyroid medication on your own, without specific guidance from your physician, based on reliable blood test results.

When to Consider Starting Thyroid Medication

On most laboratory scales, hypothyroidism is considered to begin with TSH values greater than 4 or 5, although many physicians don't treat with thyroid medication until the TSH rises over 8. In my opinion, such a rigid view overlooks the point I made earlier: In women, weight gain, increased blood pressure and cholesterol, menstrual irregularity, infertility, PMS, depression, and memory loss are occurring long before the TSH goes that high. In addition, current studies in the infertility field have found that women often have difficulty conceiving if their TSH is much above 2.0. In my view, if we wait until TSH is above 5, it allows all of these problems to get worse unnecessarily.

I prefer to begin treatment earlier, in a preventive approach. In our practice, we may start very low doses of thyroid medication when the TSH is only 3 or so, especially if thyroid antibodies are high, or if the free T3 or free T4 are lower than optimal and women are having a lot of symptoms of low thyroid. The earlier treatment is begun, the less likely you are to develop all the other adverse effects of low thyroid, such as high blood pressure, elevated cholesterol, impaired cognitive function, or serious weight gain. It will also be easier to regain optimal health if you aren't starting from rock bottom. To return to the lake analogy I used earlier, it is easier and faster to replenish the water supply if it is just low, not bone dry!

Thyroid Medication Options

If you need to take thyroid medication, or are already taking it, you may be wondering if it is better to take synthetic, pure bioidentical T4 (Synthroid, Unithroid, Levoxyl, and generic levothyroxine) or a mixed, *animal-derived* T4-T3 blend (such as Armour thyroid). Should you take "natural" or "synthetic"? And what is the difference? It is important to remember that *natural* can mean *bioidentical* to what your body makes, or it can mean coming from a biological (natural) source, which may be chemically different from the molecule made by your body. *Synthetic* can simply mean "made in a laboratory" to be identical to what your body makes, or it can also mean "chemically new" and unlike that which your body makes. It is crucial for you to know the difference and not get caught in marketing ploys.

Now that scientists have identified the exact molecular makeup of T4, they have been able to create ("synthesize") an identical copy to what the body makes. This has given us standardized commercial preparations of the T4 thyroid hormone, such as the brands Unithroid, Synthroid, Levoxyl, as well as generic tablets of L-thyroxine (T4, or levothyroxine) made by different manufacturers. All of these are identical to the human T4 thyroid hormone, even though they are made in a laboratory. These are "natural" for your body because the body can't tell the difference between this carbon-copy molecule and the T4 molecule made by your own thyroid gland. These FDA-approved commercial products have been successfully used to manage thyroid problems in millions of people worldwide over the last six decades. Don't be misled about their safety and effectiveness by all the marketing hoopla about "natural" products being "better" for you. For most people, the T4 in these products will be converted by the thyroid gland and body tissues to adequate amounts of T3. If this conversion does not take place normally, you can take natural, bioidentical T3 using either a commercial, short-acting one called Cytomel, or a specially compounded, sustained release form of T3 that is available from compounding pharmacies.

It has become quite confusing to consumers because there has recently been a lot of marketing of one brand, Armour thyroid, as a "natural" thyroid that's better for you than Unithroid, Synthroid, or Levoxyl. Armour thyroid is "natural" because it is derived from a biological source—desiccated (dried) animal thyroid tissue—and contains both T4 and T3. This blend of T3 and T4, however, is not the same, natural ratio of these two hormones that we have in our body. As a result, this product often provides more T3 than you need and not enough T4.

Since it is a fixed-dose combination, it cannot be individually fine-tuned to your needs as we can do if we use separate tablets of T4 and T3. I prefer to get the best balance that is natural for your body and not use a ratio natural to a pig or cow!

With the increasing concern about prion contaminants (viral-type particles) in livestock that can lead to lethal brain diseases, I am concerned about the safety of taking thyroid tablets made from ground-up animal glands. While the meat supply in the United States is considered safe, we don't always know the true source of animal tissue used for some of these products, especially the OTC "thyroid glandulars." This is a risk I prefer not to take when we have standardized, effective, non-animal-derived bioidentical thyroid hormone products available.

My other concern with animal-derived hormones is that they have the potential to cause our bodies to form antibodies to the hormones and to our own endocrine glands. This was one of the early problems recognized decades ago with the animal-derived insulin given to diabetics, and also with the allergies to horse serum when this was used in the past as a base for many injections. Most of these problems have been resolved with the development of synthetic human insulin and injections no longer being given in a horse serum base. Similar problems occurred with animal-derived thyroid products when they were all we had and therefore used more widely. I have seen too many women develop high levels of both types of thyroid antibodies when taking animal-derived thyroid products long-term, so I prefer not to use them for this reason. Unithroid, Synthroid, Levoxyl, and the generic brands of levothyroxine (T4) are not animal-derived, so they don't have animal residue to stimulate antibody production. This is a good example of how "natural" sources are not always better for humans.

If you need T3 in addition to T4, I have found that there are better options than Armour thyroid. Cytomel is a commercial T3 product that has been in use in the United States for several decades. It can be effective, but it has a very short duration of effect, which means people often experience too much T3 stimulation soon after taking it, and then feel a "crash" when it wears off. I have used Cytomel over the years, but my patients often don't like the "rise" and "fall" feeling they have with it. That led me to look for a longer-lasting preparation of T3.

About 1986, I asked a pharmacist if he could compound a sustained-release T3. He was able to make a very successful, long-acting T3 tablet. He uses a hypoallergenic base to help reduce the possibility of allergic reactions, which is very good for chemically sensitive people with a lot of allergies. Since that time, I have primarily used this compounded T3 whenever I have patients who need this added to a commercial T4 product. Doses can be made up to be as low or as high as needed, rather than being limited to the few commercial strengths available. Using separate tablets, I can individualize the doses of each hormone to give the right balance for each person. You can check Appendix II for pharmacy suggestions that your own doctor can use to order these sustained-release T3 prescriptions if it is something that is appropriate for you.

To Be Safe: Start Low, Go Slow

Too much thyroid, too fast, will commonly cause rapid heartbeat, palpitations, headaches, anxiousness, irritability, or insomnia. Keep in mind also that symptoms of too much thyroid are the same ones that occur if your estradiol is too low. If thyroid is added too quickly before estradiol is optimal, it is like someone pouring gasoline on a fire! Your heart races, your mind races, you are not sleeping, and your head pounds. Not much fun. So don't overdo the thyroid, thinking you can feel better faster. Start with a low dose, and increase slowly, using laboratory results and your doctor's advice, as well as your body's response, to guide the dose changes.

When I prescribe one of the T4 products, especially for women who have other hormone imbalances, I usually start at half the lowest commercial dose for about two weeks. I then work to increase the dosage gradually, based on how my patient tells me she feels and on how the TSH is responding. I'd like to see the TSH from about 0.5 to 2.0. Then, if there are remaining symptoms of low thyroid function and the free T3 is low, I may add T3 starting with a very low dose, such as 5 mcg. Again, I increase very slowly. If 5 mcg feels like too much at once, I suggest splitting the tablet, taking half in the morning and half at lunchtime. If you take T3 much later than lunchtime, it may cause restless sleep due to overstimulation of the brain pathways.

It can become complicated when working with the ovarian and thyroid hormones at the same time, since they affect each other in a variety of ways and the symptoms of being either too high or too low often mimic each other. Therefore, I prefer to stabilize the ovarian hormones with whatever approach a woman prefers, and then work with the thyroid balancing—unless the TSH is so high that the hypothyroidism simply must be treated right away. It can be quite a juggling act, and I often find I have to combine our "science" (lab tests) along with a lot of "art" (clinical judgment and listening to the person) in order to decide what to do at any given time.

Thyroid hormone replacement is a clearly a complex topic. These are the highlights of some crucial issues I think are important for you to address in working with your physicians. *I do not advocate using thyroid hormone supplements just because you feel tired all the time, or just based on low body temperature, or solely for weight loss if all of the laboratory studies are completely normal, including thyroid antibodies.* Too much thyroid can actually cause fatigue; and also weight *gain* in the early stages, by stimulating appetite to fuel the excess thyroid-induced metabolic demands. Excess thyroid can also cause significant wasting of skeletal muscles throughout the body, leading to more weakness and more fatigue that makes you incorrectly think you need thyroid. If you also have low estradiol and testosterone, this is another cause of both muscle and bone loss. It is critical to check both ovarian and thyroid hormones carefully before making treatment decisions. Serious health consequences can occur if women are given excess thyroid hormones when they don't really have a thyroid problem. Recent news headlines described several women who were hospitalized for complications of excess thyroid. Don't be tempted to take a "quick fix" approach to fatigue, low energy, or weight problems by increasing thyroid medication. Especially do not increase your medicine on your own. It is dangerous and you may end up with more problems than you bargained for.

Cortisol: What to Have Checked and How to Interpret Your Results

A serum cortisol at eight A.M. or four P.M. is the most reliable first step in checking for low or high cortisol; sometimes endocrinologists also do a twenty-four-hour urine for free cortisol. Saliva tests are not reliable measures of cortisol to diagnose Cushing's or Addison's disease.

High cortisol. An eight A.M. serum cortisol level higher than 20–25 mcg/dl is considered abnormal and suggests the need for additional tests to clarify the cause. The typical tests that are done include serum free cortisol, corticotropin binding globulin (CBG), ACTH, twenty-four-hour urine for urinary free cortisol, and dexamethasone suppression test (DST). If the DST shows morning or afternoon cortisol higher than 5 mcg/dl the day after you take 1 mg of dexamethasone, then I recommend you have a thorough evaluation for possible Cushing's disease. This will involve further tests, such as serum ACTH, both serum and twenty-four-hour urine for free cortisol. A corticotrophin releasing hormone (CRH) stimulation test may be appropriate, and this is usually done by endocrinologists. If these follow-up tests are abnormal, imaging studies (MRI, CAT scans, etc.) are usually ordered to check the adrenal glands and pituitary for possible tumors causing the excess cortisol production.

Low cortisol. An eight A.M. cortisol lower than 5 to 7 mcg/dl is suggestive of adrenal insufficiency if your electrolytes are also abnormal. If the eight A.M. cortisol is greater than 10 mcg/dl, and your serum electrolytes (sodium, potassium) are normal, this makes it very unlikely that you have adrenal insufficiency, or "adrenal exhaustion," the current buzzword. If your cortisol is low and you have low sodium and high potassium, I urge you to see an endocrinologist who has experience with these disorders. AI, also called Addison's disease, is a serious metabolic illness that can cause death if not properly evaluated and treated. It should *not* be self-treated with over-the-counter adrenal supplements.

There are additional tests that should be done to confirm the diagnosis and identify any possible causes. A serum ACTH, and ACTH (Cortrosyn) stimulation tests are generally done next to evaluate the cause of adrenal insufficiency (for example, adrenal destruction or pituitary dysfunction). If you are having fatigue, weakness, and a low energy level and your cortisol is above 10 and below 20, you should have your other hormone systems tested as I have discussed, since these symptoms have many causes in addition to adrenal problems. Remember, true adrenal insufficiency is associated with marked weight *loss* in virtually *all* people who have it, so if you are *gaining* weight, it is highly unlikely that you have adrenal insufficiency.

Make sure you see a physician experienced with the various medicines that are used to replace the inadequate adrenal production of cortisol, and knowledgeable about side effects and problems that can occur. It can be dangerous to take over-the-counter "adrenal support" supplements, or "adrenal glandulars," especially if you have only had saliva tests or "kinesiology" (muscle testing) to check for low cortisol and adrenal insufficiency. I have seen many women who have been told that they have "adrenal exhaustion" based on these unreliable tests, but then when serum cortisol assays were done at the proper times of day, they actually had *high* cortisol reflecting the stress response from other hormone imbalances and/or the excess corticosteroid medicine. Adrenal glandulars and "herbal adrenal support" products sold in health food stores are animal-derived, with the same potential problems I described for animal-derived thyroid products—allergic reactions, stimulation of antibody formation, or prion contamination. Taking these products may actually suppress your own adrenal hormones further, or could add to the problem of high cortisol.

Getting Tested for Insulin and Glucose
Chapter 13 describes the multiple health problems that occur when glucose and insulin are out of kilter. Here's how to get properly tested.

Fasting tests. First have a blood test for fasting glucose and insulin, measured first thing in the morning, at least twelve hours after your last meal. A healthy fasting glucose should be in the 65–100 mg/dl range. Normal fasting insulin is usually 6–25 micro-International Units per milliliter (mIU/ml), depending on which assay the lab uses.

Some labs show a "normal" fasting glucose as high as 115 mg/dl, but the latest diabetes research indicates that if your fasting glucose is above 100, it suggests the beginning of glucose intolerance, which can lead to insulin resistance.

These are the new diagnostic criteria for diabetes from the American Diabetes Association:

- *Fasting glucose greater than 126 mg/dl*
- *A casual (random) glucose greater than 200 mg/dl along with symptoms, or*
- *A two-hour postprandial glucose greater than 200 mg/dl*

Postprandial (after meals) tests. Another way to check for early stages of glucose intolerance, insulin resistance, or diabetes is to measure glucose and insulin two or three hours after a typical meal. This test is called a two- or three-hour postprandial glucose and insulin, and tracks how high your glucose and insulin rise in response to eating. The results are more helpful if you eat a meal that is usual for you, rather than "loading up" on protein, as some lab staff tell women.

A two-hour postprandial glucose between 140 and 200 mg/dl indicates you have impaired glucose tolerance. If your two-hour postprandial glucose is over 200, you likely have diabetes and need a thorough evaluation by your physician.

A typical two-hour postprandial insulin range is 6–35 mIU/ml. Both the fasting range above, and this postprandial range, are generally accepted, but different laboratories use different assays with different reference ranges. As a result, insulin results are not as standardized as are glucose tests, so interpretation is more difficult.

If your two-hour postprandial insulin is at the high end or above the lab's normal range, you may be insulin resistant. High fasting and postprandial insulin levels are common in young women with significant weight gain, in women with PCOS, and in perimenopausal women losing the beneficial effects of their estradiol.

Other tests. Hemoglobin A1C measures the amount of glucose incorporated into hemoglobin, the oxygen-carrying molecule in red blood cells. This test is a sensitive marker that detects glucose problems earlier and gives a picture of blood glucose levels over the past three months. If you already have diabetes, hemoglobin A1C is used to monitor the impact of diet and medications on your glucose control. The desirable goal is a hemoglobin A1C of less than 6, which indicates good glucose control.

Insulin resistance: more complete sensitive tests. One way to detect insulin resistance is the *Insulin Response to Glucose Test.* You drink a measured amount of glucose, then test glucose and insulin at regular intervals over five hours to see the pattern in the rise and fall of both, correlated with any symptoms as the levels change. Women are often told this longer test is not necessary. I disagree. So does the World Health Organization, which now recommends using the oral glucose tolerance test to identify early insulin resistance and those at higher risk for diabetes. Using only the fasting glucose means too many people with pre-diabetes are missed.

Your doctors may say, "We don't do those to diagnose diabetes," or "A three-hour test is fine, you don't need the full six hours," or "It doesn't matter when in your cycle you do a glucose tolerance test, it's all the same." I disagree on all points. We are not simply looking for diabetes; we are looking for the early change of insulin resistance, and for objective laboratory data that explains your descriptions of uncontrollable food cravings, difficulty losing weight, mood swings, and other physical symptoms.

If you only have a *three-hour* test to measure glucose-insulin response, as many doctors recommend, you miss the last two hours when additional abnormal changes often occur, such as a reactive hypoglycemia or a persistently elevated insulin value. Brain symptoms such as memory loss, concentration difficulties, and mood swings are especially likely to get worse in the last two hours, providing important clues to causes and treatment approaches.

Useful information comes from testing the week before your menstrual period, around Days 20–23, the cycle phase when women experience their worst food cravings. The rise in progesterone, and the relative balance with estradiol, affects both your symptoms and your body's insulin-glucose response. At midlife, insulin resistance often gets worse, especially if you have ovulatory levels of progesterone with decreasing estradiol and androgens "unmasked" by the decline in estradiol. These combined hormonal shifts cause more glucose changes that trigger physical and emotional symptoms.

We do these tests in the office whenever possible, for several reasons. Labs often mess up the tests and don't do what we ask. Most physicians have the patient go to a lab, then only look at the numbers for each hour of the test. If the numbers fall into the "normal" range, the patient is told "everything is normal," without being asked how she *felt* during the test. This overlooks the most crucial information of all: what the patient has to say about her symptoms as the glucose and insulin levels rose and fell.

I ask patients to log everything experienced throughout the test, and my staff makes written observations as well. We sometimes do a short cognitive assessment (to check memory, attention, concentration, etc.) at each hourly blood draw.

This integrated information allows me to correlate symptoms with "the numbers" and determine an individualized course of treatment, such as the balance of carbohydrate, fat, and protein, the spacing and number of meals, and what medications are needed.

Effective Treatment Strategies to Get Your Glucose and Insulin in Balance

Step 1: Nutrition. Your first line of defense to regulating insulin—and there is no way around it—is nutrition. Medication alone will not do it. The balance and timing of foods you eat each day is critical. Skipping meals and eating large amounts in the evening leads to more insulin and more fat storage. High carbohydrate foods increase insulin production. You need to eat smaller, balanced meals throughout the day to provide the cornerstone of your insulin-balancing program. You also need adequate protein and the right balance of healthy fats—all are the first, and most important, steps you can take to keep excess insulin from destroying your health. Detailed meal plans to improve glucose-insulin balance are described in *Women, Weight and Hormones* (see Appendix II).

Step 2: Exercise. Exercise acts like an "invisible insulin" to improve muscle use of glucose from the bloodstream so that it can be used for energy instead of floating around in the bloodstream doing damage. Lower blood glucose, in turn, decreases the insulin pouring out of your pancreas in response to all that glucose hanging around. Less insulin in the bloodstream means you burn fat for fuel more effectively, and also build more muscle, which then increases your metabolic rate. Just walking five to ten minutes a few times a day is one of the simplest, quickest, and least costly things you can do to reduce the deadly consequences of insulin resistance.

Step 3: Restore ovarian hormone balance. You need to get your estradiol, progesterone, testosterone, and DHEA back into healthy ranges. They all work together to improve your insulin response, increase your metabolic rate, and help you build healthy muscle.

If you are overweight, have glucose intolerance, insulin resistance, or actual diabetes and you need contraception, I recommend that you avoid the higher-progestin pills (Loestrin, Alesse, Mircette, and others). BCPs with less progestin and better estrogen ratios work better to improve insulin sensitivity and do not overstimulate the appetite! These include oral pills Ovcon 35, Modicon (and their generics), Yasmin, Orthocyclen, and possibly Orthocept, as well as the new non-oral, vaginal ring contraceptive called Nuvaring.

If you do not need contraception, or have had a hysterectomy, then focus on using the natural bioidentical hormone preparations. The patch form of estradiol, compared to oral, gives better results for insulin sensitivity, based on many international studies published in the last few years by renowned researchers. If you have a uterus and are not producing your own progesterone adequately, *non-oral* natural progesterone such as Crinone vaginal gel typically causes fewer adverse effects on blood sugar swings and insulin production than oral forms. Don't use over-the-counter progesterone ("wild yam") creams, since many of these contain too much added progesterone and seriously throw your insulin-glucose pathways out of whack. OTC progesterone creams have not been demonstrated to be reliable in preventing excess buildup of the lining of the uterus.

In my experience, the following hormone preparations are more likely to aggravate insulin resistance and glucose intolerance since they do not give optimal levels of estradiol and/or contain higher doses of progestins: mixed estrogens (Premarin, Estratab/Estratest, Cenestin), synthetic progestins (Provera, MPA), and progestin-dominant combination products such as PremPro, Prem Phase, CombiPatch, Femhrt. All of these can make it harder to control insulin resistance.

Step 4: Decrease your stress to lower cortisol. Remember, cortisol helps make more body fat for storage. The higher your stress, the higher your cortisol, and the more problems with insulin resistance. Take stress-busting steps now (see Chapters 18 and 19 for more information).

Step 5: Insulin "sensitizer" medications. If balancing your ovarian hormones doesn't improve insulin resistance, you may want to talk with your doctor about other medications, such as Glucophage (metformin), Actos (pioglitazone), and Avandia (rosiglitazone). All of these improve insulin sensitivity. I use these quite successfully for women of all ages, especially those suffering from PCOS. Lifestyle strategies are the first course of treatment, but many women need additional medicines to get the insulin resistance under control and facilitate healthy weight loss. Once glucose and insulin are normalized, many women are able to stop the medication and maintain the improvements with healthy eating, regular exercise, and good hormone balance.

With these medicines I prescribe a lower than usual dose and increase very gradually. This way, side effects are minimized. "Start low and go slow" is how I approach starting new medications. The American Diabetes Association and Joslin Diabetes programs recommend combination therapies of two or more of the above medications, even in younger women, to control insulin resistance early and prevent full-blown diabetes and all its complications later. The specific combination must be tailored to your body's responses by your physician, looking at all the variables described.

In Summary

It is becoming increasingly common to see younger women struggling with the early stages of hormonal imbalance. Don't waste time feeling lousy and missing out on life. There are effective medication options to help you achieve improved thyroid, cortisol, and insulin balance. Addressing these hormonal imbalances when you are young can help prevent many of the chronic weight and health problems as you get older.

If you suspect an imbalance in any of these hormone systems, get evaluated properly. Make sure your diagnoses are based upon reliable blood tests. Don't depend on saliva tests. If you are not satisfied with your physician's evaluation, don't hesitate to get a second opinion. Try to use the bioidentical human hormone formulations wherever possible, unless you need the potency of the synthetic hormones in BCPs to suppress ovarian cycles and/or provide contraception. Be careful of animal-derived products. Remember to individualize your treatment by starting with low dosages and work with your physician to gradually increase the dose depending upon your response to the medication and the results of appropriate lab tests. Keep symptom logs to help you focus on how you are feeling with each change in medication.

If these issues are addressed properly, you may not need so many antidepressant or antianxiety medicines to improve mood, decrease anxiety, and improve your energy and sleep. This will help reduce both side effects and lower your medication costs. Careful monitoring and communication with your physician is key. There is no need to wait to address the situation "later." You deserve to feel better now!

Starting Your "Clean-Up Campaign":
Get Rid of Ovarian Disruptors You Can Control

Introduction

Now that you have read about the many ways your ovaries can be damaged by the environment and your lifestyle, let's explore ways to "clean up" and improve your overall health.

Eliminating Hormone-Disrupting Habits

Cigarette Smoking

When you smoke, you don't even look healthy. I can easily spot a smoker just by her skin and her voice, regardless of age. More than just appearance, however, cigarette smoking damages your ovaries, your unborn children, your brain, and your body. It also increases your risk of both ovarian and breast cancers. And don't forget the adverse effects of secondary smoke on children and those around you.

Tobacco is a highly addictive drug that seduces, only to then steal your health. If you smoke and have hormone problems, your first clean-up prescription is to *stop smoking*!

This is easier said than done, I know. But you can do it. Your life and health depend on it. There are excellent smoking cessation strategies available to help you clean up the habit (see Appendix II). One highly effective way is the nicotine patch, in gradually decreasing doses, to help you taper off the nicotine addiction and reduce withdrawal symptoms. You must avoid smoking cigarettes while using the patch, however, or the excess nicotine can cause a serious heart rhythm disturbance from nicotine toxicity. There are also other medications, such as Zyban and some antidepressants, that help diminish nicotine withdrawal.

Alcohol

Alcohol has an ancient history in cultures around the world. Studies show that people who drink small amounts of alcohol regularly gain some health benefits, such as lower heart disease risk. Moderate use means a *glass* of wine or beer, not a whole bottle of wine in one evening. For women, however, even moderate use may increase risk of menstrual disturbances, changes in fertility, and later increased risk of breast cancer. Women react differently to alcohol than do men. We have fewer gastric enzymes to metabolize alcohol, so we absorb approximately 30 percent more alcohol into our bloodstream, even if we drink the same amount. If you have symptoms of declining hormonal levels, alcohol further suppresses poorly functioning ovaries. If you take birth control pills or prescription hormone therapy, alcohol increases liver production of estrone, the unwanted type of estrogen, and can interfere with the positive effects of hormone therapy. Daily use of alcohol, even in moderate amounts, suppresses your immune response and can aggravate allergies and chemical sensitivities. Alcohol adds significantly to daily calories, doesn't add any nutritional value, and leads to more body fat around your middle.

Enjoying wine or beer or other alcoholic beverages on special occasions may be fine, but don't drink alcohol every day, even in small amounts. It saps your brain power and your energy.

Excess Caffeine

I certainly enjoy a good cup of coffee in the morning—I love the aroma as it fills my kitchen and I enjoy the taste. Go ahead and enjoy yours too. Two or three cups of coffee or tea a day has never been shown to have any adverse health effects; in fact, tea (more so than coffee) contains modest amounts of antioxidants. There aren't any serious health problems in studies of caffeine use, as long as you keep total caffeine intake to less than 200–250 mg a day (the equivalent of three or four regular-size cups of coffee).

Like many things, caffeine becomes a problem when you overdo it. If you are chronically tired, and use caffeine as a "pickup" to get through the day, it can actually make fatigue worse. Caffeine acts as a diuretic, so it dehydrates your body, makes you lose water-soluble vitamins, and depletes calcium and magnesium needed for healthy muscle function and mood regulation, to name a few of its energy-sapping effects. By disrupting the healthy balance of serotonin and norepinephrine in the brain and nerve tissues, excess caffeine also increases pain sensations, makes you irritable, heightens anxiety, intensifies PMS, and also causes rebound headaches when it wears off.

If you drink beverages with caffeine late in the day, it disrupts your sleep cycles. Deep, Stage 4 sleep is the time your muscles repair themselves, so if you have caffeine at night, you'll wake up tired with sore, aching muscles the next morning. Then you use more caffeine to pick you up, and the cycle continues. If you want to enjoy it, limit yourself to two cups of your favorite caffeinated beverage in the morning and switch to water for the rest of the day. Many women don't realize that "fatigue" is also a symptom of dehydration from too little water intake. Don't forget to watch for "hidden" sources of caffeine in soft drinks, over-the-counter cold or headache relievers, and some of the herbal "energy boosters" now widely available.

If possible, try to purchase "organically grown" coffee and teas to avoid residual pesticides often present on the leaves of tea and coffee plants. If you can't find products locally, check the Internet for on-line and mail-order services.

Stimulant "Diet" Pills

Using stimulant diet pills on a regular basis causes some of the same problems as excess caffeine: disruption of the brain's endocrine regulating pathways, alteration of weight-regulating pathways, mood crashes when they wear off, anxiety, insomnia, and chronic fatigue from revving your body engines too fast and depleting its energy reserves. If you take these every day, talk with your physician. You may need medication to get off them safely and avoid withdrawal problems. Follow your physician's advice and stop using these drugs. Proper hormone balance, diet, and exercise are still the best way to lose weight. Sorry, there is no quick fix!

Cocaine

Even though this drug is illegal and there are stiff consequences for its use, it is still widely abused in this country. Young women are especially vulnerable to its endocrine and mood effects. Cocaine is one of the most powerful stimulant drugs of all, blasting neurotransmitters out of their nerve cell storage sites with a vengeance. Because of its potency, new studies have shown that even one "hit" can permanently alter the brain, leading to addiction. The high that follows release of this flood of chemical messengers is fleeting, which is why it triggers such intense cravings for more. The "rush" can stimulate the heart so intensely that it sometimes leads to sudden death. Avoid cocaine. If you are using it, seek professional help from an experienced addiction therapist *now*.

Cleaning Up Your Diet, Getting Rid of Excitotoxins

The typical American diet of fast foods—lots of soft drinks, high-salt, high-fat processed foods—contain significant amounts of additives and flavor enhancers, such as *monosodium glutamate* (MSG), and hydrolyzed vegetable protein (HVP). MSG is the cause of "Chinese restaurant syndrome"—headaches, palpitations, and fluid retention experienced after a meal in a Chinese restaurant. This compound imparts an "excited," intensified taste to foods, but unfortunately, it also is an excitatory amino acid (like aspartate in sweeteners found in soft drinks) that overstimulates brain cells, including pathways regulating the menstrual cycle.

MSG is ubiquitous today in frozen, canned, and processed convenience foods and difficult to avoid unless you carefully read labels. Manufacturers are clever at disguising it under other names, such as "natural flavorings" and "*hydrolyzed vegetable protein.*" HVP is a product high in three different excitotoxins—glutamate, aspartate, and cystoic acid. The amino acid glutamate is even sold as a supplement in health food stores, supposedly for memory enhancement. Don't use these supplements. They can actually damage nerve cells, including those in the memory centers. These excitatory amino acids cause an increase in free radical, or oxidative, damage to cells, particularly nerve and muscle tissue. Tabulate your total daily intake by checking labels.

Many families, especially when both parents work outside the home and time is at a premium, have difficulties preparing healthy meals. Despite your best efforts, fast-food restaurant meals seem to increase steadily with the number of children or family activities on a given day. Sales pitches aimed at kids for "fun foods" make it doubly difficult for parents to set limits and serve wholesome foods. The quick and easy convenience foods available everywhere just add to the problem. If you ever wonder why it's difficult to resist these delights, just remember there are a lot of talented, experienced marketing experts working for savvy food manufacturers whose sole goal is to make you desire these foods—most of which are high in fat, sugar, salt, and flavor-enhancer additives.

Start looking for ways to eliminate these chemicals—you may even find you have better "brain power" when you cut the excitotoxins from your diet. It takes detective work, but the results are worth the effort. For more on how these chemicals can adversely affect your health, read the book I used as a reference for the box on page 343, *Excitotoxins: The Taste That Kills,* by Russell L. Blaylock, M.D.

Take a look at the chart to see just how many different food additives contain these compounds, and start being aware of how much aspartate, glutamate, HVP, or MSG is actually in what you are eating. Work to eliminate as many as possible.

Cleaning Up the PVCs

Common everyday plastic cling wrap is another source of unwanted chemicals in your food. If it is made of clear polyvinyl chloride (PVC), an inherently brittle plastic, it contains a plasticizer, DEHA, to make it more flexible. DEHA causes reproductive system defects and other birth defects in offspring, as well as liver cancer in mature animals. This compound leaches into the food it surrounds. The molecules migrate from the packaging into the food until the wrapping is depleted of the chemical. A Consumers Union test showed that DEHA reached levels of 153 parts per million (ppm) in cheddar cheese samples wrapped in packaging containing DEHA. The Commission of the European Communities sets a limit of 18 ppm, quite a difference. PVC packaging includes plastic trays in boxed cookies or chocolates, and may also be in plastic bottles, and the lining of cans. Bottles can often be identified by the #3 recycling label on the bottom. Meat and poultry is often packaged in PVC. Be sure your cling wrap is polyethylene based, *not* polyvinyl. Check the label. Only buy products that clearly state the contents.

Cleaning Up Your Bedroom Habits

Good sleep is absolutely critical to good health. Waking up multiple times at night is also one of the earliest brain effects of declining estradiol levels. Women with hormone problems can't sleep, yet sleep is the time when our body replenishes and recharges itself for the next day's activities.

To sleep well, we also need quality mattresses and bedding. We often spend less money on a mattress than most other furniture we own. Some types of mat-

HIDDEN SOURCES OF MSG AND EXCITOTOXINS

Food Additives Always Containing monosodium glutamate (MSG)
Hydrolyzed vegetable protein (HVP; contains three different
    excitotoxins—aspartate, glutamate, and cystoic acid—that is
    converted to cysteine)
Hydrolyzed plant protein, or hydrolyzed protein
Textured protein
Plant protein extract
Hydrolyzed oat flour
Yeast extract, autolyzed yeast
Sodium or calcium caseinate

Food Additives Frequently Containing MSG
Malt flavorings or extract
Bouillon cubes, dry soup powders, canned chicken or beef stock
"Flavoring" or "natural flavoring"
"Natural spices"
"Seasoning" or "natural seasoning"

Food Additives That May Contain MSG
Carrageenan
Soy protein concentrate
Soy protein isolate
Whey protein concentrate (depends on manufacturer)
"Enzymes" (protease enzymes break food proteins into their component
    amino acids, some of which are excitatory amino acids like
    glutamate)

Other Excitotoxin Sources
Foods containing aspartate, aspartame, aspartic acid
Nutrasweet
Glutamate (glutamic acid) amino acid supplements
Cysteine (cystoic acid) amino acid supplements

Reference: Russell L. Blaylock, M.D., *Excitotoxins: The Taste That Kills,* (Santa Fe, N. Mex.:
Health Press, 1994).

tresses contain synthetic chemicals that "outgas" or emit vapors that can interfere with sleep and aggravate allergies. Check both foam and innerspring mattresses for content. Synthetic materials such as polyfoams, styrene, butadiene rubber, and toxic glues cause unsuspected problems for many people.

In addition, bedding fabrics are often made of synthetic fibers that don't "breathe," so they trap moisture that attracts dust mites and promotes growth of various microorganisms such as mold. The average human body releases up to a pint of moisture each night. Women with "night sweats" from hormone imbalance may lose even more. To help eliminate these problems, dry your bedding outside in the sunshine. If that's not possible, then use your clothes dryer, but avoid perfumed fabric softener strips that add more noxious chemicals to the mix. Sunlight helps kill troublesome microorganisms and dust mites, and the fresh air gives a fresh, natural smell that is much better than the chemicals in fragranced products.

Don't use fragranced products at all, especially if you have hormone problems and are sensitive to chemicals or have allergies. Also avoid fragranced candles, air fresheners, and other sources of petroleum-based chemicals in your bedroom. These produce combustion by-products and volatile organic compounds. Use pure, unscented candles of 100 percent beeswax or vegetable wax.

Your bedroom should be an oasis, as free of chemical contaminants as possible, an environment that promotes a restful night's sleep. Your body needs this time to recoup each day. In the box on page 345 you'll find more tips to improve sleep. If these approaches don't work, and you've restored hormones to optimal levels, talk with your doctor about formal sleep studies.

Cleaning Up Your Workaholism

You're a Type-E woman—being *every*thing to *every*body *every* day. "Just one more hour, and then I'll be finished. Just one load of wash, then I'll stop. Just one more report and then I'll take a break. Just one more room and then I'll be finished." Whatever your daily work, it is all too easy to get caught in the vicious cycle of perfectionistic workaholism, endlessly trying to do everything.

Take an inventory of your daily time sheet: How many hours do you work outside your home? How many hours do you work inside your home? How many hours do you spend on the needs of others? How many hours do you spend on your needs? Maybe you don't define yourself as a workaholic, but take a close and honest look at the hours you just totaled up . . . do you see a balance here?

Workaholism is destructive. It can rob you of your health and vitality (remember Harriet in Chapter 7). You can ignore the signals for a while, but they catch up with you. I have personally been dealt that lesson in spades many different times in my adult working life. I think my body will go on and on and on. I think I am immune. And guess what? If I push too hard at work, have too many stresses from patient load, business or family issues, and too much to accomplish in too short a time, eventually it catches up with me. Although I generally know on some level what I am doing, if I ignore early warning signs that I'm on overload, I get slapped down every time.

Like it does to me, workaholism will eventually force you to stop and listen to your body's cries for a rest. No one is immune to the destructive effects of overwork, and lack of rest and recovery. Heed your body. Spend some time on you.

SLEEP-IMPROVING STRATEGIES

1. Go to bed when you are pleasantly tired. Try not to wait until you are so exhausted you can hardly move.
2. Establish a simple routine at a consistent bedtime. Likewise, have a regular wakeup time so your body keeps its normal rhythm.
3. Do not go to bed hungry, or too full from a heavy meal.
4. If pain interferes with sleep, ask your physician about proper medication.
5. If you need a nap, take one earlier in the day, preferably before three P.M. If you nap in the evening, you may wake up restless halfway through the night and then feel tired the next day.
6. Gentle exercise (like a short walk) helps you relax and feel genuinely tired. Make it a habit but don't overdo it. Don't do an aerobic exercise routine just before retiring. It revs you up too much and makes it harder to fall asleep. On the other hand, lack of physical activity during the day makes sleep more difficult.
7. A glass of warm milk, along with a relaxing warm bath, really does help you fall asleep.
8. Avoid stimulants late in the evening (coffee, cola, tea, or chocolate) since they can keep you awake.
9. Once in bed, comfort is important. Make sure the bedroom isn't too hot; most people sleep better in cool rooms. Make sure you have a comfortable pillow and mattress.
10. Fresh air and quiet create a more conducive environment for sleep.
11. If outside traffic sounds are a problem, try playing a recording of "white noise," such as ocean surf, to mask intrusive sounds.
12. Don't take your work to bed with you. I know this is easier said than done, but bedtime is not the time to rehash the concerns of the day.
13. Keep a pad and pencil by the side of the bed. If something does come to mind, write it down. You can then dismiss it and focus on relaxing thoughts or pleasing images that help you "drift off."
14. Darkness in the bedroom is more important than most people realize; it helps the brain naturally produce melatonin, which maintains normal sleep. If your bedroom has a lot of light coming in the window, try wearing a sleep mask. It's cheaper and safer than melatonin supplements or sleeping pills.

Clean Up Endocrine-Disrupting Chemicals Around You

The National Institute of Environmental Health Sciences (NIEHS) oversees a variety of studies that suggest that many women's health problems—including autoimmune diseases, breast cancer, and reproductive cancers and dysfunctions, including infertility, premature menstruation, and premature menopause—are connected to chemical exposure from everyday products at home and work (see Chapter 5 for more detail). So, how do you reduce exposure and health risks?

Let's start with the things you use every day—cosmetics, lotions, conditioner, shampoo, soap, gel, hair spray, nail polish and remover, perfume, deodorant, toothpaste, mouthwash, among others. All of these are heavily fragranced, and most people's noses are now numb to the smells. But your brain isn't; it gets the full impact because the smells are carried along the olfactory nerve directly to the areas of the limbic system that regulate mood, sleep, memory, and other vital functions. That's one way that strong chemicals can disrupt memory and cause you to feel suddenly irritable. All of these chemicals affect your health in ways you never dreamed, including causing daily headaches. Except for very few, very expensive perfumes that use only plant-based compounds, over 95 percent of the chemicals in today's scented products are derived from *petroleum-based* compounds. These compounds are *neurotoxins,* chemicals that damage nerve cells and disrupt major pathways in the limbic system. Even the potent synthetic "musk" found in many popular perfumes, colognes, and aftershave products falls into this group of chemicals.

Studies show that these chemical fragrances can cause central nervous system disorders, immune disorders, allergic reactions, birth defects, and even cancer. This is really not new. It was reported to the U.S. House of Representatives in 1986 by the Committee on Science and Technology, based on extensive scientific evidence. These reports have been overlooked and ignored in terms of their potential to cause such varied health problems. Most of the research focus is on the cancer-causing potential of these chemicals rather than the subtle types of brain and immune system effects.

Most of you use scented products and do not notice any problems right away. Over time, and with hormone imbalances, you may develop traditional allergies, or what is known as *multiple chemical sensitivities* (MCS). The dyes, dry-cleaning solutions, laundry products, fragrances from perfumes and household products, mothballs, and a host of other products in your home environment all have the potential to further disrupt neuroendocrine pathways. I encourage my patients to eliminate as many of these scented products as possible, particularly if they have hormone and allergy problems. Many hypoallergenic home and personal care products now help relieve allergies and sensitivities (see Appendix II for helpful sources).

There are other sources of chemical vapors in our homes. Have you ever noticed the strong plastic smell when you open a new shower curtain liner? New sheets, pillowcases, carpets, and permanent press clothes are usually treated with formaldehyde, another chemical smell that causes problems for many women. Mothballs, Lysol spray, and Pine-Sol all have harsh chemicals that release noxious vapors and are severe irritants for women with hormone problems who are chemically sensitive. Advertisements bombard us with a different cleaning product for every purpose, all containing these strong chemicals. It is important to minimize these, as well as eliminate mold and mildew, which also release toxic vapors.

But how do you suppose our grandmothers got along? They used simple nontoxic remedies to handle most cleaning problems. We can reduce our household chemical overload, and save money at the same time, by following their example. I use simple white cider vinegar and tap water for cleaning just about everything from shower tiles to glass tabletops to windows to kitchen counters and floors. It works better than many commercial products, and doesn't contaminate your living and working environment with harsh chemicals. If I need an abrasive for various tasks, I add simple baking soda.

My grandmother used a concoction of vinegar, water, and a small amount of olive oil on a cloth, an excellent solution that trapped dust effectively. Lemon juice makes a fine brass polish. Instead of the strong-smelling silver polish, use Spic and Span in an aluminum foil–lined pan full of hot water. It whisks the tarnish away without the harsh chemicals and odors of the usual silver cleaners. I have used these approaches for the last thirty years since I first began having problems with sensitivity to a lot of perfumes and chemicals. These approaches are inexpensive and they work. There are additional excellent ideas in the series of healthy cleaning books by Anne Berthold-Bond, or in Carolyn P. Gorman's book, *Less Toxic Living.*

Clean Up Pesticides: They May Kill Pests, but What Do They Do to You and Your Children?

You now realize the dangers of most commercial pesticides used inside the home and outside on the yard and garden. If you must use them, be sure to follow directions and take necessary precautions. Many pesticide chemicals, as well as medicines, fragrances, solvents, and cleaners, are absorbed through the skin. If you spill any on yourself, wash the area thoroughly. Pesticides also release vapors that can adversely affect your brain if inhaled. This is a serious problem for older folks, but children (and your pets) are also vulnerable to residues from the sprays, and should not be in the area to be treated when they are being used.

There are many less toxic options for getting rid of pests, inside and outside your home. Glue traps work wonders on ants, spiders, scorpions, roaches, and other indoor pests. Boric acid solution is another nontoxic pest killer (see Appendix II for other nontoxic ideas for outdoor pest control).

Inventory your home for products—pesticides, cleaning products, paint and paint thinners—that contain potentially dangerous ingredients. Isolate them in storage areas such as a locked garage or outside shed, rather than the basement. Vapors from these chemicals can be as harmful as the product itself. If there is a warning label that the product is not safe for humans or pets, or is toxic, or if the label says that "special care" needs to be taken in the handling and application of the product, stop and ask yourself, "Is this product safe to have around?" Look for safer alternatives.

Minimize exposure to potentially toxic chemicals for you and your family. Not all of the suggestions listed on page 349 are feasible, but do what you can. Even small changes can add up over time. Remember, these are all potentially harmful endocrine disruptors. Patients say daily that they had no idea these products could cause *hormone* problems! Consumers simply are not told about potential damage. Better, safer options exist.

WAYS TO MINIMIZE YOUR BODY EXPOSURE TO ENDOCRINE DISRUPTORS

- Don't smoke. Limit alcohol to special occasions, in small amounts.
- Increase your fiber intake to help eliminate environmental chemicals from your intestinal tract.
- Reduce your fat intake. Fats are where these chemicals concentrate.
- Work to maintain optimal percent body fat (20–25 percent for women under fifty). Toxic chemicals are stored in body fat for up to thirty years.
- Exercise regularly to maintain optimal body fat and decrease your risk for breast cancer, heart disease, and osteoporosis.
- Use caution with soy and phytoestrogens that mimic and interfere with your own natural estrogen.
- Make sure any hormones you take are bioidentical to your body's own natural hormones, unless there are medical reasons (contraception, endometriosis, or fibroid suppression, among others) for which the synthetic hormones work better.
- Minimize use of processed foods containing artificial sweeteners, monosodium glutamate (MSG), hydrolyzed vegetable protein, and other excitatory amino acids.
- Take antioxidant vitamins and minerals, magnesium, and zinc to neutralize some of the cell-damaging effects of excitotoxins.
- Read labels. Don't always assume sports supplements, diet foods, energy boosters, and products from health food stores are "safe." Soymilk often has glutamate in the form of hydrolyzed vegetable protein added as a flavor enhancer. Sports drinks and diet foods often contain aspartame, another excitotoxin to avoid.
- Although hormone-disruptor chemicals and environmental chemical pollutants can be transferred from mother to baby via breast milk, most experts still feel that the positive benefits of breast-feeding outweigh potential risks.

WAYS TO MINIMIZE TOXIC CHEMICALS AT HOME

- PCBs and pesticides DDT, kepone, chlordane, Lindane, and benzene hexachlorane and benzene hexachloride (BCH) are banned in the United States but are still produced here and exported to other countries. Residential areas near these plants, working in these plants, trips to other countries, and possibly imported produce may be sources of exposure. Check your local EPA office to see what chemical producers are near your home.
- Minimize pesticide use in your home and look for alternative nontoxic products.
- Avoid using the pesticides Endosulfan, methoxychlor, and triazine herbicides altogether, even though they are still made in the United States.
- Avoid traditional pesticides contained in pet collars and dips to control fleas and ticks. This minimizes children's risk of exposure to toxic chemicals when they play with their pets.
- Avoid golf courses the day of and the day after they spray with pesticides. Call and ask when they spray, and plan your golf dates accordingly.
- Keep your kids off pesticide-covered or chemically fertilized lawns and gardens.
- Ask your grocer if their produce is sprayed with pesticides. If yes, express your concerns and let the manager know that you plan to shop elsewhere unless they offer pesticide-free produce options.
- Be aware of any local warnings to avoid fish contaminated with PCB, dioxin, or mercury.
- Call your local water company and find out what is in the water and how it is treated. If you are on a well, be particularly careful when farmers spray their crops, and periodically test your water for contamination.
- Instill a reverse osmosis water filter with carbon system that will remove chemicals and particles (regular charcoal filters generally only remove odors and chlorine and bad tastes but not all toxic chemicals). If possible, use a shower filter or whole house carbon filter to eliminate chlorine and chlorine gas from the water and air.
- Look for fresh fruits and vegetables, dairy products, poultry, and meats that have not been treated with products that contain pesticides or growth hormones and chemicals. For chicken, try to buy those labeled "free range," "no antibiotics," and "fed organic feed."
- Avoid "basted" or "self-basting" turkeys that have added fat, water, broth, and flavor enhancers containing MSG. Choose "fresh" or "fresh-frozen" birds instead.
- If there are no local resources for organic foods in your area, check the Internet for sources of healthy, antibiotic-free, and hormone-free foods.

- Avoid plastics, particularly PVC (#3). Don't store or heat foods in plastic containers, Styrofoam, or PVC cling wraps. Instead, heat foods in porcelain or glass. Avoid boxed cookies and chocolates with plastic trays, which are usually PVC plastic. Check plastic bottles to see if they are marked PVC #3. Be especially careful of plastic-wrapped cheeses.
- It is best to cook with stainless steel, cast iron, and glass. Teflon, aluminum, and copper are generally considered safe. Don't use plastic in microwave ovens.
- Avoid alkyl phenol ethoxylates (APEs) found in detergents, hair-coloring products, spermicides, and some plastics. Studies show these have estrogenic effects in mammals.
- Babies should not be given toys made of plastic. Use unpainted, unvarnished toys made of wood.
- Avoid lead-based paints in toys, dishes, or on walls. Lead accumulates to toxic levels that adversely affect the brain, especially in children.
- Remove and dispose of the plastic covers on dry cleaning, and then air dry-cleaned clothes outside before putting them in your closets.
- Know where local hazardous waste sites are. People living in residential areas near hazardous waste sites are found to have higher rates of medical problems. Public awareness has done much to identify these sites, but caution is still required as new sites are uncovered.
- Your workplace and home office should be well ventilated to prevent accumulation of fumes from toners, solvents, and cleaners.
- Try new "microfiber" cleaning cloths using only water to clean, so you can remove stains and dirt without added chemicals.
- Don't use room or bathroom fresheners at all or those particularly noxious deodorizers often used in municipal public toilets. Most of these contain formaldehyde as well as synthetic fragrances that are detrimental.
- Avoid the inexpensive particleboard or plywood furniture that is popular for offices and children's rooms. These need extensive airing to outgas the formaldehyde isocyancerates, and other chemicals used in the manufacturing process. They may also contain pesticides and create tremendous "dust wads," no matter how often you clean.
- The same formaldehyde problem occurs with much of the carpeting sold today. Tile or wood flooring is better than wall-to-wall artificial-fiber carpeting. Even wool carpeting is made with pesticides in the fibers, which can break off and become inhaled, particularly dangerous for small children and animals.
- Avoid permanent press products treated with formaldehyde, which can be irritating to eyes and skin, and cause headaches.
- Wash your hands frequently and encourage your children to do the same.

In Summary

We may not yet know all of the adverse effects these endocrine disruptors have on our bodies, but what we do know is quite alarming. Don't take these warnings lightly. Eliminate as many of these substances as you can.

Every little bit helps. Accumulation of these endocrine disruptors, not necessarily just one or two, wreaks havoc on the health of our ovaries and the rest of our bodies. Use common sense and caution. Scrutinize what you put in your mouth, on your body, and in your home, work environment, and around your children.

19

Create Your Path to Optimal Energy and Health

Introduction

Knowledge is power. I have often said this is crucial when it comes to your health and your life decisions. But let me add: *Accurate* knowledge is power. And power is freedom. Freedom to accomplish what is important to you for your health and your life, in a way that you feel best suits your needs. To do this, however, you must first have a reliable information base. As I have discussed throughout this book, there is so much information available these days, both accurate and inaccurate, it can be overwhelming, as well as confusing. What I find dismaying is that even articles from reputable sources often only scratch the surface of important issues and play it safe to avoid offending advertisers. We see this especially with the issue of estrogen.

Most information on estrogen never differentiates between the different types or the brand used in the studies. And rarely is it mentioned that we are constantly being exposed to estrogenic chemicals—in our foods, homes, water, and air—that are far more dangerous to our health than anything that has ever been found with our own body estrogens. In my view, this is a tragic oversight, and it leaves out an enormous, and perhaps even central, piece of the total hormone picture. I hope that with the science-based information I have provided in this book, you will be better equipped to ask probing questions, evaluate media stories, and make decisions about your health.

I encourage you to constantly question the information you receive. Ask what is the source, and what may be the underlying agendas. Are the studies cited funded by the industry that will profit from favorable findings? As more and more women speak out for answers to the type of complex health issues we have explored in this book, hopefully there will be more and more products brought to the market to provide solutions. Some products will be good, some will not. Some may even be harmful, but unfortunately we may not know this for decades. Look for solutions and treatments that address the underlying cause, and be wary of prescriptions, medications, and products that just treat the symptoms. If you do not, you may not only put your health at risk but you may also wind up spending a lot of money on multiple medications and over-the-counter products that may have side effects for which you will need additional medications, products, or treatments. This is when you need to stop and ask: "Am I on the right path?" If you suspect you are not, do not be afraid to act quickly. The following tips will help you get back on the right path:

- *Become proactive about getting information, explore your options, read about pros and cons of various choices, and make notes and lists of your questions before you take action.*
- *Research your family health history, write it down, and take copies with you to your medical visits.*
- *Know your health risks, write them down, and give a copy to your physician.*
- *Take an inventory of every supplement you are taking, list all the ingredients and doses and take a copy of this to every medical visit. Insist that all of your doctors keep this information in your chart. We ask our patients for this information at every visit, but I continue to be surprised at the women who say, "I don't know what I'm taking," or "I don't know what's in it."*
- *Keep a single list of all of your prescription medications and the doses of each one. This is especially important if you are seeing and receiving prescriptions from multiple physicians. Share this list with each doctor. Take a copy to every medical visit.*
- *Keep track of your past and present "health data" (we call this your "medical records"). Get copies and keep a set to take with you if you have an emergency or see a new physician.*
- *Pay attention to your "numbers" (medical test results); ask for copies of your lab reports and key test results to keep for your records and to show other physicians you may consult.*
- *Do your homework investigating resources for physicians and other health professionals who will best suit your needs for your health "team."*
- *Keep track of your symptoms (charted with your menstrual cycle, or phase of hormone therapy); take this log to your medical appointments. I ask our patients to write down, before each appointment, "What's better since last time? What's not better?"*
- *Before each appointment with your health professionals, make a list of questions you want answered. This will focus your thoughts so that important items are not overlooked in the discussion.*
- *Speak up and ask questions if you don't understand an explanation or directions. The days of passively sitting back and not saying anything are long gone. Being actively involved will help reduce risk of medical errors, and will result in your receiving better care.*

One Woman's Successful Journey

Another story I'd like to share with you is that of a young woman I have known on both a professional and personal basis. I have watched her struggle with hormonal problems even before she realized she had them. I have seen her turn disappointments into triumphs, and throughout the years gain the knowledge and confidence to work with her own physicians to positively deal with her hormonal challenges. I hope her story will inspire you and give you the courage to keep reaching for your own goals.

When I first met *Tanya* she was thirty years old and just recovering from her second exploratory laparoscopic surgery for possible uterine fibroids and unexplained infertility. She had been trying to conceive for five years and had already had several rounds of diagnostic tests and attempts at artificial insemination with accompanying fertility drugs, without success. Tanya has always been a very fit and health-conscious person. She exercised on a regular basis, ate well, and maintained her body fat within optimal levels. The only health complaint she had, other than not being able to conceive, was severe PMS. She experienced overwhelming light-headedness, sweats and chills, cramps, and nausea prior to her period. Although these episodes were usually controlled by ibuprofen if taken in time, they were early clues of premature decline in her ovarian hormones.

Over the next few years, discouraged from unsuccessful infertility treatments and tired of the hormonal roller coaster infertility drugs can cause, she and her husband decided to explore other options for starting a family. Adoption seemed the next logical step, but she quickly found out this was not an easy process either. After considering the various options, from working with an adoption agency to adopting a child from another country, they decided to become foster-adoptive parents with their state's child protective services. This seemed to fulfill their desires for a family, and also give a new chance for a better life to a child in need. This process took nearly a full year to complete.

An incredible part of this story is that one month prior to their final licensing from the state, Tanya was laid off in a downsizing from her administrative position with a health care organization she had been with for eight years. Initially devastated, she realized this was a blessing in disguise when she got a call from her caseworker at Child Protective Services asking if they could take an immediate placement. Three children, ages eleven months, three, and four years old, seriously abused, were in immediate need of a foster home. This is what Tanya and her husband had been waiting for . . . and more! Because of the severe abuse, neglect, and parental unfitness of the biological parents, and with the support of the children's biological relatives, Tanya and her husband officially adopted the three siblings nine months after the initial placement. Now, if you know anything about Child Protective Services, you know that this was a fast adoption.

Tanya firmly believes that this was a "God deal," as she likes to call it. The timing was just right, coming after her layoff so she could be home with the children. She felt it was just meant to be. Even more amazing, all three children looked just like her husband. Comparing baby pictures and snapshots of her husband at age four and five, you could barely see a difference. For a while, though, she still hoped every month that she would be surprised and find herself pregnant, but this never happened. She has now accepted this, because her life is full and she is still amazed how fortunate they are and how much happiness the children have brought them.

And now the rest of the story. Throughout the years, Tanya has been interested in my work and shared with me her own "hormonal" stories. She had a complete hormonal evaluation when she was thirty, which showed some early hormone decline but nothing so out of normal that she wanted to address it at the time. Over the years, the more she learned, researched, and we discussed, the more she saw in herself the hormone connections I have been writing about, and the work I have been doing with patients for the last twenty years.

She worked with her own physician to implement many of the treatments I have outlined in this book. Her PMS, and later cyclic acne, and menstrual headaches are improved. She would often tell me, "I am so grateful to have this knowledge. I would have just struggled through these symptoms, felt miserable, and probably wound up paying through the nose for expensive medications that I didn't like taking. I continue to be amazed how really basic all this is when you stop and think about it. Yet no one is making these hormone connections. Even when I bring it up to friends, or other doctors, it is just dismissed. I think everybody is afraid of 'hormones.' My friends' doctors are putting them on Prozac and Sarafem, or prescribing lots of other medications, or just telling them to tough it out and simplify their lives. What people don't seem to understand is that if your hormones are out of whack, you don't have a healthy foundation. Without hormones in balance it's tough to make the positive lifestyle changes that in the long run will help make a difference. You just don't feel up to it." Well, obviously Tanya "got" the message and was able to proactively take charge of her life and health.

Recently she had an unexpected "opportunity" to once again apply what she had learned. She had an unrecognized ruptured appendix, severe infection, and adhesions that ultimately caused a total hysterectomy, with removal of the uterus, both ovaries, and tubes. Tanya was prepared. She sought a second opinion with us prior to her surgery, and we were able to guide her through the hormone options for after surgery. Immediately after the surgery, she asked her surgeon to start estrogen replacement therapy. She was given an injection of estradiol. She also had a prescription for estradiol patches and applied these as the injection began to wear off. Tanya is now stabilized on a regimen of low-dose Estrace AM and PM with an estradiol patch to provide continuous stable estrogen levels. Recent blood work showed good estradiol levels, low testosterone levels, and borderline thyroid levels. Since we have successfully stabilized her estradiol levels, the next step will be to address the thyroid and restore her testosterone to optimal levels.

During her last consult she commented, "This is not what I thought I would be dealing with at age thirty-five. This was not a 'club' I wanted to join. But since I am now a full-fledged menopausal woman (although surgically induced), I am grateful that I had a knowledgeable hormone specialist to guide me through it. Except for the recovery from the surgeries, I feel like my transition has been very smooth. I have not experienced any symptoms from the estrogen drop, except when I forget to take my pills on time! I am so glad that I was able to get on top of this from the beginning. My body may be hormonally the equivalent of a fifty-one-year-old lady, but I certainly do not feel like one. I am confident that if I can keep my hormones at optimal levels, and continue to exercise and eat right, I will continue to feel like my old self, maybe even better! Thanks for being there for me."

Needless to say, this encouraged me to continue getting the message out. I encourage you to do as Tanya has done in being proactive to get her health needs met, knowledgeable about her options, and in being psychologically resilient enough to flow with the challenges and setbacks that came her way. When we are out in a sailboat, we cannot control the direction of the wind, but we can learn to adjust the sails to get where we want to go. That's what I hope this book has given you—the knowledge to "trim your sails" and make the adjustments in your health strategies as your conditions and needs change.

No one ever found a cause for Tanya's infertility, though we have often wondered if all the exposure to pesticides in the farming area in which they lived may have been a factor. She clearly had many of the early warning signs that have been reported in animals and in the few human studies that have looked at this issue: unusually early decline in her ovarian hormone levels, headaches, early onset of fibroids when she didn't have any of the usual risk factors for developing them, and mild endometriosis, again without the more common risk factors or family history. We will likely never know if she was one of the silently injured ones from the widespread endocrine disruptors in her environment.

This is why you need to pay close attention to the warnings I have described throughout this book. The very fact that we do not yet know all the ramifications and consequences of these persistent organic pollutants is itself the very reason you need to take seriously the concerns that have been raised. Take charge of your health. Know what your hormone levels are, using reliable blood tests. Get rid of as many sources of these chemicals as possible. You do not need this contamination in your home and your bodies. Do your research carefully. Check before you try something new you heard about on the evening news.

If new medicines or supplements or herbs are suggested, ask yourself: What am I taking, and why am I taking it? Are there sound reasons for me to take it? What is in it? Where does it come from? Do I really need it? What reputable scientific information backs up the claims. Who will profit from my buying this product? Who is funding the research? Ask lots of questions and don't be satisfied until you have confidence in the answers you receive.

Getting older is a fact of life. It may not be as much fun as some other times in your life, but it sure beats the alternative. What is hard to accept is the feeling that our body is betraying us, letting us down, getting old before its time. This is not how it is supposed to be. While these are natural feelings, don't let yourself get stuck in the negativity and blame. Try to understand what is going on and work to positively improve your health and fitness. Your body is telling you that you simply can no longer get away with all the things you used to get away with. You must carefully scrutinize every aspect of your lifestyle—eating habits, environment, medications, supplements, activity levels—and start using many of the tools we have discussed throughout this book. Cumulatively, they will make a difference.

Don't take your symptoms lightly. Don't fall into the trap of denial, or let others fool you into thinking you can't be experiencing hormone decline because you are not the textbook menopausal age of fifty-one. The sooner you get on top of your health problems, the better.

As you identify potential problem areas and work toward making positive changes, be gentle with yourself. Be understanding of your body, and give it time to respond, to recover, to heal, to rejuvenate. Hormone imbalance doesn't turn around after one doctor visit. Your body needs time to recover, restore, repair, and readjust. Remember to like yourself during this process. Use positive self-talk. This may sound corny, but it does make a difference. Accept where you are and what you are experiencing, while you look at ways to move forward.

Make yourself and your health your top priority—and don't feel guilty! If you don't take care of yourself, who will? You need to take care of yourself so you can be healthy enough to give to the other people in your life.

Balance is the key. The body is an exquisitely sensitive, precious instrument, and it needs the proper balance in order to function optimally. That balance will be achieved in different ways, with different techniques and medications, for different individuals, using the tools of modern medicine coupled with the options and wisdom of complementary medicine when appropriate. Each one of us is an individual with different needs. The key is to find a blend of therapeutic approaches that is right for you, with careful attention to healthy food, optimal hormonal balance, exercise, optimal vitamin and mineral supplementation, body therapies, other medications as appropriate, as well as practicing positive mental attitudes, meditation, and prayer. Slow down and take time for you. All of these help you regain and sustain your health, energy, and vitality and find the "old self" you know and miss.

It has been an inspirational journey for me as I have worked with the women who cross my doorstep in search of answers, in search of ways to feel better, restore balance, and have the energy to lead fuller lives. I don't take these responsibilities lightly. I have seen the devastation in women's lives, as well as the lives of those who love them, when there is misinformation and mistreatment. I find myself at times overcome with anger and frustration, and immense sadness, at what women have been told, at the gross misinformation in the press and books by those who only seek to be a "guru" to sell the most books, or tapes, or vitamins, or wild yam creams, or herbs, or saliva tests, or "designer" formulations . . . or whatever the latest gimmick may be. The appalling morass of myth, hype, misinformation, and distortion, along with the fear tactics frequently used in marketing and advertising, creates untold damage and suffering for the women who are seeking help. Damage is also done by those who fear to venture out of the narrow tunnel vision of their specialty, who make rigid pronouncements based on their medical training from twenty-five years ago, and do not take the time to look, to think, to learn, or even question. I don't have an easy answer for you, but I do encourage you to rely on your own wisdom and common sense, and on medical professionals who care about you; those whose knowledge you can trust because you have done your homework, and who work with you to find approaches that *help*. Look for those who are willing to admit when they *don't* know something, and will help you find someone who does, or who will help you search for the answers.

Go forward, in good health, with zest.

Appendix I: Glossary of Medical Terms

This is a list of medical abbreviations and a glossary of the medical terms I have used throughout this book. If you are going to take charge of your health, it will help if you are familiar with these terms and what they mean so you will understand your physician when he or she explains what is happening to your body.

I. List of Medical Acronyms Used in This Book

Hormones
E1—estrone
E2—estradiol
E3—estriol
CEE—conjugated equine estrogens (Premarin, PremPro)
FSH—follicle stimulating hormone
GH—growth hormone
LH—luteinizing hormone
SHBG—sex hormone binding globulin
T4—thyroxine (thyroid)
T3—triiodothyronine (thyroid)
TSH—thyroid stimulating hormone

Other Terms:
BCP—birth control pill (see also "OC")
BMI—body mass index
BMR—basal metabolic rate
BTL—bilateral tubal ligation
CHOL—cholesterol
CVD—cardiovascular disease
DA—dopamine
DEXA—dual-energy X-ray absorptiometry
EFA—essential fatty acids
EPI—epinephrine
ERT—estrogen replacement therapy
FFA—free fatty acids
GABA—gamma aminobutyric acid
GLA—gamma linolenic acid
HDL—high density lipoprotein ("good" cholesterol)
HRT—hormone replacement therapy
IUD—intrauterine device
LDL—low density lipoprotein ("bad" cholesterol)
NE—norepinephrine

NTx—N-telopeptide (bone breakdown product)
OC, or OCP—oral contraceptive pill
PCOS—polycystic ovary syndrome (also abbreviated just PCO)
PMS—premenstrual syndrome (also called PMDD—premenstrual dysphoric disorder)
POD—premature ovarian decline
POF—premature ovarian failure
POPs—persistent organic pollutants
SERMS—selective estrogen receptor modulators
ST—serotonin (also called 5-HT or 5-hydroxytryptophan)
TG—triglycerides

Measurements

cc—cubic centimeter (1 cc = 1 ml)
dl—deciliter
ɪᴜ—international units
mcg—microgram
mg—milligram
ml—milliliter (1 ml = 1 cc)
ng—nanogram
pg—picogram

II. Medical Terms Defined

Ablation: To remove, as in endometrial ablation. A surgical technique to remove as much as possible of the uterine lining (endometrium) to prevent heavy bleeding and reduce the risk of endometrial cancer.

Addison's disease: Also called "adrenal insufficiency" (AI). An uncommon but medically serious condition caused by an abnormally low production of adrenal hormones. True Addison's disease can be life-threatening if left untreated, but many conditions can cause similar symptoms in the early stages, so an endocrinology evaluation is important if this condition is suspected. There are reliable blood tests to identify the various types of adrenal disorders and distinguish them from other endocrine problems.

Adrenal glands: Two small glands situated on top of the kidneys, which secrete steroid hormones (cortisol, aldosterone, DHEA) and the stress hormones epinephrine and norepinephrine (sometimes grouped together in common usage and called "adrenaline"). Clinical conditions affecting the adrenal include hypoadrenalism or adrenal insufficiency (AI - see definition under *Addison's disease*) and hyperadrenalism or adrenal excess (see definition under *Cushing's syndrome* [disease]).

Affect (affective): A term used to mean "mood" or range of emotional expression. *Affective* refers to emotional content or to disorders of mood.

AIDS: Acquired immune deficiency syndrome, a sexually transmitted viral disease with a long incubation period; leads to a severe chronic illness that is usually fatal.

Alopecia: Loss of hair that is excessive and abnormal. There are many medical, dietary, and lifestyle causes. Anorexia, bulimia, and decline in ovarian and thyroid hormones are common causes in women.

Amenorrhea: The absence of menstrual bleeding in a woman who has not gone through menopause; may be due to prolonged stress, thyroid disorders, excessive exercise, eating disorders, premature ovarian failure, or other causes.

Amino acids: Chemical molecules found in foods that serve as the "building blocks" for the body to make its proteins. "Essential amino acids" are those that the body cannot synthesize and therefore must be included in the food we eat. Dietary protein containing all the essential amino acids is a "complete protein" and can be obtained from animal/dairy products and also by combining, at one meal, any three of the following: nuts, grains, seeds, or legumes.

Anabolic: A term meaning "to build up," as in the "anabolic" phase of metabolism, a process of using nutrients to build larger molecules that are used by the body for growth, repair, and healing. See also *catabolic* and *metabolism*.

Anabolic steroids: Hormones that stimulate the growth of bone and muscle (lean body mass) and have male ("virilizing") effects on body chemistry and shape.

Androgenic: An adjective used to describe substances (natural or synthetic) that produce masculine changes in the body: stimulating male pattern hair growth (or loss), oily skin, acne, deepening of the voice, increased appetite, increased muscle mass, increased bone mass, and increased total cholesterol with lower HDL.

Androgens: A group of hormones that produces masculine effects on the body. This group of hormones is produced by both the adrenal glands and the gonads (testes in males and ovaries in females). Androgens are produced in much smaller amounts in women compared to men. Androgens decrease with age in both men and women, but after menopause in women the levels of androgens are higher relative to the amount of estrogen that remains. This change in balance of androgens to estrogen produces the characteristic body changes (waist-area fat, hair growth on face and chin, etc.) seen in older women.

Androstenedione: An androgenic hormone produced by the ovaries, testes, and adrenal glands; excess levels in women (such as in PCOS) lead to unwanted facial hair, acne, infertility, body fat gain around the middle of the body, oily skin, and other masculinizing effects.

Angina: Pain in the arm, neck, or chest caused by lack of blood supply (ischemia) to the heart.

Antibodies: Protein substances produced by the body (or transferred from a mother to infant during pregnancy) that react with foreign substances called "antigens" as part of our immune process. Antibodies are made in response to foreign tissue such as grafts, bacteria, and viruses; antibodies may also be produced that react against our own body organs (thyroid, ovary, etc.) in the autoimmune disorders.

Antigen: A substance that triggers the formation of antibodies to stimulate an immune reaction; may be introduced from external sources (bacteria, viruses, etc.) or formed within the body.

Antioxidants: Substances such as beta-carotene, selenium, and vitamins A, C, and E, which protect the body's cells and tissues from oxidative damage caused by free radicals.

Atherosclerosis: Artery-clogging deposits formed by cholesterol, fibrin, and "sticky" platelets; a major cause of heart attacks, strokes, angina, and other cardiovascular disease.

Atrophy: Wasting or thinning of tissues or organs. An example is vaginal atrophy, or the thinning and drying of vaginal mucosa that occurs when estradiol, and to some extent testosterone, declines at menopause or is diminished in younger women from other causes.

Benign: Noncancerous or nonmalignant.

Bioavailable: A substance, often carried in the bloodstream, that is unattached to carrier proteins and therefore able to bind to special receptor sites on cells throughout the body. The amount of a compound or hormone that is bioavailable is also called "active" or "free fraction."

Bioflavinoids: Substances found in plants along with vitamin C that exert a beneficial effect upon the walls of the blood and lymphatic vessels.

Bioidentical: Referring to a molecule that has exactly the same makeup and configuration as those made by the body. Hormones that are bioidentical may be made in the laboratory from building blocks found in plants, but end up with the same chemical structure as the hormones made by body organs such as the thyroid and ovary. Bioidentical hormones are often called "natural" hormones, but "natural" may also refer to a biological source (such as a horse) that produces molecules different from those made by the human body. Bioidentical is a more correct term than "natural" when referring to types made by the human body and pharmaceuticals that are designed to duplicate those made by the body.

Bisphosphonates: A group of medications that prevent excess bone breakdown and stimulate the formation of healthy new bone. Examples are Fosamax and Actonel.

Body mass index (BMI): A scientific way of determining body composition. It is calculated according to the formula BMI = weight (kilogram)/height squared (meters). The normal BMI for women ranges from 20 to 25 kg/m² and many hormonal and menstrual problems can be overcome by keeping weight in the normal range.

Bone resorption: The normal process of bone breakdown or "remodeling" that occurs throughout our lives to allow healthy strong bone to replace older, brittle bone. Resorption can lead to osteoporosis if the bone-building process slows down too much and the breakdown (or "withdrawal") of bone exceeds bone formation.

Bound hormone: Hormone that is circulating in the bloodstream connected to a carrier protein (such as sex hormone binding globulin [SHBG] or corticosteroid binding globulin [CBG]), and therefore is not "free" to be biologically active at cell receptor sites. (See *free hormone.*)

Breakthrough bleeding (BTB): Irregular vaginal bleeding or spotting occurring in women when they are taking oral contraceptives or postmenopausal hormone therapy.

Calcitonin (thyrocalcitonin): A hormone produced in the thyroid gland that regulates calcium balance in the body.

Calcium: A crucial mineral involved in maintaining normal bone strength/density, and normal nerve and muscle function.

Cancer: A malignant growth/tumor with rapid multiplication of abnormal cells that may spread to and invade distant body parts.

Cardiovascular disease (CVD): Disease of the heart, arteries, veins, and capillaries that make up the circulatory system.

Catabolic: A term meaning "to break down," as in the "catabolic" phase of metabolism, a process of breaking nutrients into smaller molecules that are either utilized by the body for growth and repair, or excreted through the skin, lungs, kidneys, and bowels. See also *anabolic* and *metabolism.*

CAT scan: A computerized X ray of consecutive sections of the body, which is used to look for tumors, masses, and other abnormal structural changes within the body.

Cell: The basic unit of structure of all animals and plants that carries out the physical functions of life processes, either by itself or working with other cells making up organs.

Cellulite: Fatty deposit resulting in a dimply or lumpy appearance of the skin. It is gradually lost with proper fluid intake, exercise, and overall weight loss.

Cervix: The opening of the *uterus* that projects into the *vagina.* It is also called the mouth of the womb. Some women report that the penis thrusting against the cervix during intercourse leads to greater sexual stimulation and more intense orgasm, which may be a reason to leave the cervix if a woman needs to have the uterus removed.

Chlamydia: A sexually transmitted bacteria that is a common cause of pelvic infection and infertility; may lead to premature ovarian decline or failure.

Chloasma: Brownish pigmentation of the face that can occur in pregnancy (may also be caused by some types of hormonal imbalance and progestin-dominant birth control pills).

Cholesterol: An important body molecule that is needed for the body to make sex hormones, adrenal hormones, and other molecules. It is found in the blood in three forms: (1) high density lipoprotein (HDL), which protects against plaque formation in the arteries (atherosclerosis); (2) low density lipoprotein (LDL), which promotes plaque formation (atherosclerosis); oxidized LDL is the form that damages the walls of blood vessels; and (3) very low density lipoprotein (VLDL), also a plaque promoter. Cholesterol is produced in the liver even when dietary intake is lowered, and it is found in all animal fats and oils (butter, milk, meat, cheese, etc.). A risk ratio is calculated by dividing total cholesterol by HDL value, with a ratio less than 4.5 being the goal for women.

Circadian rhythm: The regular, rhythmic pattern of changes in biological activity and function that occurs over the course of a day. Examples of circadian rhythms are our sleep-wake cycle, the daily cyclic variation in cortisol and melatonin secretion, among many others.

Climacteric: The span of years in a woman's life when hormone levels are gradually decreasing, leading to changes in body shape and function, ultimately ending in the last menstrual period.

Clitoris: The female equivalent (embryologically) of the penis. It is the small bulb found at the top of the vulva, just below the pubic bone, and is covered by a hood of tissue. It contains erectile tissue and nerve endings that are very sensitive to stimulation and enhance a woman's sexual arousal and orgasm. Clitoral nerve endings become less sensitive at menopause with declining hormone levels.

Clotting factors: Substances carried in the bloodstream that promote coagulation (the process of clotting), such as prothrombin, thrombin, thromboplastin, calcium in ionic form, and fibrinogen. Clotting can be retarded by cold, smooth surfaces, and other substances. Clotting is hastened by warming or by providing a rough surface (such as plaque inside arteries). Medications may be given to promote or decrease clotting.

Cluster headache: A severe and intense headache, more common in males, which lasts several hours and may recur frequently over a six- to eight-week period.

Combined oral contraceptive pill (OC): A contraceptive pill containing both female sex hormones, estrogen and a synthetic progestin. (To contrast the combined OC, there are also progestin-only contraceptives. Micronor is an oral tablet; Norplant and Depo-Provera are long-acting implants/injectables).

Complex carbohydrates: Carbohydrates are macronutrients that provide a quick energy source. *Complex carbohydrates* refers to those found occurring naturally "complexed" with fiber, minerals, and other nutrients (such as grains, whole fruits, vegetables). They are more slowly absorbed and utilized than processed or refined carbohydrates (sweets, pasta, white bread).

Conception: The fertilization of the female egg by the spermatozoa (sperm).

Conjugated estrogens: A mixture of estrogens, chemically different from those made in the human female ovary, that may come from animals (Premarin, horse) or plants (Cenestin).

Consent form: A legal document that you are required to sign, thereby giving your consent, before undergoing a surgical operation or before taking some medications.

Contraindication: A medical condition that makes it inadvisable to use a certain medication—for example, the presence of active breast cancer would usually contraindicate taking estrogen; cigarette smoking is a contraindication for using the oral birth control pill if women are over thirty-five.

Corpus luteum: The yellow-colored, progesterone-producing sac that is formed within the ovary from the remains of the follicle after it has released its egg at ovulation.

Corticosteroid: Also called "glucocorticoid." Any of a number of steroid hormones produced by the cortex of the adrenal gland. Cortisol is an example.

Cortisol: An adrenal cortical hormone (glucocorticoid), usually referred to as our body's "stress" hormone because it prepares the body to respond to emergencies or stresses. It is closely related to cortisone in physiological effects.

Cortisone: A steroid compound made naturally by the adrenal glands and also produced synthetically in laboratories for use as a drug. It has a powerful anti-inflammatory effect, but may produce many adverse side effects with high levels over long periods of time.

Creatinine: The end product of creatine metabolism; found in muscle tissue, blood, and urine. High levels may indicate excess muscle breakdown, for example, or advanced stages of kidney disease.

Cushing's syndrome (disease): A group of symptoms and signs such as moon-shaped face, buffalo hump, and high blood pressure caused by excessive amounts of cortisone either produced by the adrenal gland or taken as medication.

Cystic acne: A skin disorder manifesting as blocked pores and pimples, many of which are blind cysts containing pus. It is a severe form of acne.

Daidzein: An isoflavone compound (also called "phytoestrogen") found in soy and other plants that has weak estrogenic effects.

DEXA, or dual-energy X-ray absorptiometry: A highly reliable means of measuring bone mineral density using very small amounts of radiation. Recommended for women with multiple risk factors for osteopenia/osteoporosis, or women who want a baseline measure before beginning menopause.

DHEA, or Dehydroepiandrosterone: One of the androgens produced in the adrenal glands and ovaries in women. Excess levels cause facial hair, scalp hair loss, oily skin, and acne, among other changes.

Disogenin: A steroid compound found in wild yams and other plants that is used by pharmaceutical companies as a "building block," or precursor molecule, to make bioidentical forms of human hormones such as progesterone and 17-beta estradiol. Disogenin in extracts of wild yam (found in skin creams) cannot be converted by the human body to progesterone or estradiol because we lack the necessary enzymes to do this.

Diuretic: A substance, whether synthetic or natural, that stimulates the kidneys to excrete salt (sodium chloride) and water, thereby relieving fluid retention.

Diurnal: Variation by time of day. For example, hormones in the body are often higher at one time of day and lower at another in a predictable pattern. Diseases may alter the normal diurnal pattern—for example, melatonin is normally highest at night (promotes sleep) and lowest in the bright sunlight of daytime. Melatonin that doesn't shut off properly in the daytime is considered a cause of seasonal affective disorder syndrome ("winter depression," or SADS).

Dopamine: A mood-elevating chemical messenger produced in the brain and body; it is also important in preventing Parkinson's disease, and as an inhibitory neurotransmitter preventing inappropriate milk secretion by the breast.

Down-regulation: A process in the brain and body in which the number (or function) of cell receptors are decreased. May occur as a natural process or due to medication effects.

Ectopic pregnancy: A pregnancy implanted in an abnormal position, usually inside a fallopian tube; may cause severe pain, hemorrhage, and infection if it ruptures into the pelvis.

Endocrine disruptor: Naturally occurring or man-made chemical compounds that may attach to hormone receptors in the body and change the way hormones work by blocking their action, intensifying their action, or causing other disruption in the normal actions. Examples of chemical compounds that have hormonelike actions in humans are the phytoestrogens found in many plants such as soy, or man-made chemicals like pesticides. See Chapter 5 for further discussion and types of compounds.

Endocrine glands: Glands that manufacture and secrete hormones.

Endocrinologist: A medical specialist in diseases of the endocrine glands and their hormones; in the United States, endocrinologists focus primarily on evaluating and treating problems of the nonreproductive endocrine glands pituitary, thyroid, parathyroid, pancreas (disorders of insulin, such as diabetes), and adrenal (Addison's, Cushing's, and disorders of androgen excess such as hirsutism), while the ovaries as an endocrine organ are primarily evaluated and treated by gynecologists.

Endocrinology: The study and treatment of disorders of the glands and the hormones they secrete.

Endometrial ablation: A surgical technique to remove as much as possible of the uterine lining (endometrium) to prevent heavy bleeding and reduce the risk of endometrial cancer.

Endometrial hyperplasia: Abnormal degree of thickening of the lining of the uterus, usually due to excess estrogen effect with insufficient progesterone or progestin effect. If left uncontrolled, may lead over time to the development of endometrial cancer.

Endometrial lining: Also called "endometrium." The lining of the uterus. This tissue grows under the influence of estrogen (*proliferative* endometrium), and thickens under the influence of progesterone each month (*secretory* endometrium) in the menstrual cycle. The fall in progesterone (or a progestin, such as Provera, Aygestin, and others), triggers the secretory endometrium to "slough" and then be shed from the uterus in the monthly bleeding.

Endometriosis: The presence of small islands (implants) of endometrium lying outside of the uterus, scattered about the abdomen and pelvic cavities and many times stuck on the outside of the intestine and bladder. Endometrium tissue is normally found only inside the uterus, and menstrual blood is released to the outside of the body via the vagina. When these implants bleed at the time of menses, they cause such severe pain because the blood is released into the abdomen and pelvis and acts as a significant irritant to other organs.

Endorphins: Also called "enkephalins." Natural pain-relieving and mood-elevating compounds (peptides) produced in the brain, spinal cord, and body to produce a morphinelike analgesia.

Enterohepatic circulation: Blood flow from the gastrointestinal tract to the liver that prolongs the action of compounds such as estrogen and other hormones by allowing them to "recirculate" rather than be excreted in the stool.

Enzymes: Proteins produced by living cells that assist body functions by acting as catalysts in specific biochemical reactions. Enzyme catalysts are not themselves consumed in the reactions.

Epinephrine (adrenaline): A chemical messenger made by the adrenal gland that prepares the body to handle emergencies; called the fight-or-flight response. Epinephrine is also made in the laboratory to be used as a drug to treat severe allergic reactions, asthma, severe bleeding, and certain types of heart rhythm problems.

Equine estrogens, equilin: Estrogens derived from **pregnant mares'** urine and used to make the animal-derived estrogen Premarin. These estrogens are chemically different from those made by the human ovary. They have some effects that are similar to human estrogens, and some effects that are quite different. See Chapters 5, 13, and 15 for detailed explanations.

Essential fatty acids: Fatty acids necessary for cellular metabolism that cannot be made by the body, so they must be supplied in the diet. Good sources are fish oil, oils from nuts and seeds, and evening primrose oil.

Estrogen: The group of three sex hormones produced by the gonads (ovaries in women, testes in men) and the adrenal gland. In women, the higher amounts of these sex hormones are responsible for the female characteristics of breasts, feminine curves, menstruation, and pregnancy.

- **Estrone (E1):** One of the human estrogens made by the ovary, adrenal gland, and body fat before menopause. It is the one found in higher amounts after menopause because it is still made by body fat and, to a lesser extent, the adrenal glands. Estrone serves as a "storage" form of estrogen for the ovary to make the more active estradiol before menopause. High estrone levels are more associated with breast and uterine cancers, a good reason to maintain a healthy percent body fat and weight.

- **Estradiol (E2, 17-beta estradiol):** The primary estrogen produced by the ovary before menopause. It is the biologically active estrogen at the estrogen receptors and the most potent of all the natural human estrogens. Estradiol is involved in over four hundred functions in a woman's body, and is the form of estrogen that is lost at menopause when the ovary follicles are depleted.

- **Estriol (E3):** The weakest of the primary human estrogens, it is produced in large amounts during pregnancy. It is barely detectable in the nonpregnant female body, so women do not normally have estriol present to a measurable degree on a continuous basis and it has not been shown to have bone-, heart-, or brain-preserving effects.

- **Estradiol valerate:** A synthetic estrogen, chemically different from the 17-beta estradiol produced by the ovary; used for menopausal hormone therapy in Europe for many years, but not used very often in the United States.

- **Ethinyl estradiol:** A more potent synthetic estrogen used in birth control pills where the higher potency is needed (with the synthetic progestins) to adequately suppress the ovaries and provide reliable contraception. Not generally used in the United States for menopausal hormone therapy.

Evening primrose oil: The oil extracted from the evening primrose plant. It is a good source of the omega-6 fatty acids, in particular the essential fatty acid know as gamma linolenic acid (GLA).

Fallopian tubes: The tubes that carry the egg (ovum) from the ovary to the uterus. Fertilization of the egg occurs in the outer part of the fallopian tube.

Feedback: The process by which products made in a series of reactions provide messages back to the beginning of the process to control further reactions. Feedback may be electrical, chemical or mechanical, or thermal. An example of a thermal "feedback" is the thermostat that controls your furnace. Chemical feedback occurs when hormone levels reach a critical level and feed back to the brain that no more is needed for a while.

Female sex hormones: The two sex hormones produced by the female ovary and placenta during pregnancy, estrogen (see above for types) and progesterone.

Fertilization: The union of the female egg (ovum) with the male sperm (spermatozoa), which occurs in the fallopian tube.

Fetus: A developing human, medically defined as from the end of the eighth week of pregnancy until birth.

Fibrocystic: Development of dense, lumpy, ropy (fibrous) changes in tissue. Sixty to 70 percent of healthy women will have "fibrocystic" changes in their breasts, and this does not indicate a disease process. Similar changes may occur in muscle tissue in chronic pain syndromes.

Fibroid (fibroma): Noncancerous growth of the uterus consisting of muscle and fibrous tissue. The medical term is *leiomyoma,* or sometimes just *myoma.* The presence of fibroids tends to cause heavy, painful bleeding and cramps. At times they cause back pain, referred pain to the hip, or bladder pain and pressure with incontinence, depending on where the fibroids are found in the uterus.

First-pass metabolism: Breakdown of chemicals, medications, hormones, and such by the liver as a first step after being absorbed into the bloodstream from the gastrointestinal tract. First-pass metabolism can eliminate as much as 70 percent or more of an oral dose of a medication or hormone. This step is omitted when medications and hormones are absorbed directly into the bloodstream from the skin (patch or cream) or muscle (injection).

Follicle stimulating hormone (FSH): A hormone secreted by the pituitary gland that reaches the ovaries via the bloodstream and stimulates the growth of ovarian follicles to form the egg that is released at ovulation. FSH levels above 10–15 indicate that the brain senses a decline in ovarian hormones; levels of FSH greater than 20 are defined as menopausal. FSH also functions in men to stimulate the sperm-producing cells in the testes; high FSH levels in men indicate low levels of testosterone, sometimes called "andropause."

Follicular (phase): The first half of the ovarian hormone cycle leading up to the release of the egg at ovulation. Estrogen (estradiol) is the dominant hormone for this part of the cycle, and there is very little progesterone present.

Free hormone: Hormone that is circulating in the bloodstream not connected to a carrier protein, and therefore "free" to be biologically active at cell receptor sites. See also *bound hormone.*

Free radicals: "Scavenger" molecules that are highly reactive, attacking body cells and tissues, causing damage leading to diseases like cancer. Free radicals are produced in the body when cells turn food into energy, and they lack an electron, so they try to "borrow" one by attaching to other molecules in cells. This sets off a chain reaction leading to cell damage. Vitamins E and C and even estradiol are called "antioxidants" because they bind up these free radicals and help prevent damage to cells.

Frigid (sexual): A negative term applied to women who are considered by their partner to be sexually unresponsive and disinterested. Hormonal, medical, and relationship factors may cause loss of sexual desire and responsiveness, and all of these should be properly evaluated to determine the cause of sexual difficulties.

Galactorrhea: The presence of milk or milky fluid in the breasts when not breastfeeding. It is usually a symptom of elevated prolactin, which may be caused by some medications (such as antidepressants) or by benign hormone-producing tumors (adenomas) of the pituitary gland.

Gamma aminobutyric acid (GABA): An inhibitory neurotransmitter in the brain and nerves throughout the body; activation of this neurotransmitter produces a calming or antianxiety effect.

Gamma linolenic acid (GLA): An omega-6 essential fatty acid that is used to synthesize prostaglandins. It has an anti-inflammatory effect in the body. Good sources are breast milk, evening primrose oil, borage plant oil, and black currant seed oil.

Genistein: An isoflavone compound (also called "phytoestrogen") found in soy and other plants that has weak estrogenlike effects. In some concentrations it acts to block estrogen receptors, while in other concentrations it may stimulate the estrogen receptors in certain tissues.

Glands: Body organs or tissues, generally soft and fleshy in consistency, that manufacture and secrete or excrete hormones, chemicals that exert their effects on target organs elsewhere in the body.

Glucocorticoid: A group of hormones produced in the adrenal cortex that are primarily active in protecting against stress and in regulating protein and carbohydrate metabolism. These compounds (such as cortisone) tend to increase blood glucose and liver glycogen, and suppress the immune response and inflammatory response. Levels that are too high over time cause bone loss.

Goitrogen: A chemical substance that can trigger formation of a goiter, or benign growth, in the thyroid gland. Goitrogens may be naturally occurring compounds or man-made. See Chapter 9 for further discussion.

Gynecology: Surgical specialty of medicine that provides surgical and medicinal treatments for problems related to women's reproductive organs.

Half-life: A measurement of how long it takes for half of a substance to be lost or removed; for example, drug half-life refers to how long it takes for the concentration of a drug or hormone to be decreased by one-half due to metabolic breakdown or excretion. It is usually estimated that it takes five half-lives for a substance to be completely gone from the body.

HDL: See *cholesterol.*

Hirsutism: A condition of excessive facial and body hair (excluding hair on the scalp) and in women is often due to excess of androgens.

Hormone receptor site: A "binding" or "docking" site in or on cells for hormones to connect in order to exert their actions. The hormone and its receptor create what is called a "receptor complex" that sends signals to the cell to carry out various functions.

Hormone replacement therapy (HRT): Technically, the administration of any hormonal preparations (natural or synthetic) to replace the loss of natural hormones produced by various glands (thyroid, ovary, testes, pancreas, adrenal, pituitary, etc.). *HRT* in common usage now refers to menopausal administration of female hormones (estrogen and progestin).

Hormones: Chemicals produced by various glands that are then transported around the body to exert their multiple metabolic effects.

Hot flash (flush): Episode of vasodilation in skin of head, neck, and chest, accompanied by sensation of suffocation, sweating, feeling suddenly hot or cold. Occurs commonly during the transition to full menopause due to falling hormone levels that trigger changes in the brain heat regulatory center.

Hyperplasia: Abnormally thickened lining of the uterus; if left untreated, may later increase the risk of uterine (endometrial) cancer.

Hyperthyroidism: A condition caused by excessive hormone secretion of the thyroid glands that will increase the basal metabolic rate, increase heart rate and blood pressure, and disrupt sleep, and may cause marked weight loss.

Hypoestrogenic: The condition of having less than optimal levels of estradiol from any cause. Estradiol decline leads to classic symptoms affecting many different body systems, such as hot flashes, insomnia, memory loss, headaches, palpitations, fatigue, thinning hair, dry skin/eyes, bone loss, rise in cholesterol and blood pressure, urinary leakage, loss of libido, vaginal dryness, muscle aches, crawly skin, and more.

Hypothalamus: The "master conductor" or "control center" situated at the base of the brain, it regulates body temperature, thirst, appetite, sex drive, and all other hormonal glands. It releases hormones that travel directly to the pituitary gland and stimulate the release of pituitary hormones, which govern the other endocrine glands.

Hypothyroidism: A slowing of overall body metabolism due to deficiency of the thyroid hormone production or function. There are many diverse symptoms, but common ones include obesity, dry skin and hair, low blood pressure, slow pulse, sluggishness of all functions, constipation, depressed mood, muscle aches/weakness, hair loss, low energy, goiter.

Hysterectomy: Surgical removal (abdominal or vaginal) of the uterus only. In common usage, women may say "hysterectomy" when both the uterus and ovaries have been removed or when just the uterus has been removed. The medical term for removal of the uterus and ovaries together is "hysterectomy with bilateral salpingo-oophorectomy (BSO)."

Immune system: The defense and surveillance system of the body that protects against infection by microorganisms and invasion by foreign tissues and substances. The immune system is made up of specialized blood cells (lymphocytes, B-cells, T-cells, etc.), blood proteins (antibodies), the spleen, thymus gland, lymph nodes, and bone marrow. Immune function is impaired with a variety of endocrine imbalances, such as menopause and thyroid disorders.

Implant: A device that is surgically implanted into a part of the body for cosmetic or therapeutic purposes. Hormone-containing implants are sometimes used for contraception or for menopausal hormone replacement therapy.

Inflammation: A condition characterized by swelling, redness, heat, and pain in any tissue as a result of trauma, irritation, infection, or imbalances in immune function.

Incontinence: Involuntary loss of urine. Several different types. See Chapter 11.

Insulin: A hormone secreted by beta cells of the pancreas that is essential for the proper metabolism of blood sugar (glucose), for maintenance of proper blood sugar level, and for promoting storage of fat. Insulin medication is used to control high blood sugar in diabetes.

Isoflavones: Chemical compounds found in a variety of plants (soy, red clover, etc.) that are weakly estrogenic in their effects and are often called "phytoestrogens" (*phyto* meaning "derived from plants"). Common isoflavones that are being studied for their health effects are genistein, daidzein, biochanin, and formononetin.

IUD: Intrauterine device, an object inserted into the uterus, typically used for contraception, but may also be a means of delivering hormones (for example, Progestasert progestin delivery system).

Laparoscope: A long thin telescopic instrument, utilizing a fiberoptic lighting system, that is inserted through a small incision in the abdominal wall. It functions like a hollow flashlight enabling the surgeon to view internal organs and insert operating instruments through a hollow tube.

Laparoscopy: Surgical technique used in gynecology, general surgery, orthopedic surgery, and others that is performed through the laparoscope in order to use smaller incisions and still visualize areas inside the body. In many cases, laparoscopic surgery means shorter recovery time.

LDL: See *cholesterol.*

Libido: Level of sexual desire, sexual energy, or drive.

Lipoproteins: Carrier proteins in the bloodstream that transport fats (cholesterol and triglycerides) in the blood.

Luteal (phase): The progesterone-dominant second half of the menstrual cycle, from ovulation until menses begin. The primary hormone of this phase is progesterone. It is also the time of the cycle when PMS occurs.

Luteinizing hormone (LH): A hormone produced by the pituitary gland that triggers ovulation and the egg release to become the corpus luteum. In men, LH stimulates production of testosterone by the testes, and LH levels will rise in men with low testosterone.

Male hormone: A hormone that promotes masculine characteristics in the body such as facial and body hair, acne, deepening of the voice, increased muscle mass, and increased libido.

Malignant: Cancer, cancerous.

Manic depression (bipolar disorder): A biological disorder of brain function that produces episodes of euphoria, delusions, and abnormally increased energy, alternating at variable intervals with severe depressions.

Melatonin: A hormone produced by the pineal gland in the brain and involved in regulating the sleep-wake cycle; levels rise during darkness and fall at daylight. Excess melatonin levels that fail to shut off during the day have been thought to cause seasonal affective disorder (SADS).

Menopause: The cessation of menstruation. The last period. May be natural (due to depletion of the ovarian follicles) or surgical removal of the uterus (with or without removal of ovaries). When the ovaries are gone or have lost their follicles, the body loses the hormones estradiol, progesterone, testosterone, and much of the DHEA. The period of time leading up to menopause, when hormone production by the ovaries is decreasing, is called "the climacteric."

Menstrual clock: A specialized part of the hypothalamus regulating the cyclical timing of the phases of the menstrual cycle.

Menstruation: Monthly bleeding from the vagina in women from puberty until menopause, caused by shedding of the lining of the womb (uterus) if there is no fertilization of an egg.

Metabolic hormones: Hormones that are involved in regulating cellular energy processes, synthesis of body proteins, and other functions involved in tissue growth and repair.

Metabolic rate: The rate at which the body converts chemical energy in foods into heat (thermal) and movement (kinetic) energy. Metabolic rate is governed by hormones from the thyroid, ovary, testes, adrenal, and pancreas.

Metabolism: Chemical processes, regulated by hormones, utilizing the raw materials of food nutrients, oxygen, minerals, vitamins along with enzymes to produce energy for body functions such as growth, repair, healing. See also *anabolic, catabolic metabolism.*

Metabolite: Any product of metabolism. Some metabolites are active and needed for other functions, and some metabolites may be toxic and need to be excreted. An example of a toxic metabolite is ammonia from the breakdown of protein; an active metabolite of progesterone has anxiety-relieving properties when it binds to the brain's GABA receptor.

Microgram (mcg): One millionth part of a gram. One thousandth of a milligram.

Milligram (mg): One thousandth of a gram. See also *picogram, nanogram.*

Milliliter (ml): One thousandth of a liter, or about 1 cc.

Micronized: Making particles, such as large steroid hormones, small enough to be well-absorbed when taken by mouth.

Mineralocorticoid: Hormones produced by the adrenal gland that primarily function to regulate electrolytes (sodium, potassium, chloride) and water balance in the body. An example is aldosterone.

Molecule: A chemical compound made up of different arrangements and types of atoms; a molecule is the smallest unit into which a substance may be divided without loss of its unique characteristics.

Myomectomy: The surgical removal of fibroids (myomas) that leaves the uterus and cervix intact. This procedure preserves fertility, but may frequently be a more complicated surgery with greater blood loss than hysterectomy. Complications and risk of damage may be similar to hysterectomy. Careful evaluation by an experienced surgeon is important to determine whether a woman is a good candidate for myomectomy.

Nanogram (ng): One billionth of a gram.

"Natural" hormones: Bioidentical hormones are often called "natural" hormones, but *natural* may also refer to a biological source (such as the horse) that produces molecules that are different from those made by the human body. *Bioidentical* is a more correct term than *natural* when referring to the types made by the human body and pharmaceuticals that are designed to duplicate those made by the body. Hormones that are "bioidentical" may be made in the laboratory from building blocks found in plants, but end up with the same chemical structure as the hormones made by body organs such as the thyroid and ovary.

Neuron: A nerve cell, the structure and functional unit of the nervous system. Neurons function in initiation and conduction of electrical and chemical "nerve" impulses.

Neurotransmitters: Chemicals that transmit messages from nerve cell to nerve cell in the brain, and between the brain and the tissues and organs of the body. Common ones referred to throughout this book are serotonin, dopamine, acetylcholine, GABA, norepinephrine.

Nonandrogenic: Not causing masculine hormone effects in the body.

Norepinephrine (noradrenaline): A hormone produced by the adrenal gland and certain areas of the brain that helps the body prepare for and cope with stress. It also has a mood-elevating effect, but levels that are too high may cause feelings of anxiety, raise blood pressure, and cause insomnia. Epinephrine (adrenaline) is another "stress hormone" produced by the adrenal gland with similar effects in some tissues and opposite effects in others.

Nucleus: The vital body inside cells that contains the genetic material (DNA) and is responsible for regulation of essential functions for cell growth, protein synthesis, metabolism, reproduction, and transmission of characteristics of a cell.

Oophorectomy (ovariectomy): Surgical removal of the ovaries.

Oophoritis: An inflammation involving the ovaries that may be caused by autoimmune disorders, bacterial infections such as chlamydia, viral illness such as mononucleosis and many others, or exposure to environmental toxins.

Oral: A substance taken by mouth that then passes through the stomach and intestines to be absorbed and undergo first-pass metabolism by the liver. This is contrasted with *non-oral,* or *parenteral,* which means that the substance delivered is absorbed directly from tissues into the bloodstream without going through the stomach and intestines and bypasses the first-pass changes in the liver. Examples of non-oral delivery include sublingual, subcutaneous, transdermal (also called "topical"), vaginal, rectal, intramuscular, and intravenous.

Orgasm: The physical and emotional release of sexual arousal tension; also called "climax."

Osteoblast: Cells that constantly function to build new bone (an easy way to remember is that "*blasts build bone.*" These cells are stimulated by estradiol and testosterone and to a mild degree by progesterone, if first primed with adequate estradiol.

Osteoclast: Cells that are responsible for breaking down old brittle bone in the process called "*remodeling*" that keeps the skeleton strong and healthy. Estradiol and testosterone both help to keep the osteoclasts from breaking down too much bone; if these hormones are diminished, the osteoclasts break down more bone than can be built back, and bone loss leading to osteoporosis occurs.

Osteopenia: Loss of bone density that is not yet severe enough to be considered osteoporosis. Osteopenia will progress to osteoporosis if active measures are not taken to maintain bone (such as calcium, magnesium, exercise, estradiol and testosterone therapy, or use of newer medications such as Actonel, Fosamax, or Miacalcin).

Osteoporosis: Loss of bone density (mass) due to loss of bone minerals and reduction of the normal bony architecture that provides strength to the skeleton. Causes bones to become porous, brittle, and more easily broken. Once osteoporosis occurs, aggressive combined treatment with calcium, vitamin D, magnesium, exercise, estradiol and testosterone therapy, and use of newer medications such as Actonel, Fosamax, Miacalcin, or Evista are needed to prevent fractures.

Ovarian blood supply: The blood carried to the ovaries via the ovarian arteries, which branch off from the uterine blood vessels. The ovarian arteries run alongside the fallopian tubes and may be injured or damaged with surgical procedures on the tubes (such as tubal ligation or hysterectomy even if the ovaries are not removed).

Ovaries: The female sex glands (gonads) located on each side of the uterus, which produce eggs and the female sex hormones (estrogen and progesterone), along with the androgens (androstenedione, testosterone, and DHEA).

Ovulation: The release of the egg from the ovary occurring around midcycle.

Ovulation pain: "Mittelschmerz" pain occurring at ovulation, which may be sharp and severe and last from a few minutes up to twelve hours.

Ovum (ova): An ovarian follicle that has released to become the egg (ovum) at ovulation. An ovum that is fertilized with sperm becomes an embryo that develops into a fetus.

Pancreas: A gland situated behind the stomach that produces pancreatic juice (contains digestive enzymes such as lipase and amylase) and also the hormones insulin and glucagon that function to regulate blood sugar and carbohydrate metabolism.

Parasympathetic nervous system: The part of the autonomic nervous system that regulates body relaxation and functions of growth and repair such as digestion. Its primary chemical messenger or neurotransmitter is acetylcholine.

Parathyroid gland: Located close to the thyroid gland, one of several small endocrine glands that secrete a hormone, parathormone, which regulates calcium and phosphorus metabolism.

Parenteral: Referring to a method of delivering substances (such as medications) directly to the bloodstream and bypassing the digestive system and first-pass liver metabolism. Parenteral routes include vaginal rings, intrauterine devices, vaginal and rectal suppositories/tablets, sublingual troches or tablets, transdermal (skin patch), subcutaneous (implant), intramuscular (IM) and intravenous (IV) injections.

Peak level: The highest level of a hormone or medication that is reached after taking a dose or being produced by the body. ("Trough" level is the lowest point reached after a medication or hormone is taken or produced by the body.)

Pelvic inflammatory disease (PID): Inflammation of the pelvic organs, particularly the uterus and fallopian tubes, caused by infectious microorganisms, typically occurring from sexually transmitted bacteria, fungi, and viruses.

Perimenopausal: Time frame of several years prior to menopause, when hormone production declines and menstrual periods start to be skipped, and continuing through menopause to the first few years just after periods stop. It has a variable age of onset and symptoms commonly include insomnia, mood changes, bone loss, cholesterol changes, disrupted sleep, hot flashes, and other phenomena. See also *premenopausal.*

Persistent organic pollutants (POPs): Man-made compounds, such as pesticides and industrial chemicals, that persist for decades or even *centuries* in the environment without breaking down as naturally occurring chemicals do. Most of the compounds in this class are damaging to the endocrine systems of living organisms, including humans, so they are included in the broader category of endocrine disruptors. POPs can adversely affect everything in the human body that is governed by hormones. See Chapter 5 for further discussion.

Pessary: An oval-shaped object designed to be inserted into the vagina for support of a prolapsed uterus or bladder; may also be used to deliver medications or hormones to vaginal tissue.

Pharmacokinetics/dynamics: Study of drug absorption, delivery to tissues of the body, metabolism, and excretion.

Physiological: Of the normal body processes and functions.

Phytoestrogens: Plant- *(phyto-)* derived chemical molecules that may attach to the body's estrogen receptors and trigger certain estrogenlike actions; some of these compounds have estrogen-blocking actions (antagonists) that may or may not be desirable. They occur naturally in several hundred different types of plants, including soy, clover, and a variety of grains.

Picogram (pg): One trillionth of a gram.

Pituitary gland: A mushroom-shaped gland connected by a vascular stalk to the base of the brain. The pituitary gland manufactures hormones (FSH, LH, TSH, ACTH, and others) that in turn control other hormonal glands, such as the thyroid, adrenals, ovaries, and breasts.

Placenta: The hormonal organ designed to provide for the nourishment of the fetus and the elimination of its waste products. It produces a number of hormones, such as progesterone, estradiol, and estriol, which have roles in sustaining pregnancy and adapting the mother's body to adjust to the increased physiological demands of pregnancy. It is formed in the uterus by the union of uterine mucous membrane with membranes of the fetus.

Plaque: A deposit of platelets, fibrin, calcium, cholesterol, and other fatty substances that build up in arteries and cause clogging that leads to reduced blood flow and may cause angina, heart attacks, or strokes. The whole process of plaque buildup and artery damage is referred to as atherosclerosis.

Plasma: The liquid part of blood and the lymph (minus the red and white blood cells) that contains proteins, clotting factors, and other chemicals such as glucose, hormones, etc.

PMS: See *premenstrual syndrome.*

Polycystic ovary syndrome (PCO or PCOS): A disorder of the ovaries in which the usual female hormonal balance is altered, and there are excessive levels of insulin and male hormones accompanied by changes in body shape and irregular menstruation. It may be hereditary, or it may also be triggered by environmental endocrine disruptors, stress, or weight gain. In PCOS, the ovaries develop multiple small follicles or "cysts," which may or may not be seen on an ultrasound scan of the pelvis. Other common features: truncal obesity, acne, glucose intolerance and insulin resistance, excess facial and body hair, thinning scalp hair, hypertension, infertility, and changes in mood related to the hormonal imbalances.

Postmenopause: The years following the end of menstruation and decline in production of ovarian female hormones (menopause).

Postnatal, postpartum: The time period after childbirth.

Precursor: A substance ("building block") that is used to make another compound, hormone, or medication. For example, cholesterol molecules are used as the building blocks for the body to make other steroid hormones, such as progesterone.

Premature menopause, or premature ovarian failure (POF): Decline of ovarian hormone production, with loss of menstrual periods and ovulation/fertility that occurs before the age of forty-two. It is characterized by high, menopausal levels of FSH and LH, and low levels of the ovarian hormones (estradiol, progesterone, testosterone, and DHEA). POF or premature menopause may have many causes, for example, autoimmune disorders, chemical exposure, bacterial or viral illnesses, surgeries that damage ovarian blood flow, cigarette smoking, or genetic factors.

Premature ovarian decline (POD): Decline in production of the normal levels of ovarian hormones that occurs prior to the age of forty-two, which is the age arbitrarily selected as the lower end of the age range for the onset of "normal" menopausal declines. Typically, estradiol declines first, while the ovary still makes healthy normal levels of progesterone, testosterone, and DHEA. Later in the process of ovarian decline, estradiol reaches a low enough level that ovulation no longer occurs regularly and progesterone then declines, followed still later by reduced testosterone production. At this time, there is no accepted medical "code" for this phase of diminished ovarian hormone levels, but doctors often use such terms as *irregular menses* or *PMS* to define hormonally related problems.

Premenopausal: The time leading up to menopause characterized by hormonal changes and irregular menstrual flow. It may begin as much as ten years before actual menopause, but more commonly occurs about four to five years before menopause. See also *perimenopause.*

Premenstrual syndrome (PMS): A collection of variable symptoms such as mood disturbance, headaches, abdominal bloating, among many more recurring on a cyclical basis in the week or two before menstrual bleeding that can at times be severe enough to interfere with quality of life and ability to function. See also *peri-menopause.*

Progesterone: A steroid hormone produced by the corpus luteum (formed from the egg released at ovulation in the ovary) or placenta during pregnancy. Small amounts are also made by the adrenal glands. Responsible for secretory changes in uterine endometrium in second half of menstrual cycle to prepare the uterus to receive and nourish a fertilized egg. Progesterone also has many metabolic functions designed to help a mother's body change in ways that will support a pregnancy (pro-*gesta*tion hormone = pro*geste*rone).

Progestin: A group of hormones that have progesteronelike effects on the uterus and body; progesterone is correctly included in this larger class of hormones, but common usage is that *progestin* usually refers to synthetic compounds that are made in the laboratory and are chemically different from the natural ovary compound progesterone.

Progestin-only pill ("mini-pill"): A contraceptive pill containing only a progestin such as norethindrone (Micronor, among others). Unless it is given with estrogen to balance the unwanted side effects, the progestin-only pills are not recommended for midlife women due to the potential for adverse effects on cholesterol, glucose control, and body weight. Progestin-only pills, implants, or injections are not recommended for women with a history of depression, diabetes, headaches, hypertension, or weight gain as progestins aggravate all of these problems unless estrogen is also given.

Progestogens: Natural or synthetic substances that have effects similar to the natural female hormone progesterone. Synthetic progestogens (called "progestins") are commonly used in birth control pills and HRT to regulate menstrual bleeding. Examples are medroxyprogesterone acetate (Provera, Cycrin), norethindrone (Aygestin, Micronor), norethisterone, norgestrel, etc.

Prolactin: A hormone secreted by the pituitary gland that stimulates milk production in the breasts. At times other than nursing, high levels of prolactin from medications or pituitary tumors may cause headaches, weight gain, depression, and breast discharge (galactorrhea).

Prostaglandins: Chemicals manufactured throughout the body that exert a hormone-like effect and influence muscular (including the uterus) contraction, circulation, and inflammation. Release of prostaglandins in the uterus at the time of menstruation is a cause of menstrual cramps.

Prostate gland: This gland is located just below the bladder in men and secretes fluid into the ejaculate of semen during male orgasm.

Psychosis: A severe biochemical disorder of brain function characterized by delusions, hallucinations, and abnormalities in thinking and reasoning. It may have many causes—schizophrenia, major depression, manic-depressive disorder, alcohol intoxication, severe endocrine illness (for example, hyper- and hypothyroidism), drug abuse (cocaine), and medication toxicity (such as atropine, digitalis, lidocaine, stimulants, and many others).

Psychosomatic: Physical symptoms that are triggered by psychological and emotional causes and not due primarily to physical disease. This term is often misused when applied to women, as in "the cause isn't known so it must be psychosomatic, or stress-related."

Psychotherapy: The process of using systematic "talking" approaches to treat stress-related problems, emotional issues, and disturbances in self-image. Many different methods may be used, depending upon the training of the therapist.

Psychotropic drugs: Drugs that act primarily on the brain to produce effects on mood, thinking, sleep, and other functions. Examples are sedatives, tranquilizers (antianxiety agents), antidepressants, antipsychotics, analgesic and anesthetic agents.

Puerperium: The period of time after childbirth required to return the reproductive organs to their prepregnant size and condition. This takes six to eight weeks.

Receptor: See *hormone receptor site.*

Receptor antagonist (blocker): A compound, hormone, or medication that binds at a cell's receptor site but blocks the normal action of that receptor system. Examples are beta-blockers, which block the normal action of the beta adrenergic receptors; Tamoxifen, which blocks the estrogen receptor of the breast and brain even though it will activate the estrogen receptors in the uterine lining (endometrium).

Rectal: Pertaining to the rectum.

Sebaceous glands: The tiny oil-producing glands in the skin. If they overproduce oil and/or become obstructed, pimples or acne will result.

Serms: An acronym for a class of medications called "*S*elective *E*strogen *R*eceptor *M*odulators." These drugs have both agonist (activating) and antagonist (blocking) actions at the body's estrogen receptors, depending on the particular organ. Examples are Tamoxifen and Raloxifen; both drugs *block* breast estrogen receptors and *stimulate* estrogen receptors elsewhere (such as in bone). Because they block important actions of estrogen, they are not a pure replacement for all of estrogen's actions in the body. Side effects of both medicines include hot flashes, formation of blood clots, pulmonary emboli, cataracts, and increased risk of uterine cancer (Tamoxifen).

Serotonin (5-HT): A potent brain chemical that regulates sleep, mood, libido, appetite, pain, and repetitive thoughts and actions. Serotonin's chemical name is 5-hydroxytryptophan and it is made by the brain and body from dietary sources of the amino acid tryptophan (milk, turkey, whole grains, etc.).

Serum: The fluid portion of the blood after coagulation has removed the cells, fibrin, and fibrinogen.

Sex hormone binding globulin: A carrier protein in the bloodstream (made in the liver) that binds or carries estrogen, testosterone, and progesterone to provide a reservoir of hormones ready for release into the free fraction to become the active form.

Sex hormones: The male and female hormones produced from cholesterol by the testicles, ovaries, adrenal glands, and body fat: testosterone, estrogens, progesterone, androgens.

Steroid drugs and hormones: The group of chemical substances that has a chemical structure consisting of multiple rings of carbon atoms. Cortisone (the drug), estrogen, progesterone, and testosterone (sex hormones).

Stress (urinary) incontinence: Loss of urine due to pressure on weakened bladder structures and supporting ligaments; this weakness occurs as a result of estrogen loss and damage during childbirth. Increased pressure on the bladder may come from coughing, sneezing, laughing, straining to lift objects, or prolonged standing.

Stroke: Brain damage resulting from diminished blood supply and oxygen (ischemia) to the brain; usually occurs as a result of a clot blocking the arteries.

Sublingual: Medication, hormones, allergy drops, etc., taken by placing under the tongue to be absorbed into the bloodstream.

Sustained (timed) release: A process in which a medication is prepared or formulated in such a way as to deliver small amounts over a longer period of time.

Sympathetic nervous system: The part of the autonomic nervous system that prepares the body for stress through effects of the stress hormones it releases (for example, by increasing oxygen to the tissues, increasing heart rate, blood pressure, and glucose release, etc.). Its primary chemical messengers (neurotransmitters) are norepinephrine and epinephrine.

Symptom: Any physical or emotional change in the body that is perceived as distressing or painful. *Symptom* usually means a change that makes a person feel unwell. *Phenomena* is a word used to describe changes that don't necessarily cause distress.

Syndrome: A group of symptoms and objective signs that typically occur together and serve to characterize a disease or disorder.

Synergistic: Substances interacting in ways that produce an effect *greater than* just adding the effects of the combined substances.

Synthetic: Made by synthesis; can be identical to a natural compound found in the body, or may be synthesized to be chemically different and have different properties. *Synthetic* simply means "made by synthesis"; it *does not* mean "artificial" (although common usage often implies "artificial" when the term is used to apply to a hormone).

Testes: The male gonads; two reproductive glands located in the scrotum that produce the male reproductive cells, or spermatozoa, and the male hormone, testosterone.

Testosterone: The major male sex hormone produced in the testes and also in smaller amounts by the female ovary; plays major role in men and women for sexual arousal, maintaining bone and muscle mass, psychological well-being.

Thymus: A gland located at the base of the neck that is important in development of immune response in newborns, with lesser activity as we get older. The cortex of the gland is composed of dense lymphoid tissue that produces the T-cells of the immune system.

Thyroid gland: The endocrine gland situated in front of the larynx that produces the major hormones of metabolism—thyroxine (T4) and triiodothyronine (T3)—as well as calcitonin, which regulates calcium balance.

Thyroid stimulating hormone (TSH): The hormone produced by the brain that regulates the production and release of thyroid hormones from the thyroid gland. TSH levels are low in *hyper*thyroidism, and high in *hypo*thyroidism.

Transdermal: Absorbed through the skin into the bloodstream from a cream or patch or an injection; this form of delivery bypasses the liver's first-pass metabolism.

Triglycerides (TG): One of the blood fats that the body can use to make cholesterol; elevated TG (from diet, alcohol intake, lack of exercise, and some drugs) are a significant and *independent* risk factor for heart disease in women and also increase the risk of diabetes. Consists of one glycerol and three fatty acids.

Tryptophan: An amino acid found in foods that is the major precursor (building block) for the body and brain to make serotonin (5-hydroxytryptophan, 5-HT).

Tubal ligation (BTL): The surgical procedure to cut or tie the fallopian tubes and prevent "eggs" released from the ovary from reaching the uterus. BTL is used as a method of contraception, considered permanent because it is difficult and expensive to reverse, with low probability of success. Some women notice worsening PMS and other symptoms of imbalance or decrease in ovarian hormones after tubal ligation, and this is thought to be due to changes in ovarian blood flow from the procedure.

Tumor: An abnormal growth; may be cancerous or benign—for example, a uterine fibroid is a benign abnormal growth in the uterus (see *fibroid*).

Ultrasound scan: A method of using very high frequency sound waves to visualize internal organs, blood vessels, and the fetus in pregnancy. The sound waves used are more than 20,000 hertz, and above the level that humans can hear. Ultrasound images do not involve using radiation sources, so there is no exposure to radiation during the procedure.

Up-regulation: The process of increasing the number or function of cellular receptors.

Urethra: A muscular tube that carries urine from the bladder to the outside of the body. Inflammation of this tube is called "urethritis," and causes painful, burning sensations on urination.

Urologist: A surgeon who specializes in diseases of the kidneys, urinary tract, and bladder.

Uterus: The womb or female reproductive organ that carries and nourishes a growing fetus; made up of an inner layer (see *endometrium*), and a thick muscular layer that undergoes rhythmic contractions during labor and delivery, during menstruation, and during orgasm (although not all women feel this).

Vagina: The "birth canal," or genital passage, leading from the uterus to the outside of the body at the vulva; it is muscular and elastic, expanding to accommodate the penis during intercourse, or to accommodate a baby during delivery.

Vaginal diaphragm: A soft rubber cap that fits snugly over the cervix and is used for contraception.

Vaginal ring: A small, soft plastic or silastic device containing hormones or other medication for direct topical delivery to the vagina and urinary system—for example, Estring, containing 17-beta estradiol, used to treat vaginal dryness, or the Nuvaring contraceptive containing estrogen and progestin.

Vasoactive hormone or drugs: Drugs or substances acting on the blood vessels to cause either dilation (estradiol, nitroglycerine) or constriction (nicotine) of the arteries.

Vasomotor: A term that refers to the way nerve cells connect at the smooth muscle wall of arteries and govern the opening (vasodilation) and closing (vasoconstriction) of blood vessels to control blood flow.

Virilization: The development of masculine physical characteristics due to presence of male hormones. Virilization may occur in women if the androgen hormones are too high.

Vulva: Female external genitalia; also known as the lips of the vaginal opening.

Wild (Mexican) yam: A root vegetable that grows in many areas and contains precursor compounds that can be extracted and used in the laboratory as building blocks to make the hormones estradiol, testosterone, and progesterone. Extracts of wild yam cannot be converted by the human body to the human forms of active hormones, since we do not have the enzymes to carry out these chemical reactions.

Appendix II: References and Resources

It is not possible to list the hundreds of medical and scientific peer-reviewed articles from reputable medical journals that I have read and studied for my clinical work and book writing. This is a list of selected *historical* and *current* articles that may be of interest for those of you who want a reference for your physician, or for your own reading of the medical literature. Many times I have included the older articles to illustrate how long this information has been available and how our current understandings have evolved from this historical foundation. The historical articles will be of particular interest to women who have known intuitively for many years that something "hormonal" is wrong. Many of the concepts I describe in this book have been described in the medical literature, but ignored, for decades. The current research articles help you see the depth and breadth of our existing science explaining these important hormone connections to the healthy function of our entire body. Each article provides additional references if you wish to pursue a topic in more depth. I have focused on medical research articles published in the major, peer-reviewed national and international medical journals. In the consumer books section, I have primarily selected carefully researched, reputable books written by physicians or by formally trained health professionals in other fields who are recognized for their professional expertise. For the most part, I have not included books by laypersons, who typically are not trained to evaluate conflicting medical information.

Author's Note: The Hormone Controversy

Genazzani AR, Gambacciani M. A personal initiative for women's health: to challenge the Women's Health Initiative, *Gynecol Endocrinol* 16: 255–257, August 2002.

Schneider, HPG. The view of the International Menopause Society on the Women's Health Initiative (WHI). *Climacteric* 5: 211–216, September 2002.

Writing Group for the Women's Health Initiative Investigators. Risks and benefits of estrogen plus progestin in healthy postmenopausal women. *J AM Med Assoc* 288: 321–333, 2002.

Chapter 1: When Ovaries Go Awry:
Women's Lives, Women's Stories

Abramowitz ES, Bakerk AH, Fleisher SF. Onset of depressive psychiatric crises and the menstrual cycle. *Am J Psych* 139: 475–478, 1982

Backstrom CT, Boyle H, Baird DT. Persistence of symptoms of premenstrual tension in hysterectomized women. *Br J Obs Gyn* 88: 530–536, 1981.

Coulam CB. Premature gonadal failure. *Fertility and Sterility* 38: 645–650, 1982.

Davis SR. Premature ovarian failure. *Maturitas* 23(1): 108, 1996.

Fourestie V, DeLignieres B, Roudot-Thoraval F, et al. Suicide attempts in hypo-oestrogenic phases of the menstrual cycle. *Lancet,* 1357–1360, Dec. 1986.

Sarrel P. Ovarian steroids and the capacity to function at home and in the workplace.

Oral presentation, North American Menopause Society, New York, September 21–23, 1989.

Vliet EL, Davis VL. New perspectives on the relationship of hormonal changes to affective disorders in the perimenopause. In *Clinical Issues in Women's Health*, vol. 2(4): Midlife Women's Health, Oct.–Dec. Philadelphia: Lippincott, 1991, pp. 453–472.

Chapter 2: Your Ovaries: An Owner's Manual

Bhatia SK, Moore D, and Kalkhoff RK. Progesterone suppression of the Plasma Growth Hormone Response. *Clin Endocrinol Metab* 35: 364–369, 1972.

Kalkoff R. Metabolic effects of progesterone. *J Obstet Gynecol* 142–6: 735–738, 1982.

Nieschlag E, Behre HM, ed. *Testosterone: Action, Deficiency, Substitution*, 2nd ed. Berlin: Springer-Verlag, 1998.

Stott CA. Steroid hormones: metabolism and mechanism of action. In *Reproductive Endocrinology: Physiology, Pathophysiology, and Clinical Management*, 4 ed., S.S., eds. Yen, R.B. Jaffe, and R.L. Barbieri. Philadelphia: W.B. Saunders, 1999, p. 124.

Chapter 3: Your Ovaries and Their Life Cycle

Aoki Y. Polychlorinated biphenyls, polychlorinated dibenzo-p-dioxins, and polychlorinated Dibenzofurans as endocrine disrupters—what have we learned from Yusho disease. *Environ Res (United States)*, 86(1): 2–11, 2001.

Chang KJ, Hsieh KH, Tang SY, Tung TC, Lee TP. Immunologic evaluation of patients with polychlorinated biphenyl poisoning: evaluation of delayed-type skin hypersensitive response and its relation to clinical studies. *J Toxicol Environ Health* 9(2): 217–223, 1982.

Christiansen C, Christiansen M. Climacteric symptoms, fat mass and plasma concentrations of LH, FSH, PRL, estradiol 17-beta, and androstenedione in the early postmenopausal period. *Acta Endo* 101: 87–92, 1982.

Cooke DJ. A psychological study of the climacteric. In *Psychology and Gynaecological Problems*, eds. A. Broome and L. Wallace. London: Tavistock Publ., 1984, pp. 243–265.

Crawford S, Casey V, Avis N, et al. A longitudinal study of weight and the menopause transition: Results from the Massachusetts Women's Health Study. *Menopause: J N Am Meno Soc* 7(2): 96–105, 2000.

Giesy JP, Verbrugge DA, Othout RA, Bowerman WW, et al. Contaminants in fishes from Great Lakes–influenced sections and above dams of three Michigan rivers. I: Concentrations of organo chlorine insecticides, polychlorinated biphenyls, dioxin equivalents, and mercury. *Arch Environ Contam Toxicol* 27(2): 202–212, 1994.

Gladen B, Rogan W, Hardy P, et al. Development after exposure to polycholorinated biphenyls and dichlorodiphenyl dichloroethene transplacentally and through human milk. *J Pediatrics* 113: 991–995, 1988.

Hagstad A, Janson P. The epidemiology of climacteric symptoms. *Acta Obst Gynaecol Scand Suppl* 134: 59–65, 1986.

Ho S, Chan S, Yip Y, et al. Menopausal symptoms and symptom clustering in Chinese women. *Maturitas* 33(3): 219–227, 1999.

Krstevska-Konstantinova M, Charlier C, Craen M, et al. Sexual precocity after immigration from developing countries to Belgium: evidence of previous exposure to organochlorine pesticides. Presented at the International Workshop on Hormones and Endocrine Disrupters in Food and Water, May 2000; published in *Human Reproduction* 16(5): 1020–1026, May 2001.

Lu YC, Wu YC. Clinical findings and immunological abnormalities in Yu-Cheng patients. *Environ Health Perspect* 59: 17–29, 1985.

Niessen, KH, Ramolla J, Binder M, et al. Chlorinated hydrocarbons in adipose tissue of infants and toddlers: inventory and studies on their association with intake of mother's milk, *Eur J Pediatr* 142(4): 238–244, 1984.

Olea N, Olea-Serrano F, Lardelli-Claret P, Rivas A, Barba-Navarro A. Inadvertent exposure to xenoestrogens in children. *Toxicol Ind Health* 15(1–2): 151–158, 1999.

Rogan W, Gladen B, McKinney J, et al. Neonatal effects of transplacental exposure to PCBs and DDE. *J Pediatrics.* 109: 335–341, 1986.

Rogan WJ, Ragan NB. Chemical contaminants, pharmacokinetics, and the lactating mother. *Environ Health Perspect* 102(Suppl 11): 89–95, Dec. 1994. Review.

Sowers MR, LaPietra MT. Menopause: its epidemiology and potential association with chronic disease. *Epidemiology Rev* 17: 287, 1987.

Vliet EL. Menopause and perimenopause: The role of ovarian hormones in common neuroendocrine syndromes in primary care. *Primary Care Clinics in Office Practice* 29: 43–67, 2002.

Wing R. Obesity and weight gain during adulthood: A health problem for United States women. *WHI* 2(2): 114–122, 1992.

Young CM, Blondin J, Tensuan R, et al. Body composition studies of "older" women, thirty to seventy years of age. *Ann N Y Acad Sci* 110: 589–607, 1963.

Chapter 4: Ovaries at Risk: Surprising Toxins in Your Diet

Allred J. Too much of a good thing? An overemphasis on eating low fat foods may be contributing to the alarming increase in overweight among U.S. adults. *J Am Dietetic Assoc* 95(4): 417–418, 1995.

Ames B. Paleolithic diet, evolution and carcinogens. *Science* 258: 1633–1634, 1997.

Cassidy A, Bingham S, Setchell K. Biological effects of isoflavones in young women: Importance of the chemical composition of soybean products. *Brit Nutrition* 74: 587–601, 1995.

Cassidy A, Milligan S. How significant are environmental estrogens to women? *Climacteric* 1: 229–242, 1998.

Coyle JT, Puttfarcken P. Oxidative Stress, glutamate, and neurodegenerative disorders. *Science* 262(5134): 689–695, 1993.

Fort P, Moses N, Fasano M, et al. Breast and soy-formula feedings in early infancy and the prevalence of autoimmune thyroid disease in children (from Dept. of Pediatrics, North Shore University Hospital—Cornell University Medical College). *J Am Coll Nutr* 9(2): 164–167, 1990.

Fotsis T, Zhang Y, Pepper M, et al. The endogenous oestrogen metabolite 2-methoxytoestradiol inhibits angiogenesis and suppresses tumour growth. *Nature* 368: 237–239, 1994.

Halliwell B. Reactive oxygen species and the central nervous system. *J Neurochem* 59(5): 1609–1623, Nov. 1992.

Hunt J, et al. High versus low meat diets: Effects on zinc absorption, iron status, and calcium, copper, iron, magnesium, nitrogen, phosphorous, and zinc balance in post-menopausal women. *Am J Clin Nutr* 62: 621–632, 1995.

Hunter B. Some food additives as neuroexcitors and neurotoxins. *Clinical Ecology* 2(2): 83–89, 1984.

Knight, DC and JA Eden. A review of the clinical effects of phytoestrogens. *Obstet Gynecol* 87(5 Part 2): 897–904, 1996.

Kronenberg F and Hughes C. Exogenous and endogenous estrogens: An appreciation of biological complexity (editorial). *Menopause: The Journal of the North American Menopause Society* 6(1): 4–6, 1999.

Nagata C, Kabuto M, Kurisu Y, Shimizu H. Decreased serum estradiol concentration associated with high dietary intake of soy products in premenopausal Japanese women. *Nutrition and Cancer* 29(3): 228–233, 1997.

Pirke K, Schweiger U, Laessle R, et al. Dieting influences the menstrual cycle: Vegetarian versus nonvegetarian diet. *Fertility and Sterility* 46(6): 1083–1088, 1968.

Simonian NA, Coyle JT. Oxidative stress in neurodegenerative disorders. *Anna Rev Pharmacol Toxicol* 36: 83–106, 1996.

Von Borstel R. Metabolic and physiologic effects of sweeteners. *Clin Nutr* 4(6): 215–220, 1985.

Whitten PL, Lewis C, Russell E, Naftolin F. Potential adverse effects of phytoestrogens. *Journal of Nutrition* 125(Suppl): S 776, 1995.

Chapter 5: Ovaries at Risk: "Gender Benders" and Endocrine Disruptors Around You

Abou-Donia MB, et al. Neurotoxicity resulting from coexposure to pyridostigmine bromide, DEET, and permitrin: Implications of Gulf War chemical exposures. *J Tox & Environ Health* 48: 35–56, 1996.

Allen RH, Gottlieb M, Clute E, et al. Breast cancer and pesticides in Hawaii: The need for further study. *Environ Health Perspect* 105(Suppl 3): 679–683, 1997.

Arnold SF, et al. Synergistic activation of estrogen receptor with combinations of environmental chemicals. *Science* 272: 1489–1492, 1996.

Barsano CP. Environmental factors altering thyroid function and their assessment. *Environ Health Perspect* 38: 71–82, 1981.

Birnbaum LS. Developmental effects of dioxins and other endocrine disrupting chemicals. *Neurotoxicology* 16(4): 748, Winter 1995.

Carpenter DO. Human health effects of environmental pollutants: New insights. *Environ Monit Assess* 53(1): 245–258, Oct. 1998.

Chester AC, Levine PH. Concurrent sick building syndrome and chronic fatigue syndrome: Epidemic neuromyasthenia revised. *Clinical Infectious Diseases* 18(Suppl 1): S43–S48, 1996.

Colborn T, Smolen MJ. Epidemiological analysis of persistent organochlorine contaminants in cetaceans. *Rev Environ Contam Toxicol* 146: 91–172, 1996.

Colborn T, vom Saal FS, Soto AM. Developmental effects of endocrine-disrupting chemicals in wildlife and humans. *Environ Health Perspect* 102(Suppl 2): 126, 1993.

Cooper RL, Kavlock RJ. Endocrine disruptors and reproductive development: A weight of evidence overview. *J Endocrinol* 152: 159, 1997.

Dello Iacovo R, Celentano E, Strollo AM, et al. Organochlorines and breast cancer. A study on Neapolitan women. *Adv Exp Med Biol* 472: 57–66, 1999.

Exon JH, Kerkvliet NI, Talcott PA. Immunotoxicity of carcinogenic pesticides and related chemicals. *Journal of Environmental Science and Health,* Part C: *Environmental Carcinogenesis Reviews* C5: 73–120, 1987.

Feeley M, Brouwer A. Health risks to infants from exposure to PCBs, PCDDs and PCDFs. *Food Addit Contam* 17(4): 325–333, 2000.

Hoffmann W. Organochlorine compounds: Risk of non-Hodgkin's lymphoma and breast cancer? *Arch Environ Health* 51(3): 189–192, 1996.

Holladay SD. Prenatal immunotoxicant exposure and postnatal autoimmune disease. *Environ Health Perspect* 107(Suppl 5): 687–691, 1999.

Kannan K, Tanabe S, Giesy JP, Tatsukawa R. Organochlorine pesticides and polychlorinated biphenyls in foodstuffs from Asian and oceanic countries (review). *Rev Environ Contam Toxicol* 152: 1–55, 1997.

Kimbrough RD. Human health effects of polychlorinated biphenyls (PCBs) and polybrominated biphenyls (PBBs). *Annual Review of Pharmacology and Toxicology* 27: 87–111, 1987.

Lindstrom G, Hooper K, Petreas M, Stephens R, Gilman A. Workshop on perinatal exposure to dioxin-like compounds. I. Summary. *Environ Health Perspect* 103(Suppl 2): 135–142, 1995.

MacIntosh DL, Spengler JD, Ozkaynak H, Tsai L, Ryan PB. Dietary exposures to selected metals and pesticides. *Environ Health Perspect* 104(2): 202–209, 1996.

MacMonegle Jr, CW, Steffey KL, Bruce WN. Dieldrin, heptachlor, and chlordane residues in soybeans in Illinois 1974, 1980. *J Environ Sci Health* B. 19(1): 39–48, 1984.

Mattison DR, Plowchalk BS, Meadows MJ, et al. Reproductive toxicity: male and female reproductive systems as targets for chemical injury. *Med Clin North Am* 74: 391, 1990.

Mattison DR, Shiromizu K, Nightingale MS. Oocyte destruction by polycyclic aromatic hydrocarbons. *Am J Ind Med* 4: 191, 1983.

Mattison DR, Takizawa K, Silbergeld EK, et al. Genetics of ovarian benzo(a)pyrene metabolism, oocyte destruction, and impaired fertility. In *Extrahepatic Drug Metabolism and Chemical Carcinogenesis*, eds. J Sydstrom, et al. Elsevier 1983, p. 337.

Miller GW, Kirby ML, Levey AI, Bloomquist JR. Heptachlor alters expression and function of dopamine transporters. *Neurotoxicology* 20(4): 631–637, 1999.

National Research Council. *Pesticides in Diets of Infants and Children.* Washington, D.C., 1993, pp. 123–157.

Oduma JA, Wango EO, Oduor-Okelo D, et al. In vivo and in vitro effects of graded doses of the pesticide heptachlor on female sex steroid hormone production in rats. *Comp Biochem Physiol C Pharmacol Toxicol Endocrinol* 111(2): 191–196, 1995.

Paumgartten FJ, Cruz CM, Chahoud I, et al. PCDDs, PCDFs, PCBs, and other organochlorine compounds in human milk from Rio de Janeiro. *Brazil Environ Res.* 83(3): 293–297, 2000.

Pittman KA, Benitz K-F, Silkworth JB, Mueller W, Coulston F. Environmental chemical-induced immune dysfunction. *Ecotoxicology and Environmental Safety* 2(2): 173–198, 1978.

Porter WP, Hinsdill R, Fairbrother A, Olson LJ, Jaeger J, Yuill T, Bisgaard S, Hunter WG, Nolan K. Toxicant-disease-environment interactions associated with suppression of immune system, growth, and reproduction. *Science* 224(ISS 4652): 1014–1027, 1984.

Porterfield S. Vulnerability of the developing brain to thyroid abnormalities: environmental insults to the thyroid system. *Environ Health Perspect* 102: 125–130, 1994.

Rao PS, Lakshmy R. Role of goitrogens in iodine deficiency disorders and brain development. *Indian J Med Res* 102: 223–226, 1995.

Smith EM, Hammonds-Ehlers M, Clark MK, et al. Occupational exposures and risk of female infertility. *J Occup Environ Med* 39: 138, 1997.

Swain, Wayland R. Human health consequences of consumption of fish contaminated with organochlorine compounds. *Aquatic Toxicology* 11: 357–377, 1988.

Tryphonas H. The impact of PCBs and dioxins on children's health: immunological considerations. *Can J Public Health* 89(Suppl 1): S49–52, S54–57, 1998.

Ward EM, Schulte P, Grajewski B, et al. Serum organochlorine levels and breast cancer: A nested case-control study of Norwegian women. *Cancer Epidemiol Biomarkers Prev.* 9(12): 1357–1367, 2000.

Weisglas-Kuperus N. Neurodevelopmental, immunological and endocrinological indices of perinatal human exposure to PCBs and dioxins. *Neurotoxicology* 17(3–4): 945–946, 1996.

Weisglas-Kuperus N, Sas TC, Koopman-Esseboom C, et al. Immunologic effects of background prenatal and postnatal exposure to dioxins and polychlorinated biphenyls in Dutch infants. *Pediatr Res* 38(3): 404–410, 1995.

Wolff M, Toniolo P, Lee E, Rivera M, Dubin N. Blood levels of organochlorine residues and risk of breast cancer. *J Natl Cancer Inst* 85(8): 648–642, 1993.

Yu ML, Hsin JW, Hsu CC, Chan WC, Guo YL. The immunologic evaluation of the Yucheng children. *Chemosphere* 37(9–12): 1855–1865, 1998.

Chapter 6: Ovaries at Risk: Toxic Effects of Cigarettes, Alcohol, Marijuana, and Other Drugs

Babor TF, Grant M. From clinical research to secondary prevention: international collaboration in the development of the Alcohol Use Disorders Identification Test (AUDIT). *Alcohol Health Res World* 13: 371–374, 1989.

Baird DD, Wilcox AJ. Cigarette smoking associated with delayed conception. *JAMA* 253: 2979, 1985.

Becker U, Tonnesen H, Kaas-Claesson N, and Gluud C. Menstrual disturbances and fertility in chronic alcoholic women. *Drug and Alcohol Dependence* 24: 75–82, 1989. Elsevier Scientific Publishers, Ireland.

Cooper GS, Baird DD, Hulka BS, et al. Follicle-stimulating hormone concentrations in relation to active and passive smoking. *Obstet Gynecol* 85: 407, 1995

Everson RB, Sandler DR, Wilcox AJ, et al. Effect of passive exposure to smoking on age at natural menopause. *Br Med J* 293: 272, 1986

Ferraroni M, Decarli A, Franceschi S, La Vecchia C. Alcohol consumption and risk of breast cancer: a multicenter Italian case-control study. *European J of Cancer* 34: 1403–1409, 1998.

Hommer DW et al. Evidence for a gender-related effect of alcoholism on brain volumes. *Am J Psychiatry* 158: 198–204, 2001.

Jick H, Porter J, Morrison AS. Relations between smoking and age of natural menopause. *Lancet* 1: 1354, 1977.

Kaufman DW, Slone D, Rosenberg L, et al. Cigarette smoking and age at natural menopause. *Am J Public Health* 70: 420, 1980.

Mattison DR, Plowchalk BS, Meadows MJ, et al. The effect of smoking on oogenesis, fertilization, and implantation. *Semin Reprod Endocrinol* 7: 219, 1989.

Mello N, Mendelson J, Teoh S. Neuroendocrine consequences of alcohol abuse in women. *Ann NY Acad Sci* 562: 211–240, 1981.

Mendelson JH, Lukas SE, Mello NK, et al. Acute alcohol effects on plasma estradiol levels in women. *Psychopharmacology* 94: 464–467, 1988.

Modugno F, et al. Cigarette smoking and the risk of mucinous and nonmucinous epithelial ovarian cancer. *Epidemiology* 13: 467–471, 2002.

Muti P, Trevisan M, Micheli A, et al. Alcohol consumption and total estradiol in premenopausal women. *Cancer Epidemiol Biomarkers and Prev* 7: 189–193, March 1998.

Nystrom M, Perasalo J, Salaspuro M. Screening for heavy drinking and alcohol-related problems in young university students: the CAGE, the Mm-MAST and the trauma score questionnaires. *J Stud Alcohol* 54: 528–533, 1993.

Pettersson P, Ellsinger B-M, Sjoberg C, Bjorntorp P. Fat distribution and steroid hormones in women with alcohol abuse. *J of Internal Med* 228(4): 311–316, Oct. 1990.

Pokorny AD, Miller BA, Kaplan HB. The brief MAST: A shortened version of the Michigan Alcoholism Screening Test. *Am J Psychiatry* 129: 342–345, 1972.

Roman P. Biological features of women's alcohol use: A review. *Public Health Rep* 103(6): 628–637, Nov.–Dec. 1988.

Russell M, Martier SS, Sokol RJ, et al. Screening for pregnancy risk drinking. *Alcohol Clin Exp Res* 18: 1156–1161, 1994.

Valimaki N, Harkonen M, and Ylikahri R. Acute effects of alcohol on female sex hormones. *Alcohol Clin Exp Res* 7: 289–293, 1983.

Van Voorhis BJ, Syrop CH, Hammit DG, et al. Effects of smoking on ovulation induction for assisted reproductive techniques. *Fertil Steril* 58: 981, 1992.

Wilsnack S, Klassen A, Wilsnack R. Drinking and reproductive dysfunction among women in a 1981 National Survey. *Alcoholism: Clinical and Experimental Research* 8(5): 451–458, 1984.

Yeh J, Barbierei RL. Effects of smoking on steroid production, metabolism, and estrogen-related diseases, *Semin Reprod Endocrinol* 7: 326, 1989.

Chapter 7: Ovary Shutdown: The Toxic Role of Stress Overload and Sleep Deprivation

Birketvedt G, Florholmen J, Sundsfjord J, et al. Behavioral and neuroendocrine characteristics of the night-eating syndrome. *JAMA* 282(7): 657–663, 1999.

Blackman MR. (editorial) Age-related alterations in sleep quality and neuroendocrine function: Interrelationships and implications. *JAMA* 284: 879–881, 2000.

Borbely AA. Processes underlying sleep regulation. *Horm Res* 49: 114–117, 1998.

Dijk DJ, Duffy JF. Circadian regulation of human sleep and age-related changes in its timing, consolidation and EEG characteristics. *Ann Med* 31: 130–140, 1999.

Ho KY, Evans WS, Blizzard RM, et al. Effects of sex and age on the 24-hour profile of growth hormone secretion in man: Importance of endogenous estradiol concentrations. *J Clin Endocrinol Metab* 64: 51–58, 1987.

Howard AD, Feighner SD, Cully DF, et al. A receptor in pituitary and hypothalamus that functions in growth hormone release. *Science* 273: 974–977, 1996.

Kramer R, Cook T, Carlisle C, et al. Role of the primary care physician in recognizing obstructive sleep apnea. *Arch Intern Med* 159: 965–968, 1999.

Leong GM, Mercado-Asis LB, Reynolds JC, et al. The effect of Cushing's disease on bone mineral density, body composition, growth, and puberty. *J Clin Endocrinol Metab* 81: 1905–1911, 1996.

McEwen BS. Stress, adaptation, and disease. *Ann NY Acad Sci.* 840: 33–44, 1998.

McEwen BS, Sapolsky RM. Stress and cognitive function. *Curr Opin Neurobiol* 5: 205–216, 1995.

Peeke P, Chrousos G. Hypercortisolism and obesity. *Ann NY Acad Sci* 771: 665–676, 1995.

Plat L, LeProult R, L'Hermite-Baleriaux M, et al. Metabolic effects of short-term elevations of plasma cortisol are more pronounced in the evening than in the morning. *J Clin Endocrinol Metab* 84: 3082–3092, 1999.

Post R. Transduction of psychosocial stress into the neurobiology of recurrent affective disorder. *Am J Psychiatry* 149(8): 999–1010, 1992.

Van Cauter E, Leproult R, Kupfer DJ. Effects of gender and age on the levels and circadian rhythmicity of plasma cortisol. *J Clin Endocrinol Metab* 81: 2468–2473, 1996.

Van Cauter E, Plat L, Leproult R, et al. Alterations of circadian rhythmicity and sleep in aging: Endocrine consequences. *Horm Res* 49: 147–152, 1998.

Van Cauter E, Plat L, Copinschi G. Interrelations between sleep and the somatotropic axis. *Sleep* 21: 553–566, 1998.

Weinstock M. Does prenatal stress impair coping and regulation of hypothalamic-pituitary-adrenal axis? *Neuroscience and Biobehavioral Reviews* 21(1): 1–10, Jan. 1997.

Yager J. Nocturnal eating syndromes (editorial). *JAMA* 282(7): 689–690, 1999.

Chapter 8: Lifestyle Habits and Cultural Issues— Unexpected Stress for Our Ovaries

Aloia, JF, McGowan DM, Vaswani AN, Ross P, and Cohn SH. Relationship of menopause to skeletal and muscle mass. *Am J Clin Nutr* 53: 1378–1383, 1991.

Bale P, Doust J, Dawson D. Gymnasts, distance runners, anorexics' body composition and menstrual status. *J Sports Med Phys Fitness* 36(1): 49–53, 1996.

Berga SL. Stress and ovarian function. *Am J Sports Med* 24(6 Suppl): S36–37, 1996.

Berkman S. Body image: Larger than life? *Women's Health and Fitness News* 4(8): 1–6, 1990.

Bullen B, Skrinar G, Beitins I, et al. Endurance training effects on plasma hormonal responsiveness and sex hormone excretion. *J Appl Phys: Respirat Environ Exercise Physiol* 56(6): 1453–1463, 1984.

Chen EC, Brzyski RG. Exercise and reproductive dysfunction. *Fertil Steril.* 71(1): 1–6, 1999.

Dionyssiou-Asteriou A, Drakakis P, Vatalas IA, Michalas S. Variations of serum hormone levels in young exercising women. *Clin Endocrinol* 51(2): 258–260, 1999. (Oxford.)

Duncan JJ, Gordon NF, Scott CB. Women walking for health and fitness: How much is enough? *JAMA* 266: 3295–3299, 1991.

Hakkinen K, Pakarinen A. Acute hormonal changes to heavy resistance exercise in men and women at different ages. *Int J Sports Med,* 16(8): 507, 1995.

Harrison RL, Read GF. Ovarian impairments of female recreational distance runners during a season of training. *Annals of Human Biology* 25(4): 345–357, 1998.

Keizer H, Janssen GME, Menheere P, and Kranenburg G. Changes in basal plasma testosterone, cortisol, and dehydroepiandrosterone in previously untrained males and females preparing for marathon. *Int J Sports Med* 10: S139, 1989.

Kyllonen ES, Vaananen HK, Heikkinen JE, et al. Comparison of muscle strength and bone mineral density in healthy postmenopausal women: A cross-sectional population study. *Scand J Rehab Med* 23: 153–157, 1991.

Lebenstedt M., Platte P, Pirke KM. Reduced resting metabolic rate in athletes with menstrual disorders. *Med Sci Sports Exerc* 31(9): 1250–1256, 1999.

Locke RJ, Warren MP. Exercise and primary dysmenorrhoea. *Br J Sports Med* 33(4): 227, Aug. 1999.

Norsigian, J. Dieting is dangerous to your health. *The Network News* 1986; May–June: 4–6

Notelovitz, M. Estrogen therapy and variable-resistance weight training increase bone mineral in surgically menopausal women. *J Bone Mineral Research* 6(6): 583–590, 1991.

Phillips SK, Gopinathan J, Meehan K, Bruce S, and Woledge R. Muscle strength changes during the menstrual cycle in human adductor pollicis. *J Physiol* 473: 125P, 1993.

Phillips SK, Rook K, Siddle N, Bruce S, and Woledge R. Muscle weakness in women occurs at an earlier age than in men, but strength is preserved by hormone replacement therapy. *Clin Sci* 84: 95, 1993.

Pirke K, Schweiger U, Laessle R, et al. Dieting influences the menstrual cycle: Vegetarian versus nonvegetarian diet. *Fertility and Sterility* 46(6): 1083–1088, 1968.

Pirke KM, Schweiger U, Lemmel W, et al. The influence of dieting on the menstrual cycle of healthy young women. *J Clin Endocrinol Metab* 60(6): 1174–1179, 1985.

Sarwar R, Beltran-Niclos B, and Rutherford O. Changes in muscle strength, relaxation rate, and fatiguability during the human menstrual cycle. *J Physiol* 493: 267, 1996.

Selby GB, Eichner ER. Endurance swimming, intravascular hemolysis, anemia, and iron depletion. New perspective on athlete's anemia. *Am J Med* 81(5): 791–794, 1986.

Shangold M. Exercise and the adult female: Hormonal and endocrine effects. *Exer & Sport Sci Rev* 12: 53–79, 1984.

Williams NI, Bullen BA, McArthur JW, et al. Effects of short-term strenuous exercise upon corpus luteum function. *Med Sci Sports Exerc* 31(7): 949–958, 1999.

Yen SS. Effects of lifestyle and body composition on the ovary (review). *Endocrinol Metab Clin North Am* 27(4): 915–926, 1998.

Chapter 9: Ovaries At Risk: Unusual Effects of Viruses and Medical Illnesses

Anaasti, JN. Premature ovarian failure: An update. *Fertility and Sterility* 70(1): 1–15, 1998.

Arafah BM. Increased need for thyroxine in women with hypothyroidism during estrogen therapy. *N Engl J Med* 344: 1743–1748, 2001; commentary 1784–1785.

Cann SA, van Netten JP, van Netten C. Hypothesis: Iodine, selenium and the development of breast cancer. *Cancer Causes Control* 11(2): 121–127, 2000.

Des Moraes Ruesen M. Autoimmunity and ovarian failure. *Amer J Obstet and Gynecol* 112: 5–8, 1972.

Eskin BA. Iodine and mammary cancer. *Adv Exp Med Biol* 91: 293–304, 1977.

Fackelmann K. Early menopause for diabetic women. *Science News* 152: 15, 1997.

Gloor HJ. Autoimmune oophoritis. *Amer J Clin Path* 81: 105–109, 1984.

Gold MS, et al. Depression and "symptomless" autoimmune thyroiditis. *Psychiatr Ann* 17: 750–757, 1987.

Gregoire AJP, Kumar R, Everett B, Henderson A, Studd JWW. Transdermal oestrogen for treatment of severe postnatal depression. *Lancet* 347: 930–933, 1996.

Hagmar L, Rylander L, Dyremark E, et al. Plasma concentrations of persistent organochlorines in relation to thyrotropin and thyroid hormone levels in women. *Int Arch Occup Environ Health* 74(3): 184–188, 2001.

Hall RCW, et al. Psychiatric manifestations of Hashimoto's thyroiditis. *Psychosomatics* 23: 337–342, 1982.

Hall RCW. Psychiatric manifestations of thyroid hormone disturbance. *Psychosomatics* 24: 7–18, 1983.

Henry CH, Hudson AP, Gerard HC, et al. Identification of chlamydia trachomatis in the human temporomandibular joint. *J Oral Maxillofac Surg* 57: 683–688, 1999.

Hetzel BS, Chavadej J, Potter BJ. The brain in iodine deficiency. *Neuropathol Appl Neurobiol* 14(2): 93–104, 1988.

Hoek A, Schoemaker J, Drexhage HA. Premature ovarian failure and ovarian autoimmunity. *Endocrinology Review* 18(1): 107–134, 1997.

Kim JG, Moon SY, Chang YS, Lee JY. Autoimmune ovarian failure. *Brit J Obstetrics and Gynaecology* 21: 59–66, 1995

Krassas GE. Thyroid disease and reproduction. *Fertil Steril* 74(6): 1063–1070, 2000.

Leer M, Patel B, Innes M, et al. Secondary amenorrhea due to autoimmune ovarian failure. *Australian and New Zealand J Obstet and Gynecol* 158: 1–5, 1988.

Longcope C. The male and female reproductive systems in hypothyroidism. In *Werner and Ingbar's the Thyroid*, 7th ed., eds. LE Braverman and RD Utiger. Philadelphia: Lippincott-Raven, 1996.

Massoudi M, Meilahn E, Orchard T, et al. Thyroid function and perimenopausal lipid and weight changes: The thyroid study in healthy women (TSH-W). *J Women's Health* 6(5): 553–558, 1997.

Meisler, Jodi Godfrey, M.S., R.D. Toward optimal health: The experts discuss thyroid disease. *Journal of Women's Health and Gender-Based Medicine* 9: 345–350, May 2000.

Muechler EK, Huang KE and Schenk E. Autoimmunity in premature ovarian failure. *International J Fertility* 36(2): 99–103, 1991.

Nakano T, Konishi T, Futagami Y, Takezawa H. Myocardial infarction in Graves' disease without coronary artery disease. *Japan Heart J* 28(3): 451–456, May 1987.

Nemeroff CB, Simon JS, Haggerty JJ, et al. Antithyroid antibodies in depressed patients. *Am J Psychiatry* 142: 840–842, 1985.

Prange AJ. L-triiodothyronine (T3): Its place in the treatment of TCA-resistant depressed patients. In *Treating Resistant Depression*, eds. Joseph Zohar, Robert H. Belmaker. New York: PMA Publishing Corp., 1987, 269–278.

Premawardhana LDKE, Parkes AB, Ammari F, et al. Postpartum thyroiditis and long-term thyroid status: Prognostic influence of thyroid peroxidase antibodies and ultrasound echogenicity. *J Clin Endocrinol Metab* 85: 71–75, 2000.

Reus, VI. Behavioral aspects of thyroid disease in women. In *The Psychiatric Clinics of North America: Women's Disorders* 12(1): 153–166, March, 1989. Philadelphia: W. B. Saunders Co.

Ridgeway EC. Hypothyroidism: The hidden challenge. Clinical Management conference proceedings, University of Colorado School of Medicine, Dec. 1996.

Seo BW, Li MH, Hansen LG, Moore RW, Peterson RE, Schantz SL. Effects of gestational and lactational exposure to PCB 77, PCB 126 or TCDD on thyroid hormones in weanling Sprague-Dawley rats. *Toxicologist* 15(1): 65–70, 1995.

Smythe PP. Thyroid disease and breast cancer. *J Endocrinol Invest* 16(5): 396–401, 1993.

Smythe PP. The thyroid and breast cancer: a significant association? (editorial). *Ann Med* 29: 189–191, 1997.

Thomas R and Reid RL. Thyroid disease and reproductive function: a review. *Obstet Gynecol* 70: 789–798, 1987.

Thyroid Disorders and Women's Health. National Women's Health Report. 22–56, 2000.

Vermuelen A. Environment, human reproduction, menopause and andropause. *Environ Health Perspect* 101 (Suppl 2): 91–100, 1993.

Viskin S, Long QT. Syndromes and torsade de pointes. *Lancet* 354: 1625–1633, 1999.

Wheatcroft NJ, Rogers CA, Metcalfe RA, et al. Is subclinical ovarian failure an autoimmune disease? *Human Reproduction* 12: 244–249, 1997.

Williams DJ, Connor P, Ironside JW. Premenopausal cytomeglovirus oophoritis. *Histopathology* 16: 405–407, 1990.

Chapter 10: Ovaries at Risk: Unrecognized Problems from Surgery, Medications, and Herbs

Backstrom CT, Boyle H, Baird DT. Persistence of symptoms of premenstrual tension in hysterectomized women. *Br J Obstet Gynaecol* 88: 530–536, 1981.

Casper R, Hearn M. The effects of hysterectomy and bilateral oophorectomy in women with severe premenstrual syndrome. *Am J Obstet Gynecol* 162: 105–109, 1990.

Casson P, Hahn PM, Van Vugt DA, et al. Lasting response to ovariectomy in severe intractable premenstrual syndrome. *Am J Obstet Gynecol* 162: 99–105, 1990.

Challen J. The problem with herbs. *Nat Health* Jan.–Feb. 1999: 56–60.

Divi RL, Chang HC, Doerge DR. Anti-thyroid isoflavones from soybean: isolation, characterization, and mechanisms of action. National Center for Toxicological Research, Jefferson, AR 72079, USA. *Biochem Pharmacol* 54(1): 1087–1096, Nov. 15, 1997.

Hirata JD, Swiersz LM, Zell B, Small R, Ettinger B. Does dong quai have estrogenic effects in postmenopausal women? A double-blind, placebo-controlled trial. *Fertil Steril* 68: 981–986, 1997.

Jellin JM, Batz F, Hitchens K. *Natural Medicines Comprehensive Database.* Therapeutic Research Faculty, Stockton, Calif., 1999.

Khastgir G, Studd JWW. Hysterectomy, ovarian failure and depression. *Menopause* 5: 113–122, 1998.

Knight DC, Howes JB, Eden JA. The effect of Promensil, an isoflavone extract, on menopausal symptoms. *Climacteric: The Journal of the International Menopause Society* 2: 79–84, 1999.

Masand P Chr. Symposium: Weight gain associated with use of psychotropic drugs. *Therapeutic Advances in Psychoses,* July 4, 1999.

Peterson HB, et al. The risk of menstrual abnormalities after tubal sterilization. *N Engl J Med* 343: 1681–1687, Dec. 7, 2000.

Sarrel P. Effects of hysterectomy without oophorectomy on menopausal symptoms. Oral presentation, North American Menopause Society, New York, Sept. 21–23, 1989.

Spector TD, Brown GC, Silman AJ. Increased rates of previous hysterectomy and gynecological operations in women with osteoarthritis. *Br Med J* 297: 899–900, 1988.

Studd JWW, Domoney C, Khastgir G. The place of hysterectomy in the treatment of menstrual disorders. *Disorders of the Menstrual Cycle* 29: 313–323, 2000. RCOG Press.

Watson NR, Studd JWW, Garnett T, et al. Bone loss after hysterectomy with ovarian conservation. *Ostet Gynecol* 86(1): 72–77, 1995.

Chapter 11: Ovaries out of Balance: Patterns in Women's Lives

Ballweg ML. Fibromyalgia/endometriosis link? . . . Endometriosis Association Newsletter 12: 3, 1991.

Barfield RJ, Glasser JH, Rubin BS, et al. Behavioral effects of progestin in the brain. *Psychoneuroendocrinology* 9: 217–231, 1984.

Brush MG. Increased incidence of thyroid autoimmune problems in women with endometriosis. Endometriosis: A Collection of Papers Written by GPs, Researchers, Specialists and Sufferers about Endometriosis. Compiled by the Coventry Branch of the Endometriosis Society, March 1987.

Campbell J. Is Reproductive Wastage and Failure Related to Environmental Pollution? Considerations of Human Data and Findings from a Rhesus Model. Presented at the Toxicological Pathology Symposium, Ottawa, Canada, September 1988.

Campbell JS, Wong J, Tryphonas L, et al. Is Simian Endometriosis an Effect of Immunotoxicity? Presented at the Ontario Association of Pathologists Forty-Eighth Annual Meeting, October 1985, London, Ontario, Canada.

Cronje WH, Studd JWW. Premenstrual syndrome and premenstrual dysphoric disorder. *Primary Care Clinics in Office Practice* 29: 1–12, March 2002.

Donnez J, Nisolle M, et al. Peritoneal endometriosis and "endometriotic" nodules of the rectovaginal septum are two different entities. *Fertil Steril.* 66(3): 362–368, Sept. 1996.

Donnez J, Nisolle M, et al. Rectovaginal septum adenomyotic nodules: a series of 500 cases. *Br J Obstet Gynaecol,* 104(9): 1014–1018, Sept. 1997.

Fanton JW, Hubbard GB, Wood DH. Endometriosis: Clinical and pathological findings in 70 rhesus monkeys. *Am J Veterinary Research* 47: 1537–1541, 1986.

Grimes DA, Lebolt SA, Grimes KRT, Wingo PA. Two-fold risk of endometriosis in hospitalized patients with lupus. *Amer J Obstet Gyneco* 153: 179–183, 1985.

Magos AL, Brewster E, Singh R, et al. The effects of norethisterone in postmenopausal women on oestrogen replacement therapy: A model for the premenstrual syndrome. *Br J Obstet Gynaecol* 93: 1290–1296, 1986.

Mayani A, Barel S, Soback S, et al. Dioxin concentrations in women with endometriosis. *Human Reproduction* 12: 373–375, 1997.

Muse KN, Cetel NS, Futterman LA, Yen SC. The premenstrual syndrome. Effects of "medical ovariectomy." *N Engl J Med* 311: 1345–1349, 1984.

Querleu D. Treatment of rectovaginal endometriosis. *Presse Med* 26(16): 774–777, May 1997.

Rier SE, Martin DC, Bowman RE, Dmowski WP, Becker JL. Endometriosis in rhesus monkeys (Macaca mulatta) following chronic exposure to 2, 3, 7, 8-Tetrachlorodibenzo-p-dioxin. *Fundamental and Applied Toxicology* 21: 433–441, 1993.

Rier SE, Wayman ET, Martin DC, et al. Serum levels of TCDD and dioxin-like chemicals in rhesus monkeys chronically exposed to dioxin: Correlation of increased serum PCB levels with endometriosis. *Toxicological Sciences* 59: 147–159, 2001.

Smith RNJ, Studd JWW, Zamblera D, et al. A randomized comparison over 8 months of 100 mcgs and 200 mcgs twice weekly doses of transdermal oestradiol in the treatment of severe premenstrual syndrome. *Br J Obstet Gynaecol* 102: 475–484, 1995.

Watson NR, Studd JWW, Savvas M, et al. Treatment of severe premenstrual syndrome with oestradiol patches and cyclical oral norethisterone. *Lancet* 2: 730–734, 1989.

Chapter 12: Ovarian Hormones and the Brain: It's Not Just Stress or Your Imagination!

Abramowitz ES, Bakerk AH, Fleisher SF. Onset of depressive psychiatric crises and the menstrual cycle. *Am J Psychiatry* 139: 475–478, 1982.

Ahokas A, Aito M, Rimon R. Positive treatment effect of estradiol in postpartum psychosis: A pilot study. *J Clin Psychiatry* (United States) 61(3): 166–169, 2000.

Ahokas A, Kaukoranta J, Aito M. Effect of oestradiol on postpartum depression. *Psychopharmacology* (Berlin, Germany) 146(1): 108–110, 1999.

Ahokas AJ, Turtiainen S, Aito M. Sublingual oestrogen treatment of postnatal depression. *Lancet* 351(9096): 109–112, 1998.

Akamatsu T, Akiyama T, Kimura T, Saito H, Yanaihara T. Menopausal Insomnia and Hormone Replacement Therapy. Third International Symposium, Women's Health and Menopause, June 1998.

Backstrom, T. Epileptic seizures in women related to plasma estrogen and progesterone during the menstrual cycle. *Acta Neurol Scand* 54: 321–347, 1976.

Ball DE, Morrison P. Oestrogen transdermal patches for post partum depression in lactating mothers—a case report. *Cent Afr J Med* (Zimbabwe) 45(3): 68–70, March 1999.

Bancroft J, Sanders D, Warner P, Loudon N. The effects of oral contraceptives on mood and sexuality: Comparison of triphasic and combined preparations. *J Psychosom. Obstet Gynaecol* 7: 1–8, 1987.

Barfield R, Glaser J, Rubin B, et al. Behavioral effects of progestin in the brain. *Psychoneuroendocrinology* 9(3): 217–231, 1984.

Becker D, Creutzfeldt OD, Schwibbe M, Wuttke W. Changes in physiological, EEG and psychological parameters in women during the spontaneous menstrual cycle and following oral contraceptives. *Psychoneuroendocrinology* 7: 75–90, 1982.

Bennett RM, Clark SC, Walczyk J. A randomized, double-blind placebo-controlled study of growth hormone in the treatment of fibromyalgia. *Am J Med* 104(3): 227–231, March 1998.

Bereiter DA, Barker DJ. Hormone-induced enlargement of receptive fields in trigeminal mechanoreceptive neurons. I. Time course hormones, sex and modality specificity. *Brain Res* 184: 395–410, 1980.

Bernardi F, Bertolino S, Luisi S, Spinetti A, Monteleone P, Giardina L, Petraglia F, Luisi M, Genazzani AR. Effects of Hormonal Replacement Therapy on Circulating Allopregnanolone Levels in Postmenopausal Women. Third International Symposium Women's Health and Menopause. June 1998.

Bhatia SK, Moore D, Kalkhoff RK. Progesterone suppression of the plasma growth hormone Response. *J Clin Endocrinol Metab* 35: 364–369, 1972.

Bloch M, Schmidt PJ, Danaceau M, et al. Effects of gonadal steroids in women with a history of postpartum depression. *Am J Psychiatry* 157(6): 924–930, 2000.

Bromm B, Desmedt JE, eds. *Pain and the Brain: From Nociception to Cognition.* Advances in Pain Research and Therapy, vol. 22. New York: Raven Press Ltd, 1995.

Brovermann DM, Klaiber EL, Kobayashi Y, et al. Roles of activation and inhibition in sex differences in cognitive abilities. *Pychol Rev* 75: 23–50, 1968.

Buterbaugh GG Postictal events in mygdala-kindled female rats with and without estradiol replacement. *Exp Neurol* 95: 697–913, 1987.

Cauley JA, Pertini AM, LaPorte RE, Sandler RB, Baylers CM, Robertson RJ, Slemenda CW. The decline of grip strength in the menopause relationship to physical activity, estrogen use and anthropometric factors. *J Chronic Dis* 40: 115–120, 1982.

Christiansen C, Christiansen MS. Climacteric symptoms, fat mass and plasma concentrations of LH, FSH, PRL, estradiol 17-beta, and androstenedione in the early postmenopausal period. *Acta Endocrinol* 101: 87–92, 1982.

Cullberg J. Mood changes and menstrual symptoms with different gestagen/estrogen combinations. *Acta Psychiatr Scand* (suppl) 236: 1, 1972.

Dawson-Basoa MB, Gintzler AR. 17-beta estradiol and progesterone modulate an intrinsic opiod analgesic system. *Brain Res* 601: 1–2, 241–245, Jan. 22, 1993.

Ditkoff EC, Crary WG, Cristo M, Lobo RA. Estrogen improves psychological function in asymptomatic postmenopausal women. *Obstet Gynecol* 78: 991–995, 1991.

Duncan A, Lyall H, Roberts R, Perera M, Petrie J, Connell J, Lumsden M. The Effect of 17 Beta Estradiol and Norethisterone on Insulin Sensitivity in Postmenopausal Women. Third International Symposium Women's Health and Menopause, June 1998.

Erlik Y, Tataryn IV, Meldrum DR, et al. Association of waking episodes with menopausal hot flushes. *JAMA* 245: 1741–1744, 1981.

Fillit H, Weinreb H, Cholst I, et al. Observations in a preliminary open trial of estradiol therapy for senile dementia-Alzheimer's type. *Psychoneuroendocrinology* 11: 337–345, 1986.

Fink G, et al. Estrogen control of central neurotransmission: Effect on mood, mental state, and memory. *Cell Mol Neurobiol* June 1996.

Finn DA, Gee KW. The significance of steroid action at the GABA receptor complex. In *The Modern Management of the Menopause: A Perspective for the 21st Century,* eds. G. Berg, M. Hammar. Carnforth, UK: Parthenon Publishing, 1994, pp. 301–314.

Fonseca E, Ochoa R, Galvan R, Hernandez M, Mercado M, Zarate A. Increased serum levels of growth hormone and insulin-like growth factor-I associated with simultaneous decrease of circulating insulin in postmenopausal women receiving hormone replacement therapy. *Menopause* 6: 56–60, Spring 1999.

Genazzani AR, Bernardi F, Spinetti A, Stomati M, Luisi S, Tonetti A, Petraglia F, Luisi M. The Brain as Target and Source for Sex Steroid Hormones. Third International Symposium Women's Health and Menopause. June 1998.

Gitlin MJ, Pasnau RO. Psychiatric syndromes linked to reproductive function in women: A review of current knowledge. *Am J Psychiatry* 146: 7–15, 1989.

Govoni, S. Estrogens as Neuroprotectants: Hypotheses on the Mechanism of Action. Third International Symposium Women's Health and Menopause, June 1998.

Gregoire AJP, Kumar R, Everett B, Henderson A, Studd JWW. Transdermal oestrogen for treatment of severe postnatal depression. *Lancet* 347: 930–933, 1996.

Hammarback S, Backstrom T, Holst J, von Schoultz B, Lyrenas S. Cyclical mood changes as in the premenstrual tension syndrome during sequential estrogen-progestagen postmenopausal replacement therapy. *Acta Obstet Gynecol Scand* 64: 515–518, 1985.

Henderson AF, Gregoire AJP, Kumar R, Studd JWW. The treatment of severe postnatal depression with oestradiol skin patches. *Lancet* 338: 816, 1991.

Hermann WM, Beach RC. The psychotropic properties of estrogen. *Pharmakopsychiat* 11: 164–178, 1978.

Herzog AG. Polycystic ovarian syndrome in women with epilepsy: Epileptic or iatrogenic? *Ann Neurol* 39: 559–560, 1996.

Herzog AG, Seibel MM, Schomer D, et al. Temporal lobe epilepsy: An extrahypothalamic pathogenesis for polycystic ovarian syndrome? *Neurology* 34(10): 1389–1393, 1984.

Honjo H, Ogino Y, Urabe M, et al. In vivo effects by estrone sulfate on the central nervous system—senile dementia (Alzheimer's type). *J Steroid Biochem* 34: 521–525, 1989.

Isojarvi JIT, Laatikainen TJ, Pakarinen AJ, Juntunen KTS, Myllyla VV. Polycystic ovaries and hyperandrogenism in women taking valproate for epilepsy. *N Engl J Med* 329: 1383–1388, 1993.

Jaussi R, Watson G, Paigen K. Modulation of androgen-responsive gene expression by estrogen. *Mol Cell Endocrinol* 86: 187, 1992.

Jensen J, Christensen C, Rodbro P. Estrogen-progesterone replacement therapy changes body composition in early postmenopausal women. *Maturitas* 8: 209–216, 1986.

Kaye SA, Folsom AR, Soler JT, Prineas RJ, Potter JD. Association of body mass and fat distribution with sex hormone concentrations in postmenopausal women. *Int J Epidemiol* 20: 151–156.

Keefe DL, Watson F, Naftolin F. Hormone replacement therapy may alleviate sleep apnea in menopausal women: A pilot study. *Menopause* 6: 196–200, 1999.

Klaiber EL, Broverman DM, Vogel W, Kobayashi T. Estrogen therapy for severe persistent depressions in women. *Arch Gen Psychiat* 36: 550–554, 1979.

Klaiber EL, Broverman DM, Vogel W, et al. Individual differences in changes in mood and platelet monoamine oxidase (MAO) activity during hormonal replacement therapy in menopausal women. *Psychoneuroendocrinology* 21: 575–592, 1996.

Kyllonen ES, Vaananen HK, Heikkinen JE, Kurttila-Matero E, Martikkala V, Vanharanta JH. Comparison of muscle strength and bone mineral density in healthy postmenopausal women: A cross-sectional population study. *Scand J Rehab Med* 23: 153–157, 1991.

Logothetis J, Harner R, Morrell F, Torres F. The role of oestrogen and catamenial exacerbations of epilepsy. *Neurology* 9: 352–360, 1959.

Magos AL, Brewster E, Singh R, O'Dowd T, Brincat M, Studd JWW. The effects of norethisterone in postmenopausal women on oestrogen replacement therapy: A model for the premenstrual syndrome. *Br J Obstet Gynaecol* 93: 1290–1296, 1986.

Magos AL, Brincat M, Studd JWW. Treatment of the premenstrual syndrome by subcutaneous oestradiol implants and cyclical oral norethisterone: A placebo controlled study. *Br Med J* 1: 1629–1631, 1986.

Majewska MD, Harrison N, Schwartz R, Barker J, Paul S. Steroid hormone metabolites are barbiturate-like modulators of the GABA receptor. *Science* 232: 1004–1007, 1986.

McEwen BS. Ovarian hormone action in the brain: Implications for the menopause. In *The Climacteric in Perspective,* eds. M. Notelovitz, P.A. Van Keep. Lancaster, UK: MTP Press, 1976, pp. 207–209.

McEwen BS, Biegon A, Davis P, et al. Steroid hormones: Humoral signals which alter brain cell properties and functions. *Recent Progress in Hormone Research* 38: 41–83, 1982. Discussion: 83–92.

McEwen BS, Rhodes JC. Gonadal hormone regulation of MAO and other enzymes in hypothalamic areas. *Neuroendocrinol* 36: 235–238, 1983.

Mizuki Y, Kajimura N, Miyoshi A, et al. Neuroendocrinological studies on patients with periodic psychosis of adolescence before and after menarche. 1990.

Montgomery JC, Brincal M, Tapp A, Appleby L, Versi E, Fenwick PBC, Studd JWW. Effects of oestrogen and testosterone implants on psychological disorders in the climacteric. *Lancet* 1: 297–299, 1987.

Muse KN, Cetel NS, Futterman LA, Yen SSC. The premenstrual syndrome, effects of medical ovariectomy. *N Engl J Med* 311: 1345–1349, 1984.

Namba H, Sokoloff L. Acute administration of high doses of estrogen increases glucose utilization throughout the brain. *Brain Res* 291: 391–394,

Norberg L, Wahlstrom G, Backstrom T. The anaesthetic potency of 3x-hydroxy-5x-pregnan-20-one and 3x-hydroxy-5B-pregnan-20-one determined with an intravenous EEG-threshold method in male rats. *Acta Pharmacol Toxicol Scand* 61: 42–47, 1987.

Ohkura T, Isse K, Akazawa K, et al. An open trial of estrogen therapy for dementia of the Alzheimer type in women. In *The Modern Management of the Menopause: A Perspective for the 21st Century,* eds. G. Berg and M. Hammar. Carnforth, UK: Parthenon Publishing, 1994, pp. 315–333.

Oppenheim G, Zohar J, Shapiro B, Belmaker RH. The role of estrogen in treating resistant depression. In *Treating Resistant Depression,* eds. Joseph Zohar and Robert H. Belmaker. New York: PMA Publishing Corp., 1987.

Paganini-Hill A, Henderson V. Estrogen deficiency and risk of Alzheimer's disease in women. *Am J Epidemiol* 140: 256–261, 1994.

Parry BL. Reproductive factors affecting the course of affective illness in women. *Psychiatric Clinics of North America* 12(1): 207–220, 1989.

Phillip S, Sherwin BB. Effects of estrogen on neuronal function in postmenopausal women. *Psychoneuroendocrinology* 17: 485–498, 1992.

Ravnikar VA, Schiff I, Regestein QR. Menopause and sleep. In *The Menopause,* ed. H. Buchsbaum. New York: Springer Verlag, 1983, pp. 161–171.

Rhoades R, Pflanzer R. The Pituitary Gland. In *Human Physiology.* Philadelphia: Saunders College Publishing, 1989. Discussion of effects of progesterone on androgen receptors, p. 403.

Sampson GA. Premenstrual syndrome: A double-blind controlled trial of progesterone and placebo. *Br J Psychiatry* 135: 209–215, 1979.

Sandyk R. Estrogen's impact on cognitive functions in multiple sclerosis. *Int J Neurosci* 86: 23, 1996.

Shabas D, Weinreb H. Preventive health care in women with multiple sclerosis. *J Wom Health and Gender Based Medicine* 9: 389–395, 2000.

Shaywitz SE, Shaywitz BA, Pugh KR, et al. Effect of estrogen on brain activation patterns in postmenopausal women during working memory tasks. *JAMA* 281(13): 1197–1202, 1999.

Sherwin BB. Hormones, mood and cognitive functioning in postmenopausal women. *Obstet Gynecol* 87: 20–26, 1996.

Sherwin BB, Tulandi T. "Add-back" estrogen reverses cognitive deficits induced by a gonadotropin-releasing hormone agonist in women with leiomyomata uteri. *J Clin Endocrinol Metab* 81: 2545–2549, 1996.

Slopien R, Warenik-Szymankiewica A, Maciejewska M, Wiza M. Serum Serotonin Level in Postmenopausal Women. Third International Symposium: Women's Health and Menopause. June 1998.

Smith R, Studd JWW. A pilot study of the effect upon multiple sclerosis of menopause, hormone replacement therapy and the menstrual cycle. *J R Soc Med* 85: 612, 1992.

Stenn PG, Klaiber EL, Vogel W, et al. Testosterone effects upon photic stimulation of the EEG and mental performance of humans. *Percept and Motor Skills* 34: 371–378, 1972.

Studd JWW, Smith RNJ. Estrogens and depression in women. *Menopause* 1: 33–37, 1995.

Thompson J, Oswald I. Effect of estrogen on the sleep, mood and anxiety of menopausal women. *Br Med J* 2: 1217–1219, 1977.

Vliet, EL. An approach to perimenopausal migraine. *Menopause Management* 4(6): 25–33, 1995.

Vliet EL, Davis VL. New perspectives on the relationship of hormonal changes to affective disorders in the perimenopause. In *Clinical Issues in Women's Health.* Midlife Women's Health, 2(4): 453–472, Oct–Dec. 1991. Philadelphia: JB Lippincott.

Watson NR, Studd JWW, Savvas M, et al. Treatment of severe premenstrual syndrome with oestradiol patches and cyclical oral norethisterone. *Lancet* 2: 730–732, 1989.

Yaffe K, Sawaya G, Lieberburg I, et al. Estrogen therapy in postmenopausal women: Effects on cognitive function and dementia. *JAMA* 279: 688–695, 1998.

Young EA. Alteration of the hypothalamic-pituitary-ovarian axis in depressed women. *Arch Gen Psych* 57: 1157–1162, 2000.

Chapter 13: The Perils of PCOS, Obesity, Syndrome X, and Diabetes

Batukan C, Baysal B. Metformin improves ovulation and pregnancy rates in patients with polycystic ovary syndrome. *Arch Gynecol Obstet* 265(3): 124–127, 2001.

Campaigne BN, Wishner KL. Gender-specific health care in diabetes mellitus. *J Gender-specific Medicine* 3: 51–58, 2000.

Chang RJ, et al. Diagnosis of polycystic ovary syndrome. *Endocrinol Metab Clin North Am* 28(2): 397–408, 1999.

Deedwania P. Hypertension and diabetes. *Arch Internal Med* 160: 1583–1594, 2000.

Escalante Pulido JM, et al. Changes in insulin sensitivity, secretion and glucose effectiveness during menstrual cycle. *Arch Med Res* 30(1): 19–22, 1999.

Ferrara A, et al. Sex differences in insulin levels in older adults and the effect of body size, estrogen replacement therapy, and glucose tolerance status. The Rancho Bernardo Study, 1984–87 *Diabetes* 18(2): 220–225, 1995.

Folsom A, Kushi L, Anderson K, et al. Associations of general and abdominal obesity with multiple outcomes in older women. *Arch Intern Med* 160: 2117–2128, 2000.

Gambacciani M, Ciaponi M, Cappagli B, et al. Climacteric modifications in body weight and fat tissue distribution. *Climacteric: The Journal of the International Menopause Society* 2: 37–43, 1999.

Ganesan R. The aversive and hypophagic effects of estradiol. *Physiol Behav* 55: 279–285, 1994.

Gaspard UJ, Wery, Scheen, et al. Long-term effects of oral estradiol and dydrogesterone on carbohydrate metabolism in postmenopausal women. *Climacteric: The Journal of the International Menopause Society* 2(2): 93–100, June 1999.

Geary, N. Estradiol and the control of eating. *Appetite* 29: 386, 1997.

Glueck CJ, Wang P, Kobayashi S, et al. Metformin therapy throughout pregnancy reduces the development of gestational diabetes in women with polycystic ovary syndrome. *Fertility and Sterility* 77: 250–255, 2002.

Godsland I, Walton C, Stevenson J. Carbohydrate Metabolism, Cardiovascular Disease and Hormone Replacement Therapy. In *The Modern Management of the Menopause,* Proceedings of the VII International Congress on the Menopause, Stockholm, Sweden. New York: Parthenon Publishing Group, 1994, pp. 231–249.

Gordon CM. Menstrual disorders in adolescents. Excess androgens and the polycystic ovary syndrome. *Pediatr Clin North Am* 46(3): 519–543, 1999.

Herzog AG. Polycystic ovarian syndrome in women with epilepsy: epileptic or iatrogenic? *Ann Neurol* 39: 559–560, 1996.

Herzog AG, Seibel MM, Schomer D, et al. Temporal lobe epilepsy: an extrahypothalamic pathogenesis for polycystic ovarian syndrome? *Neurology* 34(10): 1389–1393, 1984.

Heymsfield S, Gallagher D, Poehlman E, et al. Menopausal changes in body composition and energy expenditure. *Exp Ger* 29(3/4): 377–389, 1994.

Isojarvi JIT, Laatikainen TJ, Pakarinen AJ, Juntunen KTS, Myllyla VV. Polycystic ovaries and hyperandrogenism in women taking valproate for epilepsy. *N Eng J Med* 329: 1383–1388, 1993.

Kaye S, Folsom A, Soler J, Prineas R, et al. Association of body mass and fat distribution with sex hormone concentrations in postmenopausal women. *Int J Epidemiol* 20: 151–156, 1991.

Ley C, Lees B, Stevenson J. Sex and menopause-associated changes in body-fat distribution. *Am J Clin Nutr* 55: 950–954, 1992.

Nestler J, et al. Dehydroeplandrosterone: The "missing link" between hyperinsulinemia and atherosclerosis? *FASEB J* 6: 3073–3075, 1992.

Niki E, Nakano M. Estrogens as antioxidants. *Methods Enzymol* 186: 330, 1990.

Peiris A, et al. Relationship of body fat distribution to the metabolic clearance of insulin in premenopausal women. *Int J Obesity* 11: 581–589, 1985.

Pownall H, Ballantyne C, Kimball K, et al. Effect of moderate alcohol consumption on hypertriglyceridemia. *Arch Intern Med* 159: 981–987, 1999.

Rosano G. Syndrome X in women is associated with estrogen deficiency. *Eur Heart J* 16: 610–614, 1995.

Schmidt MI, Watson RL, Duncan BB, et al. Clustering of dyslipidemia, hyperuricemia, diabetes, and hypertension and its association with fasting insulin and central and overall obesity in a general population. *Metabolism* 45 (6): 699–706, 1996.

Stoll BA. Perimenopausal weight gain and progression of breast cancer precursors. *Cancer Detect Prev* 23(1): 31–36, 1999.

Tchernof A, et al. Menopause, central body fatness, and insulin resistance: Effects of hormone-replacement therapy. *Coron Artery Dis* 9(8): 503–511, 1998.

Vandermolen DT, Ratts VS, Evans WS, et al. Metformin increases the ovulatory rate and pregnancy rate from clomiphene citrate in patients with polycystic ovary syndrome who are resistant to clomiphene citrate alone. *Fertil Steril* 75(2): 310–315, 2001.

Visser M, Bouter L, McQuillan, G. Elevated C-Reactive Protein Levels in Overweight and Obese Adults. *JAMA* 282(22): 2131, 1999.

Chapter 14: The Many Faces of Infertility: Overlooked Factors

Cassidy A, Bingham S, Setchell K. Biological effects of isoflavones in young women: Importance of the chemical composition of soyabean products. *Br J Nutrition* 74: 587–601, 1995.

Coyle JT, Puttfarcken P. Oxidative stress, glutamate, and neurodegenerative disorders. *Science* 262(5134): 689–695, 1993.

Divi RL, Chang HC, Doerge DR. Anti-thyroid isoflavones from soybean: Isolation, characterization, and mechanisms of action. National Center for Toxicological Research, Jefferson, AR 72079, USA. *Biochem Pharmacol* 54(1): 1087–1096, Nov. 15, 1997.

Gray LE Jr, Ostby J, Marshall R, Andrews J. Reproductive and thyroid effects of low-level polychlorinated biphenyl (Aroclor 1254) exposure. *Fundamental and Applied Toxicology* 20(3): 288–294, 1993.

Knight, DC, Eden JA. A review of the clinical effects of phytoestrogens. *Obstet Gynecol* 87(5 Part 2): 897–904, 1996.

Kronenberg F, Hughes C. Exogenous and endogenous estrogens: An appreciation of biological complexity (editorial). *Menopause: The Journal of the North American Menopause Society* 6(1): 4–6, 1999.

Nagata C, Kabuto M, Kurisu Y, Shimizu H. Decreased serum estradiol concentration associated with high dietary intake of soy products in premenopausal Japanese women. *Nutrition and Cancer* 29(3): 228–233, 1997.

Ondrizek RR, Chan PJ, Patton WC, King A. An alternative medicine study of herbal effects on the penetration of zona-free hamster oocytes and the integrity of sperm deoxyribonucleic acid. *Fertil Steril* 71(3): 517–522, 1999.

Sharara FI, Seifer DB, Flaws JA. Environmental toxicants and female reproduction. *Fertil Steril* 70(4): 613–622, 1998.

Thomas R, Reid RL. Thyroid disease and reproductive function: A review. *Obstet Gynecol* 70: 789–798, 1987.

Whitten PL, Lewis C, Russell E, Naftolin F. Potential adverse effects of phytoestrogens. *J Nutrition* 125 (Suppl): S 776, 1995.

Chapter 15: The Ovaries and Your Other Body Systems

Abitbol J, Abitbol B. The voice and menopause: The twilight of the divas. *Contracept Fertil Sex* 26(9): 649–655, Sept. 1998.

Abraham GE, Flechas JD, Hakala JC. Effect of daily ingestion of tablet containing 5 mg iodine and 7.5 mg iodide as the potassium salt for a period of three months on thyroid function tests and thyroid volume by ultrasonometry in ten euthyroid Caucasian women. Submitted for publication, 2002.

Aloia JF, McGowan DM, Vaswani AN, Ross P, Cohn SH. Relationship of menopause to skeletal and muscle mass. *Am J Clin Nutr* 53: 1378–1383, 1991.

Arden NK, Lloyd ME, Spector TD, Hughes GR. Safety of hormone replacement therapy (HRT) in systemic lupus erythematosus (SLE). *Lupus* 3: 11–13, 1994.

Bolognia JL, Braverman IM, Rousseau ME, Sarrle PM. Skin changes in menopause. *Maturitas* 11: 295–304, 1989.

Brincat M, Kalaban S, Studd JWW, et al. A study of the decrease in skin collagen content, skin thickness, and bone mass in the postmenopausal woman. *Obstet Gynecol* 70: 840–845, 1987.

Brincat M, Moniz CF, Kalaban S, et al. Decline in skin collagen content and metacarpal index after the menopause and its preventions with sex hormone replacement. *Br J Obstet Gynaecol* 94: 126–129, 1987.

Brincat M, Versi E, Moniz CF, et al. Skin collagen in postmenopausal women receiving different regimens of estrogen therapy. *Br J Obstet Gynecol* 70: 123–127, 1987.

Brocklehurst JC, Fry J, Griffiths L, et al. Urinary infections and symptoms of dysuria in women aged 45–64 years: Their relevance to similar findings in the elderly. *Age Ageing* 1: 41–47, 1972.

Cardozo L. Role of estrogens in the treatment of female urinary incontinence. *J Am Geriatr Soc* 38: 326–330, 1990.

Castelo-Branco C, Duran M, Gonzalea-Merlo J. Skin collagen changes related to age and hormone replacement therapy. *Maturitas* 15: 113–119, 1992.

Chen Y, Dales R, Tang M, Krewski D. Obesity may increase the incidence of asthma in women but not in men: Longitudinal observations from the Canadian National Population Health Survey. *Am J Epidemiol* 155(3): 191–197, 2002.

Claude F, Allemany VR. Asthma and menstruation. *Presse Med* 38: 755–762, 1938.

Cohen A, Dubbs AW, Myers A. The treatment of atrophic arthritis with estrogenic substance. *N Engl J Med* 1222: 140–142, 1940.

Cornell Bell A, Sullivan D, Allansmith M. Gender-related difference in the morphology of the lacrimal gland. *Invest Ophthal and Vis Sci* 26: 1170–1175, 1985.

Da Silva JA, Hall GM. The effects of gender and sex hormones on outcome in rheumatoid arthritis. *Clin Rheumatol* 6: 196–219, 1992.

Davidsonn MH, Maki KC, Maryx P, et al. Effects of continuous estrogen (17-beta estradiol) and estrogen-progestin (norethindrone) replacement regimens on cardiovascular risk markers in postmenopausal women. *Arch Int Med* 160: 3315–3325, 2000.

Elia G, Bergman A. Estrogen effects on the urethra: Beneficial effects in women with genuine stress incontinence. *Obstet Gynecol Sur* 48: 509–513, 1993.

Eliasson O, Scherzer HH, De Graff AC. Morbidity of asthma in relation to the menstrual cycle. *J Allergy Clin Immunol* 77: 87–94, 1986.

Gharagozloo Z, Brubaker R. The correlation between serum progesterone and aqueous dynamics during the menstrual cycle. *Acta Ophthalmol* 69: 791–795, 1991.

Gibbs CJ, Courts II, Lock R, et al. Premenstrual exacerbation of asthma. *Thorax* 39: 833–836, 1984.

Goldberg VM, Moskowitz RW, Rosner IA. The role of estrogen and oophorectomy in immune oophoritis. *Semin Arthritis Rheum.* 11(Suppl.): 134–139, 1981.

Guttridge NM. Changes in ocular and visual variables during the menstrual cycle. *Ophthalmic Physiol Opt* 14(1): 38–48, 1994.

Hall GM, Daniels M, Huskisson EC, Spector TD. A randomized controlled trial of hormone replacement therapy in postmenopausal rheumatoid arthritis. *Ann Rheum Dis* 53: 112–116, 1994.

Hall GM, Spector T. The use of estrogen replacement as an adjunct therapy in rheumatoid arthritis. In *The Modern Management of the Menopause: A Perspective for the 21st Century,* eds. G. Berg and M. Hammar. Carnforth, UK: Parthenon Publishing, 1994, pp. 369–375.

Hall GM, Spector TD, Studd JWW. Carpal tunnel syndrome and hormone replacement therapy. *Br Med J* 304: 382–386, 1992.

Hanley SP. Asthma variation with menstruation. *Br J Dis Chest* 75: 306–308, 1981.

Harju T, Keistinen T, Tuuponen T, Kivela T. Hospital admissions of asthmatics by age and sex. *Allergy* 51: 693–696, 1996.

Hassager C, Jensen LT, Podenphant J, et al. Collagen synthesis in postmenopausal women during therapy with anabolic steroids or female sex hormones. *Metabolism* 39: 1167–1169, 1990.

Holmdahl R, Carlsten H, Jansson L, Larsson P. Oestrogen is a potent immunomodulator of murine experimental rheumatoid disease. *Br J Obstet Gynaecol* 99: 325–328, 1989.

Holzer G. Ovarian failure and joints. In *The Modern Management of the Menopause: A Perspective for the 21st Century,* eds. G. Berg and M. Hammar. Carnforth, UK: Parthenon Publishing, 1994, pp. 359–367.

Horwitz BJ, Fisher RS. The irritable bowel syndrome (review). *N Engl J Med* 344: 1846–1850, 2001.

Hsu JT, Kim CH, O'Conner MK, et al. Effect of menstrual cycle on esophageal emptying of liquid and solid boluses. *Mayo Clin Proc* 68: 753–756, 1993.

Hu F, Stampfer M, Manson J, et al. Trends in the incidence of coronary heart disease and changes in diet and lifestyle in women. *N Engl J Med* 343: 530–537, 2000.

Jackson S, Shepherd A, Brookes S, Abrams P. The effect of oestrogen supplementation on post-menopausal urinary stress incontinence: A double-blind placebo-controlled trial. *Br J Obstet Gynaecol* 106(7): 711–718, 1999.

Karpel JP, Wait JL. Asthma in women, part 3: Perimenstrual asthma, effects of hormone therapy. *J Crit Illness* 15(5): 265–272, 2000.

Katz PO, Castrell DO. Gastroesophageal reflux disease during pregnancy. *Gastroenterology Clin North Amer* 27(1): 153–167, 1998.

Kiely PM, Carney LG, Smith G. Menstrual cycle variations of corneal topography and thickness. *Am J Optom Physiol Opt* 60(10): 822–829, 1983.

LaCharity LA. The experiences of younger women with coronary artery disease. *J Women's Health & Gender-Based Medicine* 8: 773–785, 1999.

Latman NS. Relation of menstrual cycle phase to symptoms of rheumatoid arthritis. *Am J Med* 73: 947–950.

Leach N, Wallis N, Lothringer L, et al. Corneal hydration changes during the normal menstrual cycle—a preliminary study. *J Reprod Med* 6: 15–18, 1971.

Lindholm P, Vilkman E, Raudaskoski T, Suvanto-Luukkonen E, Kauppila A. The effect of postmenopause and postmenopausal HRT on measured voice values and vocal symptoms. Department of Otolaryngology and Phoniatrics, Oulu University Hospital, Finland. *Maturitas* 28(1): 47–53, Sept. 1997.

Marrero JM, Goggin PM, de Caestecker JS, et al. Determinants of pregnancy heartburn. *Br J Ostet Gynaecol* 99: 731–734, 1992.

Mathias JR, Clench MH, Abell TL, et al. Effect of leuprolide acetate in treatment of abdominal pain and nausea in premenopausal women with functional bowel disease: a double-blind, placebo-controlled, randomized study. *Digestive Diseases and Sciences* 43: 1347–1355, 1998.

Matthews KA, Meilahn E, Kuller LH, et al. Menopause and risk factors for coronary heart disease. *N Eng J Med* 321: 641, 1989.

McClung MR, et al. Effects of risedronate on the risk of hip fracture in elderly women. *NEJM* 344: 333–340, 2001.

Metka M, Enzelsberger H, Knogler W, et al. Ophthalmic complaints as a climacteric symptom. *Maturitas* 14: 3–8, 1991.

Nilas L, Christensen C. The Pathophysiology of peri- and menopausal bone loss. *Br J Obstet Gynaecol* 96: 580–585, 1989.

Pattie MA, Murdoch BE, Theodoros D, Forbes K. Voice changes in women treated for endometriosis and related conditions: The need for comprehensive vocal assessment. *J Voice* 12(3): 366–371, Sept. 1998.

Pector TD, Campion GD. Generalized osteoarthritis: A hormonally mediated disease. *Ann Rheum Dis* 48: 523, 1989.

Punnonen R, Jokela H, Aine R, et al. Impaired ovarian function and risk factors for atherosclerosis in premenopausal women. *Maturitas* 27: 231–238, 1997.

Redmond, GP. *Androgenic Disorders.* New York: Raven Press, 1995.

Rees L. An aetiological study of premenstrual asthma. *J Psychosomatic Res* 7: 191–193, 1963.

Rejula K, Haahtela T, Klaukka T, Rantanen J. Incidence of occupational asthma in young adults has increased in Finland. *Chest* 110: 58–61, 1996.

Riss B, Binder S, Riss P, Kemeter P. Corneal sensitivity during the menstrual cycle. *Br J Ophthalmol* 66(2): 123–126, 1982.

Riss B, Riss P. Corneal sensitivity in pregnancy. *Ophthalmologica* 183(2): 57–62, 1981.

Rosano GMC, Sarrel PM, Poole-Wilson, PA, Collins P. Beneficial effect of oestrogen (17-beta estradiol) on exercise-induced myocardial ischaemia in women with coronary artery disease. *Lancet* 342: 133–136, 1993.

Rosner IA, Manni A, Malemud CJ, et al. Estradiol receptors in articular chondrocytes. *Biochem Biophys Res Commun* 106: 1379–1382, 1982.

Scholes D, et al. Injectable hormone contraception and bone density: Results from a prospective study. *Epidemiology* 13: 581–587, 2002.

Schneider HPG. The International Menopause Society Report on the 10th World Congress on the menopause. *Climacteric* 5: 219–228, 2002.

Serrander AM, Peek KE. Changes in contact lens comfort related to the menstrual cycle and menopause. *J Am Optom Assoc* 64(3): 162–166, 1993.

Shames RS, Heilbron DC, Janson SL, et al. Clinical differences among women with and without self-reported perimenstrual asthma. *Ann Allergy Asthma Immunol* 8: 65–72, 1998.

Shuster S, Black MM, McVitie E. The influence of age and sex on skin thickness, skin collagen, and density. *Br J Dermatol* 93: 639–643, 1975.

Skobeloff EM, Spivey WH, Silverman R, et al. The effect of the menstrual cycle on asthma presentations in the emergency department. *Arch Int Med* 156: 1837–1840, 1996.

Smith, P. Estrogens and the urogenital tract. Studies on steroid hormone receptors and a clinical study on a new estradiol-releasing vaginal ring. *Acta Obstet Gynecol Scand* 1: 157–160, 1993.

Smith P, Heimer G, Lindskog M, and Ulmsten U. Oestradiol-releasing vaginal ring for treatment of postmenopausal urogenital atrophy. *Maturitas* 16: 145–149, 1993.

Spector TD, Hochberg MC. The protective effect of the oral contraceptive pill on rheumatoid arthritis. *J Clin Epidemiol* 43: 1221–1230, 1990.

Ter RB. Gender differences in gastroesophageal reflux disease. *J Gender Specific Med* 3(2): 42–44, 2000.

The Writing Group for the PEPI Trial. Effects of estrogen or estrogen/progestin regimens on heart disease risk factors in postmenopausal women: The postmenopausal estrogen/progestin intervention (PEPI) trial. *JAMA* 273: 199–208, 1995.

Van Thiel DH, Gravaler JS, Stremple GJ. Lower esophageal sphincter pressure during the normal menstrual cycle. *Am J Obstet Gynecol* 134: 64–67, 1979.

Van Thiel DH, Gavaler JS, Stremple GJ. Lower esophageal sphincter pressure in females using sequential oral contraceptives. *Gastroenterology* 71: 232–234, 1976.

Viskin S. Long QT. Syndromes and torsade de pointes. *Lancet* 354: 1625–1633, 1999.

Vliet EL. Hormone connections in urinary incontinence in women. *Top Ger Rehab* 15(4): 16–30, 2000.

Ward M, Stone S, Sandman C. Visual perception in women during the menstrual cycle. *Physiol and Behav* 20: 239–243, 1978.

Watts NB, Notelovitz M, Timmons MC, et al. Comparison of oral estrogens and estrogens plus androgen on bone mineral density, menopausal symptoms, and lipid-lipoprotein profiles in surgical menopause. *Obstet Gynecol* 85: 529–537, 1995.

Wenger NK. Cardiovascular disease in menopausal women: The benefits of HRT are not restricted to improving lipid profiles. *Medicographia* 21: 223–228, 1999.

Yamanishi T, Yasuda K, Suda S, et al. Effect of functional continuous magnetic stimulation for urinary incontinence. *J Urology* 163: 456–459, 2000.

Chapter 16: Balancing Ovarian Hormones for Optimal Health

Akamatsu T, Akiyama T, Kimura T, Saito H, Yanaihara T. Menopausal insomnia and hormone replacement therapy. Third International Symposium, Women's Health and Menopause, June 1998.

Araujo DAC, Farias MLF, Andrade ATL. Effects of transdermal and oral estrogen replacement on lipids and glucose metabolism in postmenopausal women with type 2 diabetes mellitus. *Climacteric* 5: 286–292, 2002.

Benyon HL, Garbett ND, Barnes PJ. Severe premenstrual exacerbations of asthma: Effect of intramuscular injection of progesterone. *Lancet* 2: 370–372, 1988.

Bjorn I, Backstrom T. Drug-related side effects is a common reason for poor compliance in hormone replacement therapy. *Maturitas* 32: 77–86, 1999.

Bush TL, Whiteman MK. Hormone replacement therapy and risk of breast cancer (editorial). *JAMA* 281: 2140–2142, 1999.

Cucinelli F, Soranna L, Murgia F, Muzj G, Perri C, Cinque B, Mancuso S, Lanzone A. Differential effect of transdermal estrogen plus progestagen replacement therapy on insulin metabolism in postmenopausal women related to their insulinemic secretion. Third International Symposium Women's Health and Menopause, June 1998.

Cullberg J. Mood changes and menstrual symptoms with different gestagen/estrogen combinations. *Acta Psychiatr Scand* (suppl) 236: 1, 1972.

Davidsonn MH, Maki KC, Maryx P, et al. Effects of continuous estrogen (17-beta estradiol) and estrogen-progestin (norethindrone) replacement regimens on cardiovascular risk markers in postmenopausal women. *Arch Int Med* 160: 3315–3325, 2000.

Davis SR, Burger HG. Use of androgens in postmenopausal women. *Curr Opinion Obstet Gynecol* 9: 177–180, 1997.

De Lignieres B, Dennerstein L, Backstrom T. Influence of route of administration on progesterone metabolism. *Maturitas* 21: 251–257, 1995.

Dickey, MD, Richard P. *Managing Contraceptive Pill Patients,* 9th ed., 2002. Available from: Essential Medical Information Systems, Inc., P.O. Box 1607, Durant, OK 74702-1607.

Ditkoff EC, Crary WG, Cristo M, Lobo RA. Estrogen improves psychological function in asymptomatic postmenopausal women. *Obstet Gynecol* 78: 991–995, 1991.

Duncan A, Lyall H, Roberts R, et al. The effect of 17-beta estradiol and norethisterone on insulin sensitivity in postmenopausal women. Third International Symposium Women's Health and Menopause, June 1998.

Falkeborn M, Lithell H, Persson I, et al. Lipids and antioxidative effects of 17-beta estradiol and sequential norethisterone acetate treatment in a 3-month randomized controlled trial. *Climacteric* 5: 240–248, 2002.

Fitzpatrick L, Pace C, Wiita B. Comparison of regimens containing oral micronized progesterone or medroxyprogesterone acetate on quality of life in postmenopausal women: A cross-sectional survey. *J Wos Hlth & Gender Based Med* 9(4): 381–387, 2000.

Gaspard UL, Wery OJ, Scheen AJ, et al. Long-term effects of oral estradiol and dydrogesterone on carbohydrate metabolism in postmenopausal women. *Climacteric* 2(2): 93–100, 1999.

Gelfand MM. Estrogen-androgen hormone replacement therapy. *European Menopause Journal* 2: 22–26, 1995.

Genazzani, AR (president of the International Menopause Society). HRT and breast cancer: Is there any news? A clinician's perspective (editorial). *Climacteric: The Journal of the International Menopause Society,* 3: 13–16, 2000.

Genazzani AR, Gadducci A, Gamnacciani M. Controversial issues in climacteric medicine II: Hormone replacement therapy and cancer. International Menopause Society Expert Position Paper. *Gynecol Endocrinol* 15: 453–465, 2001.

Godsland IF, Crook D, Wynn V. Clinical and metabolic considerations of long-term oral contraceptive use. The Wynn Institute for Metabolic Research. *Am J Obstetrics Gynecology* 166(6) Part 2: 1955–1966, June 1992.

Grabrick DM, Hartmann LC, Cerhan JR, et al. Risk of breast cancer with oral contraceptive use in women with a family history of breast cancer. *JAMA* 284: 1791–1798, 2000. (Editorial comment, pp. 1837–1838.)

Grady D, Herrington D, Bittner V, et al. for the HERS Research Group. Heart and estrogen/progestin replacement study follow-up (HERS II): Part 1: cardiovascular outcomes during 6.8 years of hormone therapy. *J Am Med Assoc* 288: 49–57, 2002.

Halbreich, U. Menopause and psychopharmacology: Signs, symptom and treatment. Third International Symposium Women's Health and Menopause, June 1998.

Henderson AF, Gregoire AJP, Kumar R, Studd JWW. The treatment of severe postnatal depression with oestradiol skin patches. *Lancet* 338: 816, 1991.

Holst J, Backstrom T, Hammerbach S, et al. Progestogen addition during oestrogen replacement therapy—effects on vasomotor symptoms and mood. *Maturitas* 11: 13–19, 1989.

Hulley S, Grady D, Bush T, et al. Randomized trial of estrogen plus progestin (HERS) for secondary prevention of coronary heart disease in postmenopausal women. *J Am Med Assoc* 280: 6–5 613, 1998.

Jensen J, Christensen C, Rodbro P. Estrogen-progesterone replacement therapy changes body composition in early postmenopausal women. *Maturitas* 8: 209–216, 1986.

Klaiber E, Broverman D, Vogel W, et al. Relationships of serum oestradiol levels, menopausal duration and mood during hormone replacement therapy. *Psychoneuroendocrinology* 22: 549–558, 1997.

Kritz-Silverstein D, Barrett-Conner E. Long-term postmenopausal hormone use, obesity, and fat distribution in older women. *JAMA* 275(1): 46–49, Jan. 3, 1996.

Low biologic aggressiveness in breast cancer in women using hormone replacement therapy. *J Clin Oncol* 16(9): 3115–3120, 1998.

Lloyd T, et al. Oral contraceptive use by teenage women does not affect body composition. *Obstet Gynecol* 100: 235–239, 2002.

Magos AL, Brewster E, Singh R, O'Dowd T, Brincat M, Studd JWW. The effects of norethisterone in postmenopausal women on oestrogen replacement therapy: A model for the premenstrual syndrome. *Br J Obstet Gynaecol* 93: 1290–1296, 1986.

Magos AL, Brincat M, Studd JWW. Treatment of the premenstrual syndrome by subcutaneous oestradiol implants and cyclical oral norethisterone: A placebo controlled study. *Br Med J* 1: 1629–1631, 1986.

Montgomery JC, Brincal M, Tapp A, Appleby L, Versi E, Fenwick PBC, Studd JWW. Effects of oestrogen and testosterone implants on psychological disorders in the climacteric. *Lancet* 1: 297–299, 1987.

O'Meara ES, Rossing MA, Daling JR, et al. Hormone replacement therapy after a diagnosis of breast cancer in relation to recurrence and mortality. *J Nat Cancer Inst* 93: 754–762, 2001.

Polo-Kantola P, Erkkola R, Irjala K, Polo O. When does oestrogen replacement therapy improve sleep quality? Third International Symposium Women's Health and Menopause, June 1998.

Powers MS, Schenkel L, Darley PE, et al. Pharmacokinetics and pharmacodynamics of transdermal dosage forms of 17-beta estradiol: Comparison with conventional oral estrogens used for hormone replacement therapy. *Am J Obstet Gynecol* 152: 1099–1106, 1985.

Prang AJ. Estrogen may well affect response to antidepressant. *JAMA* 219: 143–144, 1972.

Raudaskoski T, et al. Insulin sensitivity during postmenopausal hormone replacement with transdermal estradiol and intrauterine levonorgestrel. *Acta Obstet Gynecol Scand* 78(6): 540–545, July 1999.

Reubinoff B, Wurtman J, Adler D, et al. Effect of hormone replacement therapy on body composition fat distribution and food intake in early postmenopausal women: A prospective study. *Fertil Steril* 64(5): 963–968, 1995.

Ripley HS, Shorr E, Papanicolaou GN. The effect of treatment of depression in the menopause with estrogenic hormone. *Amer J Psychiat* 96: 905–915, 1940.

Rosano GMC, Sarrel PM, Poole-Wilson, PA, Collins P. Beneficial effect of oestrogen (17-beta estradiol) on exercise-induced myocardial ischaemia in women with coronary artery disease. *Lancet* 342: 133–136, 1993.

Sayegh RA, Kelly L, Wurtman J, Deitch A, et al. Impact of hormone replacement therapy on the body mass and fat compositions of menopausal women: A cross-sectional study. *Menopause* 6(4): 312–315, 1999.

Schneider HPG. The view of the International Menopause Society on the women's health initiative (WHI). *Climacteric* 5: 211–216, 2002.

Selby PL, Peacock M. Dose dependent response of symptoms, pituitary and bone to transdermal oestrogen in postmenopausal women. *Br Med J* 293: 1337–1339, 1986.

Sellers TA, Mink PJ, Cerhan JR, et al. The role of hormone replacement therapy in the risk for breast cancer and total mortality in women with a family history of breast cancer. *Ann Intern Med* 127: 973–980, 1997.

Seumeren I. Weight gain and hormone replacement therapy: Are women's fears justified? *Maturitas* 34(Suppl 1): S3–S8, 2000.

Sherwin BB, Gelfand MM. Differential symptom response to parenteral estrogen and/or androgen administration in surgical menopause. *Am J Obstet Gynecol* 151: 153–158, 1985.

Speroff L. Postmenopausal estrogen-progestin therapy and breast cancer: A clinical response to epidemiological reports. *Climacteric: The Journal of the International Menopause Society* 3: 3–12, 2000.

Sulak PJ, et al. Acceptance of altering the standard 21-day/7-day oral contraceptive regimen to delay menses and reduce hormone withdrawal symptoms. *Am J Obstet Gynecol* 186: 1142–1149, 2002.

Sulak P. Using OCs to manage perimenopause. *OBGyn Management* 41–50, 2000.

Talone EP, Lello S, Caporali M, Sotgia T, Pasqua C, Guardianelli F, Romanini C. Postmenopausal depressive symptoms: Psychopharmacological treatment and hormonal replacement therapy. Third International Symposium Women's Health and Menopause, June 1998.

Tchernof A, et al. Menopause, central body fatness, and insulin resistance: Effects of hormone-replacement therapy. *Coron Artery Dis* 9(8): 503–511, 1998.

Van Vollenhoven RF, McGuire JL. Estrogen, progesterone and testosterone: Can they be used to treat autoimmune diseases? *Cleve Clin J Med* 61: 276–284, 1994.

Vassilopoulou-Sellin R, et al. Estrogen replacement therapy after localized breast cancer: Clinical outcome of 319 women followed prospectively. *J Clin Oncol* 17: 1482–1487, 1999.

Vintamaki T, Tuimala R. Can climacteric women self-adjust therapeutic estrogen doses using symptoms as markers? *Maturitas* 199–203, 1998.

Watson NR, Studd JWW, Savvas M, et al. Treatment of severe premenstrual syndrome with oestradiol patches and cyclical oral norethisterone. *Lancet* 2: 730–732, 1989.

Whitehead M. Oestrogens: Relative potencies and hepatic effects after different routes of administration. *J Obstet Gynecology* 3(suppl): S11–16, 1982.

Wren BG, McFarland K, Edwards P, et al. Effect of sequential transdermal progesterone cream on endometrium, bleeding pattern, and plasma progesterone and salivary progesterone levels in postmenopausal women. *Climacteric* 3: 155–160, 2000.

Chapter 17: Test-and-Treat Strategies for Optimal Thyroid, Adrenal, and Glucose-Insulin Balance

Batukan C, Baysal B. Metformin improves ovulation and pregnancy rates in patients with polycystic ovary syndrome. *Arch Gynecol Obstet* 265(3): 124–127, 2001.

Boscaro M, Barzon L, Sonino N. The diagnosis of Cushing's syndrome. *Arch Int Med* 160: 3045–3053, 2000.

Bunevicius R, Kazanavicius G, Zalinkevicius R, et al. Effects of thyroxine as compared with thyroxine plus triiodothyronine in patients with hypothyroidism. *N Engl J Med* 340(6): 424–429, 1999.

Chen Y, et al. Why do low-fat high-carbohydrate diets accentuate postprandial lipemia in patients with NIDDM? *Diabetes Care* 18(1): 10–16, 1995.

Coulston A, et al. Persistence of hypertriglyceridemic effect of low-fat high-carbohydrate diets in NIDDM patients. *Diabetes Care* 12(2): 94–101, 1989.

Coulston A, et al. Plasma glucose, insulin and lipid responses to high-carbohydrate low-fat diets in normal humans. *Metabolism* 32(1): 52–56, 1983.

DeFronzo RA, Ferrannini E. Insulin resistance: A multifaceted syndrome responsible for NIDDM, obesity, hypertension, dyslipidemia, and atherosclerotic cardiovascular disease. *Diabetes Care* 14(3): 173, 1991.

De Leo V, La Marca A, Ditto A, et al. Effects of metformin on gonadotropin-induced ovulation in women with polycystic ovary syndrome. *Fertil Steril* 72(2): 282–285, 1999.

Despres JP, Lamarche B, Mauriege P, et al. Hyperinsulinemia as an independent risk factor for ischemic heart disease. *N Engl J Med* 334: 952–957, 1996.

Dimanti-Kandarakis E, Louli C, Tsianateli T, Bergiele A. Therapeutic effects of metformin on insulin resistance and hyperandrogenism in polycystic ovary syndrome. *Eur J Endocrinol* 138(3): 269–274, 1998.

Dong B, Hauck W, Gambertoglio J. Bioequivalence of generic and brand-name levothyroxine products in the treatment of hypothyroidism. *JAMA* 277(15): 1205–1213, 1997.

Fogelholm M, Kukkonen-Harjula K, Nenonen A, et al. Effects of walking training on weight maintenance after a very-low-energy diet in premenopausal obese women. *Arch Intern Med* 160: 2177–2184, 2000.

Goodwin FK, Prange AJ, Post RM, et al. Potentiation of antidepressant effects by L-triiodothyronine in tricyclic non-responders. *Amer J Psychiat* 139: 34–38, 1982.

Kaplan NM. The deadly quartet: upper-body obesity, glucose intolerance, hypertriglyceridemia and hypertension. *Arch Int Med* 149: 1514–1520, 1989.

Kocak M, Caliskan E, Simsir C, Haberal A. Metformin therapy improves ovulatory rates, cervical scores, and pregnancy rates in clomiphene citrate-resistant women with polycystic ovary syndrome. *Fertil Steril* 77(1): 101–106, 2002.

Lipworth B. Systemic adverse effects of inhaled corticosteroid therapy. *Arch Internal Med* 159: 941–955, 1999.

Ludwig D, et al. Relation between consumption of sugar-sweetened drinks and childhood obesity: A prospective, observational analysis. *Lancet* 1187: 505–508, 2001.

Manson J, Hu F, Rich-Edwards J, et al. A prospective study of walking as compared with vigorous exercise in the prevention of coronary heart disease in women. *N Eng Med* 341(9): 650–658, 1999.

Moller D, ed. *Insulin Resistance.* Chicester: John Wiley and Sons, 1993.

Morin-Papunen LC, Koivunen RM, Rukonen A, Martikainen HK. Metformin therapy improves the menstrual pattern with minimal endocrine and metabolic effects in women with polycystic ovary syndrome. *Fertil Steril* 69(4): 691–696, 1998.

Vandermolen DT, Ratts VS, Evans WS, et al. Metformin increases the ovulatory rate and pregnancy rate from clomiphene citrate in patients with polycystic ovary syndrome who are resistant to clomiphene citrate alone. *Fertil Steril* 75(2): 310–315, 2001.

Chapter 18: Starting Your "Clean-Up" Campaign: Get Rid of Ovarian Disruptors You Can Control

Abt AB, Oh JY, Huntington RA, Burkhart KK. Chinese herbal medicine induced acute renal failure. *Arch Intern Med* 155: 211–212, Jan. 1995.

Davis SR, et al. The effects of Chinese medicinal herbs on postmenopausal vasomotor symptoms of Australian women: a randomized controlled trial. *Med J Australia* 174: 68–71, 2001.

Koff RS. Herbal hepatotoxicity: Revisiting a dangerous alternative. *JAMA* 273: 502–503, Feb. 1995.

Milewicz A, Mikulski E, Bidzinska B. Satiety and appetite stimulating peptides in ageing women. Third International Symposium Women's Health and Menopause, June 1998.

Prior J, Vigna Y, Alojada N. Conditioning exercise decreases premenstrual symptoms. *Eur J Appl Physiol* 55: 349–355, 1986.

Racette S, et al. Effects of aerobic exercise and dietary carbohydrate on energy expenditure and body composition during weight reduction in obese women. *Amer J Clin Nutr* 61: 486–494, 1995.

Yudkin J. Dietary fat and dietary sugar in relation to ischaemic heart-disease and diabetes. *Lancet* 4–5, 1964.

Yudkin J. Sucrose, coronary heart disease, diabetes, and obesity: Do hormones provide a link? *Am Heart J* 115(2): 493–498, 1988.

MEDICAL TEXTBOOKS

While there are many excellent medical textbooks, I recommend these because they provide well-researched, up-to-date information from the worldwide literature on women's reproductive hormones and health. They are useful for health professionals and further reading for interested consumers:

Brain: Source and Target for Sex Steroid Hormones, The. A. R. Genazzani, F. Petraglia, and R. H. Purdy (eds.). New York and London: Parthenon Publishing Group, 1996.

DHEA: A Comprehensive Review. J.H.H. Thijssen and H. Nieuwenhuyse (eds.). New York and London: Parthenon Publishing Group, 1999.

Endocrine Disruptors: Effects on Male and Female Reproductive Systems. Rajesh K. Naz, Ph.D. (ed.). New York and London: CRC Press, 1999.

Gender Differences in Metabolism: Practical and Nutritional Implications. Mark Tarnopolsky, M.D., Ph.D., FRCP(C). New York and London: CRC Press, 1999.

Hormone Therapy and the Brain: A Clinical Perspective on the Role of Estrogen. Victor W. Henderson, M.D., M.S. New York and London: Parthenon Publishing Group, 2000.

Menopause and the Heart. M. Neves-e-Castro, M. Birkhauser, T. B. Clarkson, P. Collins (eds.). New York and London: Parthenon Publishing Group, 1999.

Prescriber's Guide to Hormone Replacement Therapy, The. M. Whitehead (ed.). New York and London: Parthenon Publishing Group, 1998.

Testosterone: Action, Deficiency, Substitution, 2nd edition. E. Nieschlag, H. M. Behre (eds.). Berlin: Springer-Verlag, 1998.

RESOURCES

Consumer Books, Organizations, Compounding Pharmacies

Section I

Screaming to Be Heard: Hormone Connections Women Suspect and Doctors Ignore (revised edition), Elizabeth Lee Vliet, M.D. (New York: M. Evans and Co., 2000). Describes in more detail how the ovarian hormones are linked to brain-body function and a wide array of symptoms and syndromes that are more common in women—from migraines to chronic fatigue to fibromyalgia—as well as in-depth discussion of heart disease, osteoporosis, and women's cancers. Discusses the differences among various types and ways to deliver estrogen, progesterone, progestins, and testosterone to help women work with their physicians to individualize ways of achieving hormone balance and improved health.

Women, Weight and Hormones, Elizabeth Lee Vliet, M.D. (New York: M. Evans and Co., 2001). Discusses in depth a woman's hormonal systems and how changes or imbalances affect weight and metabolism. References from peer-reviewed international medical literature are included to support the medical information presented. Easy-to-follow meal plans are included to give women with middle-body weight gain the proper balance of carbs, fat, and protein to reduce excess insulin and yet maintain enough carbs to keep the thyroid working well. There is also a detailed chapter on getting tested, which outlines the major hormones to be checked and guidelines for optimal ranges.

Woman's Body: A Manual for Life, Dr. Miriam Stoppard (London and New York: Dorling Kindersley, 1994). Compiled by a team of health experts from many fields, this book covers physical and emotional concerns of women throughout the life span and is illustrated with hundreds of color charts, graphs, and photos. It is one of the most comprehensive and practical women's health books I have found.

The Good News About Women's Hormones, Geoffrey Redmond, M.D. (New York: Warner Books, 1995). There are many parallels in the work Dr. Redmond has done to identify and treat women's hormone problems and the hormone connections I have been addressing in my own work. Dr. Redmond has been president of the Foundation for Developmental Endocrinology and has also edited medical texts on hormone disorders. This book is written for consumers, is easily understandable, and has excellent sections on androgenic disorders (excess hair growth, acne, and other problems), alopecia (hair loss), as well as many other hormone problems. He gives a balanced view of benefits and risks of hormone treatments, and a logical approach to helping women decide about hormone use and how to get reliable lab tests.

The Red Tent, Anita Diamant (New York: Picador, 1997). This novel, told in the voice of Dinah, one of Jacob's daughters, vividly describes the traditions, turmoil, and struggles of women in biblical times. The "red tent" is the menstrual tent where women stayed during their menstrual times, and this story helps us to understand how the ancients saw menstruation and what the world of women was like as they experienced together the uniqueness of the female body. It is a compelling, intense, earthy novel that gives a glimpse into entirely different perspectives on women, and is perhaps even more relevant in the twenty-first century as we read the news stories of similar struggles of women in Afghanistan.

The Premature Menopause Book, Kathryn Petras (New York: Avon Books, 1999). This is a good book written by a layperson sharing her own story about struggling with premature menopause. This book provides an abundance of resources and other helpful consumer information including websites and support groups for women finding themselves in menopause at an early age.

The Silent Passage: Menopause, Gail Sheehy (New York: Pocket Books, 1998). The bestselling book that brought the *M* word out of the closet and into the mainstream. Although it originally came out in hardcover in 1991, it is still a good overview of what to expect and offers other women's experiences.

Sections II–III

Excitotoxins: The Taste That Kills, Russell L. Blaylock, M.D. (Santa Fe, N. Mex.: Health Press, 1994). Excellent resource for understanding the damaging effects of glutamate and other excitatory amino acids in degenerative processes that affect nerve tissue, the brain, and possibly muscle function. While Dr. Blaylock is a neurosurgeon focusing on age-related degenerative neurological diseases rather than the ovaries, I have applied these concepts to potential damaging effects on ovarian function as well, based on known neuroendocrine pathways. Dr. Blaylock has included in this book an outstanding annotated bibliography for those who wish to pursue this connection further using well-documented medical studies. I am impressed with the quality of this book and its references. Dr. Blaylock has treated many patients with various degenerative neurological disorders, and is on the medical faculty at the University of Mississippi. His book is a layperson's version of his numerous scientific publications in this field.

In Bad Taste: The MSG Syndrome, George R. Schwartz, M.D. (Santa Fe, N. Mex.: Health Press, 1988). An excellent review of the health issues related to flavor enhancers, and a subject sadly overlooked by health professionals today.

Lights Out: Sleep, Sugar and Survival, T. S. Wiley with Bent Formby, Ph.D. (New York: Pocket Books, 2000). A review of the extensive research on the damaging effects of sleep deprivation and its serious consequences: obesity, diabetes, hypertension, heart disease, depression, and cancer. This book will help you understand the ways that lack of sleep interferes with all of your hormone systems, but for women in particular, the ovarian disruption can be profound. But a word of caution: Not all of the hormone explanations of the functions of estradiol and progesterone are correct, which may lead to confusion when comparing what I have described in my books with what is written in *Lights Out.*

Living Downstream: An Ecologist Looks at Cancer and the Environment, Sandra Steingraber, Ph.D. (New York: Addison Wesley Publishing Co., 1997). An outstandingly researched and well-written book about the effects of pesticides and other toxic chemicals on our risk of developing cancer. I highly recommend it.

Our Stolen Future: Are We Threatening Our Fertility, Intelligence and Survival?, Theo Colborn, Dianne Dumanoski, and John Peterson Myers (New York and London: E. P. Dutton, 1996). This well-written and fascinating scientific detective story by two environmental scientists and an environmental journalist discusses the worldwide research showing alarming damage to wildlife and humans from many types of environmental contaminants that disrupt our critical hormone systems. It provides a much more in-depth treatment of issues than I have been able to address only briefly in my book, and should be required reading for all women concerned about their health and the health of children to come.

For more information on pesticides being used in schools, workplaces, and other places in your community, contact:

Pesticide Watch
450 Geary Street, Suite 500
San Francisco, CA 94102
www.pesticidewatch.org

National Coalition Against the Misuse of Pesticides
701 E Street, SE, Suite 200
Washington DC, 20003
Phone: 202-543-5450
info@beyondpesticides.org

Overcoming Endometriosis: New Help from the Endometriosis Association, Mary Lou Ballweg (Lincolnwood, Ill.: Contemporary Books, 1987). This is an excellent resource book, even though it was published a number of years ago. See also the newer resource book listed below.

PCOS: The Hidden Epidemic, Samuel S. Thatcher, M.D., Ph.D. (Indianapolis, Ind.: Perspective Press, 2000). Dr. Thatcher is a renowned expert in reproductive endocrinology and brings to this book many years of clinical experience as one of the early advocates for increased understanding of this complex and serious metabolic disorder. The book gives an overview of what PCOS is, our current understanding of causes, and information on helpful treatments based on research findings. This is an excellent resource, recommended by the Polycystic Ovarian Syndrome Association. The phone order line for Perspective Press is 317-872-3055, or their website www.perspectivespress.com.

PolyCystic Ovarian Syndrome Association, Inc. An excellent resource for educational materials, support groups, Web discussions of PCOS. The organization also hosts an outstanding annual conference on PCOS, with presentations from many of the leading experts in the field. Check out their website www.pcosupport.com, or call 630-585-3690. Mailing address is P.O. Box 7007, Rosemont, IL 60018.

Taking Charge of Your Fertility, Toni Weschler, M.P.H. (New York: HarperCollins Publishers, 1995). This is an excellent resource for women struggling with infertility by the founder of Fertility Awareness Counseling and Training Seminars (FACTS). It teaches women about the normal menstrual cycle, natural methods of birth control, and pregnancy achievement, particularly in helping women understand how to assess their individual differences with regard to the fertile window. It is well-researched and endorsed by many fertility specialists as well. My one area of caution is the outdated and limited discussion of PMS and menopause with respect to the patterns of hormone change and treatment options. But this book achieves its primary focus on fertility extremely well, and I highly recommend it to help women understand this complex topic.

The Endometriosis Sourcebook, Mary Lou Ballweg and the Endometriosis Association (Lincolnwood, Ill.: Contemporary Books, 1995). In the words of the author, this is "the definitive guide to current treatment approaches, the latest research, common myths about the disease, and coping strategies—both physical and emotional." It has much more detail about the dioxin research than I have been able to provide, and also goes into other cutting-edge research, as well as integrated treatment options and a wide range of additional resources. I highly recommend this book.

The Thyroid Solution, Ridha Arem, M.D. (New York: Ballantine, 1999). An excellent reference book on thyroid disorders, written by an endocrinologist with solid credentials and clinical experience. Dr. Arem validates what I have seen in my practice for my entire career: Many women in particular have subclinical forms of thyroid disorders that affect mood, fertility, and weight, and create a host of other problems. In addition, Dr. Arem goes into more depth on the value of adding T3 to a thyroid medication regimen, as I have espoused and used for many years as well. I do not think Dr. Arem's information on estrogen therapy is either comprehensive or up-to-date, and I am concerned about his emphasis on the use of Premarin and Provera based on the issues I have described in *Screaming to Be Heard,* and the newer HERS and WHI studies. I do, however, think his information on thyroid is outstanding, and there is also an excellent section on thyroid effects and the brain. See also websites: www.glandcentral.com and www.thyroid.org.

Why Zebras Don't Get Ulcers, Robert M. Sapolsky (New York: W.H. Freeman & Co., 1998). Excellent and humorous review of the adverse effects over time due to high cortisol levels from stress. If you've ever wondered just how "stress" affects your entire body, this is a terrific and well-written book.

Section IV
Organization Resources

American Medical Association, www.ama-assn.org. Professional organization for physicians in all specialties, and publisher of *JAMA,* one of the leading U.S. medical journals. The AMA has many consumer educational resources on its website and is a valuable resource for articles on all aspects of women's health. The AMA also has a special section, Women's Health Information Center, that pulls together significant articles on women's health from several major medical journals.

American Society of Reproductive Medicine, 1209 Montgomery Highway, Birmingham, AL 35216; 205-978-5000; www.asrm.org. This is a professional organization of physicians and health professionals who specialize in various aspects of reproductive medicine, from infertility to menopause. ASRM publishes the medical journal *Fertility and Sterility,* which contains peer-reviewed cutting-edge research in this field; they also host medical conferences and provide educational resources for consumers.

Eating disorders: The following organizations are excellent resources for information and support for women with eating disorders. All of them have websites you can access for information, questions, and chats with other sufferers.

> The American Anorexia and Bulimia Organization: 212-575-6200
>
> Anorexia Nervosa and Related Eating Disorders, Inc. (ANRED): 847-831-3438
>
> Something Fishy, www.SFWED.org, or www.something-fishy.org
>
> Treatment Centers: The Renfrew Center, Remuda Ranch

Endometriosis Association, Mary Lou Ballweg, executive director, 8585 North 7th Place, Milwaukee, WI 53223; 800-992-3636. The organization has a wealth of patient educational materials available, as well as information about support groups and health professionals who specialize in the treatment of endometriosis. It is an excellent comprehensive resource for women with this painful condition. I highly recommend it.

H3 Environmental Corp., www.h3environmental.com. This organization was founded by Mary Cordaro, a respected environmental consultant to builders, engineers, architects, and consumers, advising on ways to create a healthy home environment free of common damaging chemicals. This site provides many resources for people who suffer from chemical sensitivities and multiple allergies.

Hysterectomy Education Resources and Services (HERS Foundation), 422 Bryn Mawr Ave., Bala Cynwyd, PA 19004; 610-667-7757; http://www.frii.com/˜geomanda/endo/hers.html. This organization provides a variety of support services for women who are contemplating a hysterectomy, as well as resource information for women who have had this surgery.

International Menopause Society, Monique Boulet, executive director, Maitre M. Steyaert, Av. des Cattleyas, 3, Box 1, 1150 Brussels, Belgium; 32.2.772.2183; imsociety@Filink.net, www.imsociety.org. This organization is an international group of health professionals involved in basic and clinical research and patient care for women (and men) in the climacteric and menopausal years, as stated in their mission: "The aim of the International Menopause Society (IMS) is to promote knowledge, study and research on all aspects of aging in men and women; to organize, prepare, hold, and participate in international meetings and congresses on menopause and climacteric; and to encourage the interchange of research plans and experience between individual members."

The IMS publishes *Climacteric,* one of the leading medical journals devoted to cutting-edge research from around the world in this field. The editors have refused to take advertising for products that have not been proven effective in properly designed, controlled clinical trials. In my opinion, it is the best available for a balanced, noncommercial resource, presenting studies of hormone effects on brain and body, as well as comparison studies of different types of hormone preparations.

International Society of Gynecological Endocrinology, www.gynecologicalendocrinology.org. The professional organization for physicians and health professionals worldwide who specialize in the evaluation and treatment of various gynecologic endocrine disorders, from precocious puberty to infertility to menopause. Their journal, *Gynecological Endocrinology,* is an excellent and very broad-based resource for articles on research being conducted worldwide in this field.

National Cancer Institute, Bethesda, MD 20892; 1-800-4-CANCER. This government-sponsored organization has a wealth of resources, educational materials, and lists of clinical trials for cancers of all types.

National Clearinghouse for Alcohol and Drug Information, P.O. Box 2345, Rockville, MD 20847; 800-729-6686 (TDD # 800-487-4899). This government-sponsored organization has a wealth of resources and educational materials, many of which are free.

National Institute on Drug Abuse, www.nida.nih.gov. This government-sponsored organization has a wealth of resources and educational materials on all aspects of substance abuse.

National Osteoporosis Foundation (NOF), 2100 M Street NW, Suite 602, Washington, DC 20037; 800-223-2226; www.nof.org. An excellent source of cutting-edge information about osteoporosis prevention and treatment. Join NOF and become an advocate in your community. I highly recommend their educational materials.

National Sleep Foundation, 729 Fifteenth Street, NW, Washington, DC 20005; www.sleepfoundation.org. This organization can steer you to an accredited sleep center or an organization related to a specific type of sleep disorder—for example, sleep apnea, narcolepsy, restless legs syndrome, and others.

North American Menopause Society (NAMS), 2074 Abington Rd., Cleveland, OH 44106; 216-844-3334; www.menopause.org. The professional organization of physicians, psychologists, nurses, and other health professionals who are interested in the health issues of menopause and perimenopause. They provide resources for consumers as well as health professionals.

Pesticide Issues: For more information on pesticides being used in schools, workplaces, and other places in your community, contact Pesticide Watch and the National Coalition of Pesticides, listed on page 410, and also:

> *International Workshop on Hormones and Endocrine Disrupters in Food and Water.*
> www.growth-reproduction.dk/referencer.htm
> www.nature.com/fertility/content/pdf/n

Resolve, Inc., 1310 Broadway, Somerville, MA 02144; 617-623-1156; www.resolve.org. This is a national organization that focuses on the problems of infertility. They have many educational resources available and also maintain a list of physicians who specialize in infertility treatment.

Sans Uteri Hysterectomy Forum, www.findings.net/sans-uteri.html. This Internet resource provides a variety of on-line information and website links for women who have had a hysterectomy.

Consumer Books

Alternative Therapies in Women's Health (published by American Health Consultants, a Medical Economics company) is a reliable resource for sound, balanced reviews of the literature and specific products. For those interested in science-based information on alternative medicine therapies in women's health, I recommend this newsletter because it does not appear to accept product advertising or to be sponsored by product manufacturers. I have found it helpful to better answer patient questions about supplements and alternative therapies. I have no financial involvement with this publication. Call 800-688-2421 for subscription information.

40-30-30 Fat-Burning Nutrition, Joyce and Gene Daoust (Del Mar, Calif.: Wharton Publishing, 1996). An excellent, easy-to-read, practical, and easy-to-follow meal plan that helps you reduce the fat-storing insulin excesses caused by our current high-carbohydrate, low-fat diets. The Daousts have done a terrific job of providing healthy meal plans for both vegetarians and nonvegetarians, and they have also provided a list of prepared foods that fit well into the 40-30-30 balance. Our patients have found this book helpful, and they have lots of lost pounds to back them up!

Cooking Low Carb, Brenda Laughlin and Kelly Nason (Littleton, Mass. Two N's Publishing, 1999). Order from www.cest-bon.com. A practical and easy-to-follow cookbook written especially for sufferers of PCOS, but useful for anyone with problems managing waistline weight gain.

CPSI/Nutrition Action Health Letter, 1875 Connecticut Avenue, NW, Suite 300, Washington, DC 20009; www.cspinet.org/nah. A hard-hitting, scientifically based newsletter that exposes frauds and fads in all the nutrition-supplement hype abounding today. An excellent resource to get reliable information since it is *not* supported by advertising.

Harvard Women's Health Watch Newsletter. In my opinion, of all the many women's health newsletters that have been started since the first edition of my book, this is by far the best in terms of quality and depth of information. It is published monthly by Harvard Health Publications, 10 Shattuck Street, Suite 612, Boston, MA 02115. The authors provide timely, well-researched information on many topics of interest to women of all ages, and the content is provided in enough depth to make it useful to guide your discussions with your own health professionals. I have subscribed to a number of other women's health newsletters so that I could evaluate their material. After detailed review, I am not recommending any other women's health newsletters because in my professional opinion, they either (1) push supplements and other products, (2) have unreliable medical information, (3) have too much "fluff" without enough depth to their content to be overly useful, or (4) push a narrow point of view without sufficient balance to be objective.

Healing Words: The Power of Prayer and the Practice of Medicine, Larry Dossey, M.D., (San Francisco: Harper, 1993). A meaningful book about the ways that modern medicine has overlooked the crucial role of prayer in healing, and how to help you reconnect with your spiritual needs as you face life's challenges. I have read most of Dr. Dossey's books and have found they are inspiring and encouraging of the steps we need to take to make medicine and healing more focused on the whole person.

Journal Watch: Women's Health. This monthly newsletter for health professionals summarizes relevant articles from major medical journals; it is published by the Massachusetts Medical Society, publishers of the *New England Journal of Medicine.* It is an excellent resource for interested consumers as well as health professionals, since there is a commentary by physician reviewers for each study that is abstracted each month. To order call 800-843-6356.

Menopause and Midlife Health, Morris Notelovitz, M.D., and Diana Tonnessen (New York: St. Martin's Press, 1994). Written by a pioneer in osteoporosis and menopause, this book presents accurate and up-to-date information about managing your health, including the role of healthy lifestyle habits. Discusses hormone therapies, pros and cons of gynecological procedures, issues about breast cancer, and other concerns of importance to women.

Menopause, Miriam Stoppard, M.D. (London and New York: Dorling Kindslerly, 1994). A beautifully illustrated book that addresses the total woman during this important transition and the years beyond. Because of all the color charts and graphs that make it easier to understand difficult medical concepts, I still think this is one of the best overall books on menopause to help women manage this transition in optimal ways.

Natural Medicines Comprehensive Database, J. M. Jellin, F. Batz, and K. Hitchens (Stockton, Calif.: Therapeutic Research Faculty, 1999). This reference book is prepared and updated regularly by research pharmacists, based on their review of well-designed medical studies from around the world and then compiled with summaries of uses, side effects, and symptoms of overdose for thousands of supplements. It is one of the most comprehensive, reliable, scientifically based compilations of information on natural medicines that I have found anywhere. It is not supported by advertising, is objective and medically sound. For more information on how to subscribe to their newsletter or purchase a copy of the reference book, call 209-472-2244 or visit their website: www.naturaldatabase.com.

Nutrition Applied to Injury Rehabilitation and Sports Medicine, Luke R. Bucci, Ph.D. (Boca Raton, Fla.: CRC Press, 1994). This book covers nutrition and the healing of injuries, arthritis, surgical wounds, and other musculoskeletal injuries in a thorough, scholarly fashion; it also has over 1,300 references for the scientific evidence on these issues.

Once-a-Month Cooking: A Proven System for Spending Less Time in the Kitchen and Enjoying Delicious, Homemade Meals Every Day, (revised edition), Mimi Wilson and Mary Beth Lagerborg (New York: St. Martin's Griffin, 1999). An excellent resource for making a month's worth of meals ahead and then having them quickly available when you are ravenous and too tired to make something healthy. Highly recommended by a close friend and mother of two active teenagers who said this book really works!

Pharmacist's Letter/Prescriber's Letter, J. M. Jellin, F. Batz, and K. Hitchens. Therapeutic Research Faculty, 3120 W. March Lane, Stockton, CA 95208. This group publishes a newsletter for health professionals with the latest information on prescription medications, including new uses and recently identified warnings or cautions about side effects and drug interactions. This reference is prepared by research pharmacists who have reviewed the medical studies from around the world and then compiled summaries of uses, side effects, and symptoms of overdose for thousands of medications. In my opinion, it is a reliable, scientifically based, valuable compilation of information useful to consumers and health professionals alike. It is not supported by advertising, is objective, and is medically sound. For more information on how to subscribe to their newsletter or purchase a copy of the reference book call 209-472-2244 or visit their website: www.prescribersletter.com.

Sacred Journey. An inspirational journal of readings, prayers, and reflections on life written by contributors of all faiths and published by the interfaith organization A Fellowship in Prayer, Inc., 291 Witherspoon St., Princeton, NJ 08542. This little journal is a wealth of short, inspiring readings that will help facilitate your daily meditation and spiritual awareness.

Sounds of Healing: A Physician Reveals the Therapeutic Power of Sound, Voice, and Music, Mitchell L. Gaynor, M.D. (New York: Broadway Books, 1999). We have all experienced in one way or another the power of sound to energize or relax us. This book shows how sound therapy (chanting, healing tones using crystal bowls, types of music, etc.) can be used to stimulate the self-healing response or simply to help find relief from stress of daily life. Written by an oncologist who has been using sound therapy as part of an integrated program for cancer treatment, it provides the science behind the theory, as well as practical suggestions for incorporating these approaches into your own life.

Strong Women Stay Young, Miriam E. Nelson, Ph.D. (New York: Bantam-Doubleday-Dell, 1998). An excellent book outlining the benefits of both aerobic- and strength-training for women to preserve and build healthy bone and muscle. I highly recommend it.

Syndrome X: The Complete Nutritional Program to Prevent and Reverse Insulin Resistance, Jack Challen, Dr. Burton Berkson, and Melissa Diane Smith (New York: John Wiley and Sons, 2000). An excellent resource for understanding the role that elevated insulin plays in causing heart disease, hypertension, elevated triglycerides, abnormal cholesterol patterns, and diabetes. Gives helpful information on nutritional approaches to correct these problems and reduce later risk of diabetes and cardiovascular disorders.

Take Charge of Your Hospital Stay, Karen Keating McCann (Cambridge, Mass.: Perseus Books, 1994). A must-read before you go in for tests, outpatient surgeries, or other procedures or find that you have to be hospitalized for anything. It may be difficult to find in bookstores, but is available through Amazon.com.

The Bodywise Woman: Reliable Information About Physical Activity and Health, written by the staff and researchers of the Melpomene Institute for Women's Health Research (New York; Prentice Hall Press, 1990). Well-researched and specific to the needs of women of all ages. Write to this organization for updates of their consumer materials.

Women's Moods: What Every Woman Must Know About Hormones, the Brain, and Emotional Health, Deborah Sichel, M.D. (New York: William Morrow and Co. 1999). This book extends what I have written in 1991 and 1994, as well as in *Screaming to Be Heard,* about the crucial hormone effects on mood syndromes in women. Dr. Sichel has included additional material on postpartum mood syndromes that many readers will find helpful. Although her emphasis is more on the serotonin connections than on the ovarian hormones, the book does provide validation for women experiencing these bewildering mood shifts.

Women & Self-Esteem—Understanding and Improving the Way We Think and Feel About Ourselves, Linda Tschirhart Sanford and Mary Ellen Donovan (New York: Penguin Books, 1992). An excellent overview of issues affecting women, still relevant today. Helps women understand cultural sources of low self-esteem and provides practical approaches for building an enhanced self-esteem; a valuable resource.

Resources for Natural Hormones

Disclaimer: I have no financial interest in any of these pharmacies or their products. I provide this information as a service to you and your physician because reliable information on these topics has been difficult for the average consumer to obtain. Compounded and "natural" hormones are not new, in spite of the recent marketing of such products. Many of these options have been around for forty years or more. I have been a long-standing advocate for the use of bioidentical, "natural" human forms of hormone preparations, and I have seen over the many years of my practice the marked positive difference that occurs when women change from the animal-derived, conjugated estrogens and synthetic forms of progestins.

> **Belmar Pharmacy, Charles Hakala, R. Ph., Lakewood, Colorado**
> (Denver area)
> Phone: 800-525-9473
> Fax: 303-763-9712

Charles Hakala has been a pioneer in compounding prescriptions for patients with challenging medical problems such as chemical sensitivities and multiple allergies to dyes/binders, in addition to his outstanding reputation in the field of compounding natural, bioidentical hormone preparations for thyroid, ovary, and adrenal hormones. For those with thyroid problems, Belmar Pharmacy is the one I have used since about 1985 for individualized sustained-release T3 preparations. Most commercial preparations containing T3 are fixed-dose combinations that don't allow adequate flexibility in dose, and also may contain dyes, binders, or animal proteins that adversely affect people with allergies and chemical sensitivities. Charles is also knowledgeable about important differences between the more reliable serum methods of hormone testing versus methods such as saliva and urine that commonly give misleading results. He will discuss these issues with both consumers and physicians. He uses micronized natural forms of estradiol, testosterone, progesterone, and DHEA derived from soybeans and wild yams, and will make prescriptions in whatever form is needed for best results. Although I don't recommend estriol and estrone as desirable forms of hormone therapy, Charles does make these compounded prescriptions for those women who wish to use these types of estrogen. Belmar pharmacists will make up prescriptions using lactose-free hypoallergenic formulations with no dyes; they also make vaginal creams that are hypoallergenic and omit some of the common irritants found in most commercial products.

> **Spence Pharmacy, Daryl Spence, R.Ph., Ft. Worth, Texas**
> (Dallas–Ft. Worth Metroplex)
> Phone: 800-209-7364
> Fax: 817-625-8103

Daryl Spence is another reliable compounding pharmacist who has created innovative topical pain-relief medications, in addition to his work with bioidentical, natural micronized hormones such as estradiol, testosterone, progesterone, DHEA.

General Comments

Both Belmar and Spence Pharmacies are full-service pharmacies with the ability to fill all of your prescription needs, not just compounded prescriptions. Both pharmacies also work with many major health insurance plans. In addition, I have found that both of these pharmacies often have better prices on common commercial prescriptions (such as estradiol patches) than my patients find at the big chain drugstores. I encourage you to do a little price comparison to decide where you want your prescriptions filled before you automatically assume the big chain drugstores are cheaper.

There are many pharmacies around the country that are now providing compounding services. There are several important reasons I have continued to collaborate primarily with Belmar and Spence pharmacies on prescriptions for my patients. First, both of these pharmacists have many years' experience in the art and science of compounding and are not just starting these services in the wake of current interest. Second, each compounding pharmacist has his or her own formula for making the various forms of prescription hormones, and each formulation will vary in how it is metabolized in the body. Therefore, each formulation will act somewhat differently in a given person and adds yet another variable to the equation of trying to solve the problem when a person has side effects. It is difficult enough clinically to sort out individual differences in metabolism and response when I know the pharmacology of a given preparation. If the preparation also varies, it can become almost impossible to sort out the Gordian knot of factors that could alter a person's response. That's why I prefer to work with brand-name products instead of generics, and to limit my prescriptions to just a few compounding pharmacists upon whose preparations I can rely for consistency.

Third, I am increasingly concerned at the degree to which some pharmacists are now practicing medicine by adjusting women's hormone doses based on questionable test methods, such as saliva and urine hormone levels, without having access to other laboratory measures that need to be included in decision making about appropriate hormone dose and route. Pharmacists are not supposed to determine hormone doses and adjustments. Pharmacists are not licensed to determine the dose that is correct for you; that function is by law the task of the physician. I have treated too many patients who have been significantly overdosed on hormones when getting their information from pharmacists making the dose changes, and I have chosen to put my prescriptions at pharmacies where the pharmacists do not engage in this practice.

Comments About FDA Approval

Women often ask, "Are these compounded hormones FDA-approved?" The answer is no, because the individual compounded prescriptions are not manufactured and distributed for sale in quantities that would require FDA approval. At reputable compounding pharmacies, the ingredients used are pharmaceutical-grade (U.S.P.) bases that are then made up into tablets or creams or suppositories to your individual needs. Individual pharmacists operate within their training and state licenses when they prepare (compound) individual prescriptions based on your own physician's decision about dose and type of medication best for you. Although many types of medications used to be compounded individually, it is no longer advantageous to do so with the current quality of manufactured products widely available. Much of the current use of individual compounding is for patients with allergies, marked sensitivities to dyes and binders in commercial preparations, patients who need smaller doses, and in particular, women who want to take natural, bioidentical human forms of hormones that aren't yet available in commercial products at regular drugstores.

Natural ovarian hormones have been in widespread use in Europe, Australia, Canada, Japan, and other countries for many years, generally with better clinical response and fewer side effects than the synthetic progestins, conjugated equine estrogens, and synthetic methyltestosterone compounds used in the United States. When these natural, or bioidentical, forms of hormones are not available commercially at the chain drugstores, the compounding pharmacies can make up ones similar to those available in Europe and other countries. For estrogen, however, there are several brands of the natural human form, 17-beta estradiol, available in the United States that are FDA-approved and made by commercial pharmaceutical companies (which means they are more likely to be covered by your health insurance plan as well as having the health benefits of being what your own body has always made): Estrace and Gynodiol tablets, Estrace vaginal cream, Vagifem vaginal tablets, Estring vaginal ring, VivelleDOT, Climara, Alora, Esclim and Estraderm transdermal (skin) patches. All of these products contain the same natural, bioidentical form of 17-beta estradiol that our ovaries made before menopause. These products are made with the precursor, or building block, molecules that come from soybeans. The primary difference in the various patches is the type of adhesive (which may affect frequency of skin rash and how well it stays on your body) and the duration of effect from the patch. We prescribe whatever brand a woman likes best.

There are also now available several generic versions of 17-beta estradiol tablets since Estrace has gone off patent. Unfortunately, I have found that the quality and potency varies widely from one generic manufacturer to another, and the dose you need may be more than what is required with Estrace to achieve the same effect. If you have been stabilized on one brand, it can lead to recurrence of your symptoms or to more side effects if you don't realize a pharmacist has switched your tablets to another manufacturer. For these reasons, I don't usually recommend the generic estradiol tablets. I have had many patients who had marked relapse of their symptoms when switched to a generic form of estradiol.

In addition to the commercial estradiol products, there are now two new FDA-approved commercial products for natural progesterone: Prometrium tablets and Crinone vaginal gel. You no longer have to turn to compounded natural progesterone products that are often not covered by insurance plans. Both Prometrium and Crinone are available through regular drugstores and are usually covered by most health plans that provide prescription plans. Both of these commercial products are made from yam and soybean precursors and are micronized for optimal absorption. They both work well for endometrial protection, so the choice of which product is appropriate for you depends on such aspects as personal preference and side effects, which will vary depending on whether progesterone is taken orally or is absorbed vaginally and therefore bypasses the liver "first-pass" metabolism.

No major pharmaceutical company in the United States has yet developed a natural micronized testosterone preparation approved by the FDA for widespread consumer use. A testosterone patch for women is in development by several companies and is currently in clinical trials, but it is not yet available on the market in the United States. *Do not try to use the men's testosterone patch—the dose is far too high for women to use.*

It is my hope that as we understand more about the important differences between the native human forms for hormones and the synthetic or animal-derived ones, the women of this country will have better options widely available. Until that time, you may ask your physician to work with reputable pharmacists to compound the natural testosterone to suit your needs. It can be made up in creams, pills, capsules, and suppositories.

Acknowledgments

My deepest thanks and appreciation to all who have made this book possible—from the dedicated researchers and clinicians worldwide who have led the way in providing the science to show how women's bodies function differently from men's, and clarified our understandings of these hormone issues in metabolism, weight gain and loss, to my medical practice teams and our patients. I am grateful to all of you.

I thank the many health professionals—physicians, nurse practitioners, registered nurses, psychologists, physical therapists, and others—who have read my books and thought they made sense and were scientifically "sound" to the point that they have sent patients for hormone evaluations. I thank you for your trust in my knowledge and approaches, and I thank you for the validation that your comments have given me. You then become "missionaries" for this crucial message in your communities and for the women whose lives you touch in your professional work. Together, we make a difference, and make positive changes toward a truly *woman-centered* health care model.

My deepest gratitude to my husband, Gordon Cheesman Vliet, a quiet strength and soul mate, who has shared this journey of helping others, blessing my life richly. You are, and have always been, the best support and encouragement I could have, truly "the wind beneath my wings."

Kudos and thanks also to Kathy Kresnik, once again laboring long hours, "above and beyond," working with me to keep the offices going and also assisting with the research, writing, and *rewriting* tasks to bring this book into being—I couldn't have done it without you!

My thanks to my clinical colleague James Talmadge Boyd, M.D., F.A.C.O.G., who has provided caring and capable patient care in our offices, thus allowing me to do my writing to broaden our work beyond our office walls.

Special thanks to Becky Johnson, Erin Lynch, Samia Yasmin, and other staff in both offices who have blossomed in their roles in caring for our patients and overseeing daily office operations. Your dedication and commitment to support my work in women's health, and to be a caring presence for our patients, have been invaluable.

Thanks also to Tom Wadkins, computer whiz magna cum laude, who has always willingly been available to solve my technical challenges and glitches to keep the projects moving ahead.

My appreciation to my business advisers David Cohen, Kim Paskal, Tony Rickert, and his A-1 assistant Debbie White, who guide me through the complexities of accounting and the legal aspects of running the business.

Gail Ross, literary agent extraordinaire, whose holiday greeting card "books change lives" illustrates her belief in the power of books to make a difference, and her dedication as an agent to get authors' messages to the broadest audience. Gail believed in this book from the outset and has been a strong advocate for me in dealing with the challenges of the publishing world. I am grateful for her wisdom, expertise, and guidance . . . and creativity for the title!

Susan Moldow, publisher, who trusted her own instincts about the crucial importance of women's hormones and pushed to have this book accepted for publication. I am grateful for her support and commitment throughout, but I especially appreciate that she has been willing to listen to and heed the input from my patients, the women dealing with these health challenges "on the front lines," about the best ways to effectively reach our readers.

Thanks to Jane Rosenman and Beth Wareham, the editors who guided my writing, and helped refine this book to make it helpful to readers, yet keep the scientific grounding that women need to understand complex issues. They both understand the trials and tribulations of the "hormonal challenges" women face and have been dedicated to making this book the best possible voice for these overlooked problems in young women.

Thanks to the friends and colleagues who reviewed the early stages of the manuscript and gave me important guidance to make this book even better. Most especially, my heartfelt thanks to Margaret Jordan, eighty and going strong, retired librarian and volunteer editor par excellence, who labored long hours, reading and rereading this manuscript to help me hone my message and make it more accessible to lay readers. Without her dedication, interest, and suggestions, I doubt I would have made my deadlines! She is an inspiring example that women of all ages can learn more about their bodies, master complex material, and use it to take steps to feel better.

And I also thank you, the women who have honored me by sharing your experiences and have allowed me to help guide you on the journey to health. We are students and teachers of one another in this "marvelous and maddening hormone journey" through our lives as women. Your insights and observations have taught me much that goes beyond the textbooks of medicine. This book becomes part of your legacy, too, as I pass on your experiences so that they can touch and help others.

Index

abdomen, 15
ablation, 360, 365–66
abortions, 115, 162
Abou-Donia, Dr., 95
acetylcholine (ACh), 71–72, 126
acne, 41, 42, 126, 248
   cyclic, xix, 202–4
   cystic, 364
Adderall, 164
Addison's disease, 173–74, 292, 360
adenocarcinoma, 100–101
adenomyosis, 205–6
ADHD (attention-deficit hyperactivity
   disorder), 163–64, 181
adrenal corticosteroid excess (Cushing's
   syndrome), 172–73, 360, 364
adrenal glands, xvi, xvii, 6, 12, 13, 125, 360
   autoimmune disorders and, 168–74
   hormones made in, 17, 25, 27, 29, 30, 34,
     36, 71, 75
   overactive or underactive, 172–74
adrenaline, 134, 366
adrenal insufficiency (AI), 173–74, 292, 360
adrenalitis, 169
adrenarche, 40, 42
adrenocorticotropin hormone, (ACTH), 34,
   36
advanced glycosylation end-products
   (AGEs), 80
affect (affective), 360
age-related macular degeneration (ARMD),
   275
aging, xvii, 10, 11, 356–57
Ahokas, Antti, 227
AIDS (acquired immune deficiency
   syndrome), 360
air pollution, 10
albumin, 156
alcohol, 6, 114–17, 273, 339–40
   binge drinking and, 114–16
   disease risks and, 115–17, 119–20
   menstrual irregularity and, 6, 114–16,
     120, 140, 339
aldosterone, 34, 35, 146
Aldrin, 91
allergies, xix, 5, 8, 10, 126, 289–90
alopecia, 360
Alora, xiii
ALS, *see* amyotrophic lateral sclerosis
Alzheimer's disease, 54, 57, 68, 72, 73, 149, 236

Ambien, 21, 133, 134
amenorrhea, 361
   hypothalamic, 142–43
American Cancer Society, 98
American Diabetes Association, 338
amines, 36
amino acids, 66–69, 71, 72, 80, 81, 361
amyotrophic lateral sclerosis (ALS; Lou
   Gehrig's disease), 68, 72
anabolic, 361
androgenic, 361
androgens, 13, 17, 25, 35, 42, 161, 361
   blockers of, 88, 255–56
   definition of, 29
   effects of, 30, 45
   receptors of, 29
androstenedione, 25, 161, 361
anger, 125, 136–39, 152
Angier, Natalie, 23
angina, 361
animal studies, xx, 9, 10, 45, 65, 67, 74, 75,
   101
anorexia nervosa, 45, 60, 140, 143, 144
antianxiety medication, 32
antibiotics, 154, 185
antibodies, 361
   adrenal, 169
   ovaries, 169
   thyroid, 7, 159, 162, 165–66
anticonvulsants, 182, 183, 256
antidepressants, xiv, 4, 30, 32, 38, 57, 126,
   152, 166, 181–83, 184, 256
antidiuretic hormone (ADH), 34, 37
antigens, 361
antinausea medication, 183
antioxidants, 127, 361
antipsychotic medication, 166, 167–68, 183
anxiety, xiv, xvi, xvii, xxv, 32, 51, 71, 218,
   220
   postpartum, 223–26
   triggers of, 74, 83, 119, 228–29
Aoki, Dr., 44–45
apigenin, 118
appetite, xv, 26, 70, 195, 197, 361
aromatase, 24–25
arsenic, 104, 105–6
arteries, 12
   blockage of, 32, 119
   clotting in, 118
   spasm of, 32–33, 119

About the Author

Elizabeth Lee Vliet, M.D., founded and is medical director for *HER Place®: Health Enhancement and Renewal for Women, Inc.* in Dallas–Fort Worth, Texas, and Tucson, Arizona. These programs focus on comprehensive evaluations of hormonal changes with physical, emotional, and social aspects of women's lives. Her clinical-research interests and publications include the effects of hormone changes in migraines, fibromyalgia/chronic pain, PMS, PCOS, depression and anxiety phenomena, osteoporosis, and cardiovascular risks. A nationally recognized speaker on women's health issues, she has presented numerous scientific papers and keynote addresses at regional, national, and international conferences and regularly teaches CME courses on women's health for physicians and other health professionals.

Dr. Vliet is the author of *Screaming to Be Heard* and *Women, Weight and Hormones*. She is a member of the International Menopause Society, the International Society of Gynecologic Endocrinology, American Society of Reproductive Medicine, the North American Menopause Society, the American Medical Association, and is currently on the advisory board for the Alliance for Better Bone Health. Dr. Vliet received her M.D. degree and did her internship in internal medicine at Eastern Virginia Medical School. With her interest in the integration of mind and body, she completed further specialty training in psychiatry and behavioral medicine at Johns Hopkins School of Medicine and is a Diplomate of the American Board of Psychiatry and Neurology, as well as a Diplomate of the American Academy of Pain Management. She received her B.S. and M.Ed. degrees from the College of William and Mary in Virginia.

Dr. Vliet served for two years as co-coordinating editor for the CME publication *Practical Reviews in Women's Health,* program chair of the Southern Medical Association Preventive Medicine Conference from 1993 to 1995, and served on the Part III Test Development Committee for the National Board of Medical Examiners. Dr. Vliet's appointments include clinical (adjunct) associate professor in family medicine at the University of Arizona College of Medicine, assistant professor in family medicine at Eastern Virginia Medical School; women's health physician at Canyon Ranch, where she developed their hormone and bone-density assessment program, as well as specialty consultations and seminars in pain management, women's health, and sexual health enhancement; medical director for the Women's Program at Maryview Hospital; associate medical director of the Pain Management Program at Maryview Hospital; director of the Behavioral Medicine Division in family medicine at Eastern Virginia Medical School; and director of consultation-liaison services at the University of Kansas School of Medicine, and consultant to the Kansas Regional Diabetes Center, where her clinical research studied glucose control on cognitive function and mood in diabetics. Dr. Vliet's approach integrates careful evaluation of hormonal changes through the life cycle with preventive and complementary medicine strategies to assist women and men in developing individualized health enhancement plans for optimal physical, emotional, and spiritual well-being.